Doctors' Secrets

The Miracle of
Antioxidants

National Library of Canadian Cataloguing in Publication

McLeod, Donald M., 1953-
        Doctors' secrets : the miracle of antioxidants / [Donald M. McLeod
Philip A. White].

Includes bibliographical references and index.
ISBN 0-9689877-1-0

        **1. Antioxidants--Health aspects. 2. Free radicals (Chemistry)--
Pathophysiology. 3. Medicine, Preventive. I. White, Philip A., 1945-
II. Title**

RM666.A555M33 2002   **616.07**   **C2002-904028-0**

Cover photo by Theo Wagner Foto Studio/Invent Ad Communications
Book produced by Invent Ad Communications

Dedication

To our beautiful and patient lifelong partners, Christine and Marlies. They have been the 'free radicals' stimulating the pursuits of our passionate research.

CONTENTS

DISCLAIMER

The contents of this book are the opinions of the authors and may not represent the consensus of opinion of the medical profession at this time. The contents of this book are not intended to be used to treat, cure, mitigate or diagnose any medical condition. The readers should consult their doctors before embarking on any changes that could affect their health.

*"Today, everyone requires supplements
for optimal health."*

–Don McLeod

*"All truth passes through three stages. First, it
is ridiculed. Second, it is violently opposed.
Third, it is accepted as being self-evident."*

–Arthur Schopenhauer

"It takes ages to destroy a popular opinion."

–Voltaire

*"Somewhere, something incredible is
waiting to be known."*

–Carl Sagan

*"Proper use of hormones and antioxidants
are our best chance of sustaining
health and longevity ."*

–Philip White

SECTION I

Introduction

DUST

"For dust thou art, and unto dust shalt thou return." Chapter 3, verse 19 of Genesis in the Holy Bible expresses eloquently this central truth of the human condition: We are mortal.

From earliest times we have known this. Life is fleeting. Life is fragile. Life is ephemeral. Life is short. It does not go on forever.

And this knowledge, this awareness, is the price we pay for the miraculous consciousness we possess as human beings: the knowledge that one day we will die. It is inevitable, it is certain, and we know it but we try not to dwell on the fact.

And yet... and yet for all of its troubles and travails, life is sweet. We do not want it to end. We want to keep it going. We want to extend this time between the dust from which we came and the dust unto which we shall return. If die we must, then we would – at the very least – like to lengthen our time alive, to expand to the maximum this inter – dust sojourn.

And that is precisely the central topic of this book – to set forth a course that allows us to lengthen our time here on earth or at least to improve it and then stave off the moment at which we once more become a lifeless part of it.

In our earlier book "Doctors' Secrets: The Road to Longevity" we focused our attention principally on hormone replacement therapy. And although we did touch upon the subject of antioxidants, the treatment was cursory and brief. In this book we would like to amend that, and accord the subject of antioxidants, the full attention it deserves. Because in addition to maintaining youthful hormonal levels, keeping the antioxidants in our bodies at optimal levels is the best way we know of currently for strengthening life and lengthening life.

AN OVERVIEW

The Enemy

Picture a large apartment building. Then picture one of the apartments within. Inside are a number of dark figures clad in hooded capes, armed with sledge hammers, chisels, axes. And now let this still image come alive like in a movie, each of the figures begins hammering chunks out of the walls, chiseling away shards from between the walls, chopping at the exposed plumbing and electrical wiring. The images continue to roll and we see these dark hooded vandals as they bludgeon the furniture, the fireplace, the stove and fridge. They smash appliances on the counter, the thermostat on the wall, the computer in the den. Fragments are flying like shrapnel and a murky dust hangs in the air.

The camera zooms back and the scene shifts. We see these same hooded vandals in every room in the building, smashing at the walls, the ceilings, the floors. Like automatons they are smashing everything. The main furnace in the building is being chopped and smashed, and the elevators, the corridors – even the main computer that runs the entire complex. Fragments are flying everywhere. The murky dust is everywhere.

As the camera zooms back still further we see nearby buildings undergoing similar attack. And as the camera pans around in a circle, we see every building in view under attack by the hooded vandals, every building exuding a murky dust through broken windows.

Admittedly, the scene pictured above is highly melodramatic, but it serves as a vivid analogy of how the human body comes under attack in its daily existence. If we look at the apartment building as the human body, each apartment in the building is an organ, each room in the building becomes a cell in the body, with items in the room representing various parts within a cell. And the marauding vandals, then, represent the physiological vandals within us called free radicals. They are the enemy and we need defence.

Free Radicals

A free radical is an atom, molecule, or compound that contains an unpaired electron. The free radicals that we will be concerned with here mostly consist of oxygen, or have an oxygen component to their makeup. Because these free radicals have an unpaired electron they are very reactive, and very electrophyllic. That is, they seek out electrons with which to complete their pairing, in keeping with the dictates of quantum mechanics. Just as nature abhors a vacuum, or north magnetic poles attract south magnetic poles, so too it is in the nature of things that electrons seek to be paired up. And it is this high degree of electrophyllic reactivity that make free radicals our enemy.

Free radicals, because of their electron imbalance, strive to achieve balance by ripping electrons – or suitable atomic bits - from various parts of the cells that make up the tissues and organs in the body. Just as little was spared by the attacks of the vandals in the foregoing melodrama, so, too, little is spared by the attacks of free radicals in the body's cells. The cell walls, the mitochondria, the lysosomes – even the nuclei and the DNA are subject to attack. And this goes on throughout the entire body. And it goes on in everyone's body, all day, every day. Nothing is spared and no one is spared.

Decay And Decline

Although it may take but an instant to die, very often the final moment has a painful and lengthy prologue. But the beginnings of this prologue are subtle and slight. We do not notice them. At first.

We do not notice when the free radicals first begin to get the upper hand, when the decay they cause to cell walls occurs more quickly than it can be repaired. We do not notice when cross linkages first begin to form between strands of protein, diminishing their flexibility and function. We do not notice the early impairment free radicals cause in the mitochondria, the power plants of our cells. We do not notice the initial damage free radicals cause to the genetic material – the DNA – in the nuclei of our cells, or the misinformation they may then pass on instead of their original information. We do not even notice when first our youthful hormone levels begin to drop.

We do not notice any of this initial decay because it is still in its early stages. It is hidden away inside. And we are young.

But in time we do notice the decline brought on by this decay.

We notice when we get out of bed in the morning and there is an odd stiffness in the bones, and we cannot recall doing any exercise the day before. We notice when we finish a squash match or our laps around the track, and feel a little more drained afterward, a little more tired. We notice when, during a particular winter, we find ourselves just a bit more susceptible to colds and flu. We notice when we feel a little more creaky in the joints after a baseball game. And we have only been sitting watching it from the stands!

For some of us there is a particular moment, that first shocking awareness, when we realize that we are already past our high point, the apogee of our youth, and we are now on the way down. These moments may take many forms. Sometimes it is something like a difficult dance step that for years we have been able to execute with ease, and now for the first time we don't quite pull it off. Or some move in gymnastics, like flipping up to our feet from a supine position on the floor, and it takes another two or three tries before we manage it, and even then it is sloppy.

Very often these moments are not recognized for what they are at the time. We pass them off as a one time thing: we were just having a bad day; or we had eaten too much beforehand, or drunk too much through the evening. The full significance of these moments comes usually in retrospect, after we have tried these moves on some future occasion, and they were still difficult to execute, or totally impossible. And then it is still some time after that, perhaps while taking a quiet walk along the ocean, or driving at night on a deserted highway, or strolling through a park on a somber autumn evening – possibly even while making our way pensively through throngs of unheeding people along a busy sidewalk – when the realization strikes us, and we experience that dismaying moment of epiphany: We are in decline. We are beginning to age. Our youth is behind us.

We are now growing old!

We do not notice the beginnings of the decay wrought by free radicals because it is within, and during our youth we are so much better able to fend it off. But later we do notice the decline.

As we move toward our forties and beyond, we notice the physical aspects of the decline through changes in the body – things like that unwanted layer of flab around the abdomen, with the belly button funneling in deeper now, making a bit of a hole. And in our skin, which is losing that youthful elasticity; so when we pinch it with our fingers the little fold takes longer to come back to smooth, and the heightened pinky color takes longer to fade to normal, and it no longer has that taut sheen it had before. We are losing elastin and the architecture of our skin collagen is changing. The muscles no longer look as though they might at any moment burst through the skin, but instead merely hang there in place. And the lustre in the hair is growing dull. And – and we now have the beginnings of a list that will only grow longer with our advancing years and many of us intensify our search for the panacea in the cosmetic industry.

Disease

Intruding on this list that will come to catalogue our decline are items that are particularly worrisome – the incidence of disease.

As the free radicals wreak further and further damage to the cells throughout the body, for many of us, various organs and body parts will in turn become weakened and damaged. Virtually every cell in the body is vulnerable to, and will sustain, free radical damage. This idea was slow in coming, slow in gaining attention, and even slower in gaining acceptance. The data supporting this concept began as a trickle, but it has now become a flood. So much so that today, even the most entrenched mainstream medical practitioners have come (reluctantly for some) to accept the concept that free radical damage is a major factor in the aging and disease process. Further, it is now commonly accepted that free radical damage is a factor in the onset or the progression of many serious diseases.

Cancer, atherosclerosis leading to heart attack and stroke – all have free radical damage as a factor in their development. The same for diabetes, arthritis, kidney disease, liver disease, lung disease, skin disease, cataracts, Alzheimer's, and weakened immune systems. All have free radical damage as an underlying common denominator. All have a greater likelihood of occurring as the damage from free radicals accumulates and increases.

It all makes sense on the face of it. If free radical damage is occurring throughout the body, if cells are being weakened in all parts of the body, then the organs comprised of these cells will be weakened too. And as this damage accumulates over the years, these various tissues and organs will each, in its own way, be adversely affected as well. Over time these adverse effects will in themselves come to constitute a disease, or at the very least, they will lay the body open to disease as the function of each organ declines. Maybe the decreasing hormone production discussed in our other books is mainly a result of neuroendocrine cell damage by free radicals as we age.

Where cells are weakened and where DNA in the nucleus has also been damaged, the daughter cells will then be more likely to exhibit anomalies after cell division. Where this ultimately results in a sufficient number of cells running amok, we then have an instance of a disease such as cancer.

Where low density lipoproteins (LDL cholesterol) in the blood are oxidized by free radicals, we will then have the gooey raw materials of plaque. And where the walls of blood vessels have been attacked by free radicals this will result in a weakened blood vessel, offering sites ideal for the development of plaque. Where this occurs in the carotid artery, or in arteries in the brain, we encounter the heightened possibility of stroke.

Where the oxidized LDLs bring about plaque that attaches to the walls of coronary arteries, we see the increased likelihood of heart attack or angina.

Where free radicals have been instrumental in bringing about ongoing inflammation, we see – amongst other things – the multifarious forms of arthritis looming.

And on and on.

Because these free radicals are able to bring their physiological sledgehammers, chisels, and axes to bear on all parts of the body, what the body needs is something that can protect it in all of its many parts. And because free radicals, if left unchecked, would tear us apart atom by atom and molecule by molecule, what the body needs is some kind of physiological warrior to do battle against them, to disarm them and repel their attacks. And such warriors exist for us in the form of antioxidants.

The Warriors

Antioxidants are the body's warriors against free radicals. They are the body's defenders.

Antioxidants are constituted such that they excel at neutralizing free radicals, at "quenching" free radicals. Just as a bodyguard is programmed to take a bullet for his or her country's leader, so too an antioxidant is "programmed" to take a bullet for us (or a sledgehammer, chisel or axe). Antioxidants possess the chemical configuration needed to take the business end of a free radical – its electrophyllic oxidizing part – and join onto it or alter it, thereby nullifying the part of it that would otherwise be engaged in ripping at the cells of the body. To mix our metaphors still further, we might liken the functioning of an antioxidant to that of a bodyguard getting between a knife-wielding assailant and the target, so that the knife becomes embedded in the bodyguard and then cannot be used on the target.

Antioxidants come from many sources, take on many guises, and battle the many faces of decrepitude and decay. They are varied and versatile. They have to be.

Free radicals exist in a number of forms as well, and arise in a number of ways. And just as a vandal with just one kind of weapon can cause many different kinds of damage to a building, so too a single form of free radical can cause a whole variety of damages. For either form of marauder, much depends upon where it is located and what it is ripping at.

Fortunately, because antioxidants exist in such variety – and possess differing properties one from another – they are able as a group to handle just about anything that free radicals can throw at them. For example, vitamin E is an admirable antioxidant, and it is fat soluble as well. This allows it to operate in fatty environments and thereby combat free radicals where many other antioxidants cannot. Vitamin C, another prominent antioxidant, is able to assist in "recycling" vitamin E molecules that have already taken a free radical "into custody". Vitamin C takes the free radical from vitamin E, thereby freeing up the vitamin E to go back for more free radicals. Then in subsequent reactions the vitamin C molecules are often able, through their own particular biochemical pathways, to rid themselves of the free radical sometimes with alpha lipoic acid and start all over. Enzyme antioxidants are able to nullify processes in the body that give rise to free radicals, preventing them from even beginning their rampage.

In so many of their operations, antioxidants are pure magic!

The one drawback that may exist in the realm of antioxidants can perhaps be better appreciated by the use of the following analogy, involving the defense of the McLeod castle. The defenders of this castle may consist of archers with longbows, soldiers with pikes, defenders with battle axes, swords, and all manner of weaponry known at the time. But having this assortment of defenders matters not if they do not exist in sufficient numbers. If there are, say, only ten of each, while the advancing army is a host of thousands, no matter how nobly the defenders fight, the castle is lost. By the sheer weight of numbers the advancing army will prevail and the defenders will be overwhelmed.

And so too it is in the case of antioxidants battling the free radicals. They may exist in a variety of forms, but where they are insufficient in number they too will be overwhelmed. Their defense will be inadequate and the body will sustain damage. The damage will accumulate. And before its time the body will fall. Atom by atom. Molecule by molecule.

As Aleksandr Solzhenitsyn put it: "It is not the ocean we drown in, it is the puddle."

A Brief History

*"True science teaches, above all,
to doubt and be ignorant."*

–Miguel de Unamuno

The central role played by antioxidants in the body has only recently gained recognition by the mainstream medical community, and even now there is skepticism as studies continue to challenge some of the suppositions we made earlier about antioxidants. Even more recent is the value placed upon

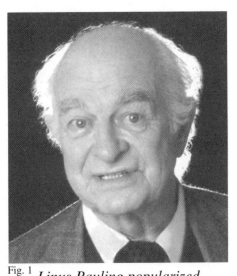

Fig. 1 *Linus Pauling popularized vitamin C in his time.*

antioxidants, both in staving off the aging process and staving off disease.

A great deal of research over the past decade or two has brought the field of antioxidants to the fore. Many have confirmed and corroborated the early findings concerning the many ways that antioxidants can fortify the body. And today the research proceeds apace to learn ever more about these wonderful anti-aging substances. Because antioxidants play such a pivotal role in the health of the body, and because they are at the basis of keeping the body in good working order, the interest today is huge.

But it has not always been so.

The beginning of the antioxidant story – well, there never is any real beginning to anything. Everything comes from something prior, something before. As Carl Sagan expressed it: "If you would bake an apple pie from scratch, first you must invent the universe."

However, a good place to jump in would be with Bert's research, done well over a hundred years ago. His experiments in 1878 were probably the first to demonstrate the toxic effects of oxygen at high tension, effects which led to convulsions and death in sparrows. Bert also noted that increased oxygen tension produced harmful effects, as well, in insects, earthworms, and other laboratory animals.

Now, although Bert's research does not deal directly with free radicals or antioxidants, it does point up the fact that there is a definite toxic side to oxygen. Prior to this finding, since its discovery (independently) by Priestly and Scheele, oxygen had been looked upon largely as a benign substance, like air or water. We know, however, that if we get two or three cupfuls of water in the lungs while swimming, water is not so benign, but can be deadly. Bert's experiments showed that oxygen, too, had not only a benign face, but a toxic face as well.

In 1889, Lorrain Smith, a pathology lecturer in Belfast, Ireland, carried out a series of experiments that corroborated Bert's observations. These experiments demonstrated that increased oxygen tension (1.7 – 1.8 atmospheres) over varying periods of time brought on severe pulmonary congestion combined with symptoms of pneumonia in mice, rats, and guinea pigs.

These experiments underscored still further the fact that oxygen did indeed have its harmful side. It also underscored – albeit tacitly – the fact that a problem is always recognized long before its solution. It would be decades before clinicians would take these, and other findings concerning oxygen's potential toxicity, into account.

During this period experiments were also taking place in the chemistry labs of the world. In 1894, in what was probably the first recorded reaction involving a free radical, a simple experiment was carried out by a researcher named Fenton. Using ferrous sulfide, hydrogen peroxide, and an aqueous solution of tartaric acid as reagents, he produced – amongst other products – the hydroxyl free radical ($OH\cdot$). This has since come to be known as the Fenton Reaction.

In 1900 another researcher by the name of Gomberg reported the first organic molecule to be recognized as a free radical – the triphenylmethyl radical.

Over the next three decades a number of researchers looked into the toxic effects of increased oxygen tension on animals, with the results being almost wholly ignored by clinicians.

In 1927, following a series of further experiments, Binger reported that "oxygen in concentrations of over 70 per cent of an atmosphere is poisonous to dogs, rabbits, guinea pigs and mice." In these experiments the lungs of the animals, not unlike those in Smith's experiments, displayed congestion, edema, hypertrophy, desquamation of alveolar cells, and mononuclear cell infiltration.

In 1945 Comroe demonstrated the toxic effect of oxygen inhaled in high concentrations by men both at sea level and at a simulated altitude of 18,000 feet.

Throughout these many decades there was little connection made at the clinical level between prolonged high concentrations of oxygen inhaled and the negative effects it produced in both animals and humans. Because of the failure to make the connection one result was an estimated 10,000 cases of blindness in premature newborns from retrolental fibroplasias (Terry's syndrome) during the late 1940's and early 1950's, when high concentrations of oxygen were used to improve chances of survival in incubators.

It was only in 1967, after Nash demonstrated a strong positive correlation between the duration and concentration of oxygen inhaled and the negative effects on the human body, that there came to be a general acceptance regarding the toxic aspects of oxygen.

As for the destructive capacity of oxygen as a component of a free radical, it was not until 1954 that a major indictment was lodged. That was the year that Dr. Denham Harman proposed his revolutionary free radical theory of aging.

Dr. Harman, commissioned by the U.S. government during the cold war, was charged with the task of coming up with an antidote to radiation poisoning. One major mechanism which made nuclear radiation so deadly was that it unleashed in the body a torrent of lethal hydroxyl radicals. The flood of hydroxyl radicals came about as the result of water undergoing ionization when subjected to the radiation.

A major observation made by Dr. Harman was that the effects of lower levels of radiation on humans were not that unlike the effects of aging, and in fact might have been regarded as something of a premature aging. He was also aware of a particular biochemical process in the body, wherein the oxidation of sugar to produce energy also produces free radicals. Dr. Harman made the connection between these two circumstances, and thereby had the key to his theory. In his milestone publication in 1954, Dr. Harman proposed that free radical formation in the cells of the body, and their effects on the cells of the body, constituted a major factor in the aging process.

Sadly this idea went largely ignored for years, and his was a voice crying in the wilderness.

Somewhat after this period, particularly in the sixties and beyond, Dr. Linus Pauling became an active proponent of another prominent antioxidant, vitamin C. Now, although Dr. Pauling did not encourage the use of vitamin C specifically as an antioxidant, he did encourage its use, and did so vociferously. And although the dosages he recommended may have been high, the fact that he was instrumental in bringing vitamin C to the fore was of great value. For one thing, multitudes benefited by supplementing their diets with vitamin C, thereby increasing their antioxidant levels on this front. For another, the controversy generated by Dr. Pauling was undoubtedly responsible for increased research into vitamin C, and into antioxidants in general. But like Dr. Harman, he was largely discounted by mainstream medical opinion. A recent publication from the Linus Pauling Institute in Portland, Oregon has lent credence to the fact of vitamin C's potential to prevent hardening of the arteries.

In 1969, Dr. T. L. Dormandy proposed that there was a correlation between biological rancidification (oxidation of lipids), and the degeneration or aging of a cell.

In that same year, Dr. J. M. McCord and Dr. I. Fridovitch discovered the antioxidant enzyme called superoxide dismutase, which has the ability to neutralize the superoxide free radical. This was the breakthrough that was needed.

Bit by bit the floodgates were beginning to open.

Over the next decade research into free radicals and antioxidants steadily increased. By the 1990's research into antioxidants was taking place in countless labs around the world. The field has currently become so important and so prominent that new information is coming forth almost daily. Parker, Ames, Tritchler, Arora are but a few of the names that have been at the forefront of this informational deluge, all adding more and more data concerning the biochemistry of antioxidants.

That free radicals play an immense role in the aging process is no longer ignored or contested by many of the mainstream medical community. That antioxidants are the most important combatants of free radicals is likewise no longer contested. However, whether we can combat aging by reducing the action of free radicals is still the subject of skepticism, but we are not sure why. People like Dr. Harman and Dr. Pauling are no longer voices crying in the wilderness. Rather, they are now accorded the recognition they richly deserve.

All of which again underscores the words of Schopenhauer: "All truth passes through three stages. First it is ridiculed. Second, it is violently opposed. Third, it is accepted as being self-evident."

Interesting Times

"May you live in interesting times." This ancient wish has the greatest chance of being fulfilled by people living today because the present day and age may well come to be looked upon as the most interesting period in history. So much is taking place around us.

We have the improved Hubble telescope bringing us improved images of our universe, along with new concepts of the universe, more discussion and conjecture about dimensions and refinements of string theory cosmologies.

We have an international space station above the earth currently nearing completion. Besides serving as a lab for conducting experiments that could never be carried out here on earth, it will almost certainly serve as a jumping off point for future space exploration – Mars, Europa, Io, Titan and beyond. And it will be that work on this station by astronauts from around the world that will bring a new sense of cooperation and comity to nations here on earth.

We have a burgeoning internet, new computers, new electronic gadgets. There is no end to the list of new things, new discoveries coming at us each year.

But the field that offers the greatest excitement these days is in the area of the life sciences. New drugs, new surgical techniques, genome manipulation, new equipment. And most importantly, we are arriving at a new and more complete understanding of the body's basic biochemistry. It is the elegance of this biochemistry and our heightened understanding of the complexity of longevity medicine that continues to inspire us, the authors.

The reason why this new understanding is so important is that it has already begun to extend the human life span. More telling yet, it is now pointing the way to extending the lifespan still further, and to a much greater degree. In areas as diverse as hormones, antioxidants, telomeres, genetics – research is going forth at a furious pace with scientific knowledge doubling every 7 years. That is because all are yielding marvelous insights into the aging process, and providing the means and stratagems of extending the lifespan still further yet. The optimism in the field is so strong that there are some of us even discussing – unabashedly – the possibility of living forever. Immortality!

Now, this is not to say that we are on the threshold of immortality, or even that immortality is in fact possible. We can all recall back in the 60's when physicists were claiming that controlled fusion reactions were just around the corner. So it does not hurt to temper optimism with a pinch of caution.

That being said, it still remains that giant steps have been taken in the last decade in discovering ways to extend our time here on earth. And one of these giant steps involves optimizing the levels of antioxidants in the body.

There is considerable agreement by researchers in this field, who hold that by maintaining these optimal levels of antioxidants we may extend our lives by a good ten or fifteen years. With the emphasis on good. Because there is also research to support the thesis that if we come into old age in good shape, then we will, at the end, have a diminished period of debilitation. Let us compress our morbidity (sickness) into the shortest time of our lives!

Besides the life-extending strategies that we have at our disposal today, there are areas of research that portend even greater lifespan extensions in the near future, as well as extensions by quantum leaps in the intermediate and distant future. Hormone replacement therapy is already improving and perhaps lengthening people's lives, and with widespread research still ongoing, many in the field believe that the greatest discoveries here are yet to come. Research into telomeres (the tips on the ends of chromosomes), and into the genes that make up the chromosomes themselves – both exemplify fields that hold huge potential for the intermediate future.

While we await these new discoveries we will, in the meantime, wish to maintain our health at the highest levels possible. One simple way to stay healthy – and to thereby stay alive long enough to take advantage of these future discoveries – is to become knowledgeable about antioxidants, and thereafter to maintain optimal levels of antioxidants in the body. By doing so we cannot say you will come into future discoveries that will allow you to live forever. But you will at least be there to avail yourselves of whatever benefits these future discoveries are able to confer. Because, by maintaining high levels of antioxidants you will, with virtual certainty, strengthen your life and lengthen your life. And this will help take you to the time when you will then be able to use future discoveries to extend your life still further. And on and on, one stage at a time.

As for immortality...well, it never hurts to dream a little.

And while we dream we will explore the realm of antioxidants, and see in more detail how they can help us to improve our lives. It is a fascinating realm and we, the authors, invite you to explore it with us, as we begin our journey with the antioxidant miracles.

"Oxidative stress can damage proteins, lipids, DNA and carbohydrates."
–Barry Halliwell D.Sc. University of London

SECTION II

Free Radicals

"Oxidative stress occurs when there is an imbalance between oxygen derived free radical production and scavenging by antioxidants."

–Canadian Longevity And Anti Aging Academy (CLA4)

"Scientists now believe that free radicals are causal factors in nearly every known disease, from heart disease to arthritis to cancer to cataracts. In fact, free radicals are a major culprit in the aging process itself."

–Dr. Lester Packer

"If you have enough antioxidants (good guys), they win and you stay healthy. If you don't have enough of the right antioxidants, the "bad guy" free radicals win and can cause a long list of diseases."

–Dr. James F. Balch

"The supreme excellence is not to win a hundred victories in a hundred battles. The supreme excellence is to subdue the armies of your enemies without even having to fight them."

–Sun Tzu

Free Radicals

UNITY, DICHOTOMY

The universe, by definition, is all one thing. However, it does appear to hold a certain innate dichotomy in its perceived makeup. Thus it appears that we cannot have thesis without antithesis, negative without positive, matter without antimatter, good without bad. And so it is that here on earth friction retards motion, and yet without it we could not walk. And so it is also that, although we cannot live without oxygen it will eventually kill us.

Not surprising, then, that to some extent this dichotomy concerning oxygen plays out still further, where we have the harmful oxidizing free radicals on the one hand, counterpoised with the beneficial antioxidants on the other.

Morality Play

It would not be altogether absurd to regard the interactions in the body between free radicals and antioxidants as something of an old time morality play. In this morality play the antioxidants represent the forces for good, while the free radicals represent the forces of evil. Only here, in contrast with the morality plays of old, these forces are not battling for dominion over the soul. They are battling for dominion over the body (which of course houses the soul).

Another difference lies in the fact that in days of old, usually just one force of evil – lust or envy, for example – was portrayed in the play. In the drama taking place in the

human body we find a number of entities that make up our
evil cast of characters. Also, in days of old, whichever force
of evil was being portrayed, it was definitely pure evil. There
was nothing good about it. In the case of free radicals, however, there is some good to them.

An Ill Wind

It is an ill wind that blows no good. So goes the old
adage, and there is a lot of truth to it. There is little in life that
is all good or all bad. And that is indeed the case for free radicals. The fact is, some of them benefit the body, are even
necessary for its proper functioning.

For example, some free radicals serve as signalling
agents in the body, affecting the expression or non expression
of particular genes. Free radicals such as nitric oxide and
superoxide are used as toxins by cells of the immune system
to destroy viruses and bacteria, and free radicals are used as
well to kill cancer cells. Further, nitric oxide is also necessary
to the body in helping regulate blood vessel dilation, and
thereby, the circulation of blood.

Now, having said this, the fact remains that most free
radicals – especially in higher concentrations – do wreak
damage upon our bodies. And whatever their limited saving
graces, free radicals are the villains in the piece.

The Villains

Throughout folklore and history, we have come to know
many different villains, and different kinds of villains. King
John (against whom Robin Hood battled) was a different
kind of villain when compared to Jack the Ripper. Jack the
Ripper was very different from John Dillinger (a bank robber
in the 1930's who, when asked why he robbed banks replied:

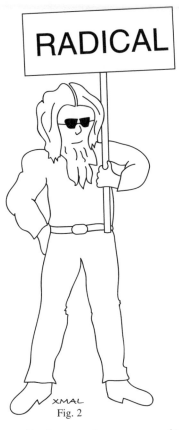

Fig. 2

Free radicals can destroy your life!

"Because that's where the money is."). And John Dillinger was different from Charles Manson.

So it is in the case of free radicals: they are different from one another – different in how they are generated, different in chemical composition, and different in their propensities for destruction.

The Cast of Characters

We might also refer to these oxygen-toting villains as Reactive Oxygen Species (ROS). ROS is a broader, more inclusive term, and as such encompasses more fully the range of free radicals we will be looking at – because, some of the "free radicals" in our list are not actually free radicals. However, these substances do readily give rise to free radicals, and since the term "free radical" is the less cumbersome of the two, it is the one we will generally employ. Also, in referring to true free radicals by common chemical notation, we will adhere to convention and include the superscript dot that accompanies this notation. The dot will also serve admirably as a symbol for the unpaired electron.

A list of the free radicals we will be dealing with most often is as follows.

• Hydroxyl radical	$HO\cdot$
• Superoxide anion radical	$O_2^-\cdot$
• Singlet oxygen	$O\cdot$
• Hydrogen peroxide	H_2O_2
• Lipid peroxyl free radical	$LOO\cdot$
• Nitric oxide	$NO\cdot$
• Alkoxyl radical	$RO\cdot$
• Peroxyl radical	$ROO\cdot$
• Peroxynitrite	$ONOO^-$

The Generation of Free Radicals

Free radicals may be generated in any of three ways.

1. The homolysis of covalent bonds.

$$A:B \rightarrow A\cdot + B\cdot$$

2. The addition of a single electron to a neutral atom.

$$A + e^- \rightarrow A^-\cdot$$

3. The loss of a single electron from a neutral atom.

$$A \rightarrow A^+\cdot + e^-$$

A great deal of our body chemistry – particularly in the production of energy – involves the transfer of electrons in oxidation-reduction reactions. In these complex reactions there may at times be some electron leakage, with the occasional electron going astray. It is not surprising then that the most common mode of free radical formation is the second one, where an electron is added to a neutral substance. Where this neutral substance is molecular oxygen we then have the generation of the superoxide anion radical.

$$O_2 + e^- \rightarrow O_2^{-\cdot}$$

A common instance of superoxide formation occurs during "respiratory bursts". Respiratory bursts entail an increased and rapid uptake of oxygen in a particular area, which also brings on a rapid generation of superoxides.

This can occur where cells of the immune system (phagocytes such as neutrophils, monocytes, or macrophages) go into battle on our behalf against invading bacteria. Some of their weaponry will often include free radicals, which these cells employ in battling the invaders. The collateral damage, however, often consists of increased levels of errant superoxide radicals, with which the body will then have to contend.

Respiratory bursts may also occur in areas of injury and inflammation. Here blood flow is increased as the body tries to clear away physiological debris. In so doing the collateral damage is once more the generation of heightened levels of superoxide radicals.

A similar situation arises where reperfusion injury occurs, immediately following a stroke. When blood flow is cut off in one area of the brain due to a blood clot, or from plaque debris that has come loose somewhere else and lodged in an artery feeding the brain, oxygen deprivation and consequent brain damage may occur. Surprisingly, however, much of the damage to brain cells occurs after blood flow is restored. With the renewed rush of blood – accompanied by a rapid upsurge in the production of superoxide radicals – the result is yet further damage to brain tissue caused by the free radicals.

Superoxide radicals may be generated by the autoxidation of reduced transition metals:

$$Fe^{2+} + O_2 \rightarrow Fe^{3+} + O_2^{-\cdot}$$

And as well, superoxide radicals may be generated by a number of reactions involving catalyzing enzymes – enzymes such as flavin oxidase and xanthine oxidase.

If the most commonly generated free radical is the superoxide radical, the most harmful free radical is the hydroxyl radical.

We have already looked at one way hydroxyl radicals are generated when we considered Dr. Harman 's early work, and his initial hypothesis that hydroxyl radicals were produced in the body by the homolytic dissociation of water under the action of ionizing radiation:

$$H_2O \rightarrow HO\cdot + H\cdot$$

Hydroxyl radicals may also come into being via conversion from superoxide radicals, a reaction in which hydrogen peroxide is involved and where ferrous and ferric ions serve as mediators.

$$O_2^{-\cdot} + Fe^{3+} \rightarrow O_2 + Fe^{2+}$$

$$Fe^{2+} + H_2O_2 \rightarrow HO\cdot + OH^- + Fe^{3+}$$

These reactions reduce to:

$$O_2^{-\cdot} + H_2O_2 \xrightarrow{\text{iron catalyst}} HO\cdot + HO^- + O_2$$

We mentioned above that some of the reactive oxygen species (ROS) were not actually free radicals. That is the case for singlet oxygen, $^1O_2$ which, although not a true free radical, behaves like one, and is extremely injurious to cells in the body.

One way in which singlet oxygen is generated is by the action of sunlight, particularly the ultraviolet part, whereby it breaks the bonds of normal diatomic oxygen, O_2. Normal oxygen is generally very stable. However, when sunlight strikes the skin, any diatomic oxygen that is present may be broken down into singlet oxygen.

Although not technically a free radical, singlet oxygen is highly reactive, and has the potential for quickly oxidizing a great many molecules in the body. Some of the more important among these are the polyunsaturated fatty acids. Where this occurs, these fatty acids (as well as phospholipids) become degraded to lipid hydroperoxides. This is particularly harmful when the oxidizing attack takes place in the fatty acids that are part of the cell membrane. When such an attack occurs it can set off a chain reaction of an autocatalytic nature. What this means is that a sequence of reactions ensues such that more free radicals are generated from the initial attack, which then continue the chain reaction until it is finally brought under control. Thus, a single "hit" by singlet oxygen (or any other destructive free radical) may set in motion the generation of hundreds of free radicals, as well as other by-products. The upshot is that the cell may sustain sufficient damage to bring about its eventual destruction and demise. It has been calculated that 80% of vitamin C stores in the skin are depleted after just 1/2 hour in the sunshine. This leaves the skin with less antioxidant to prevent free radical damage from the sun that may progress on to solar keratoses and skin cancers that we see in our medical practices every day. Weigh the benefits of attracting the opposite sex with a tan now versus the preservation of youthful skin for future interactions.

Singlet oxygen is also strongly implicated in the formation of cataracts, and in macular degeneration, which involves damage to the retina. Remember to have sunglasses with glass lenses (not plastic) to block out damaging ultraviolet sunlight.

Like singlet oxygen, hydrogen peroxide (H_2O_2) is another ROS that is not a true free radical. However, we have seen from the Fenton reaction that, in the presence of transitional metal ions such as Fe^{2+} and Cu^+, that hydrogen peroxide can readily give rise to the destructive hydroxyl radical.

$$Fe^{2+} + H_2O_2 \rightarrow Fe^{3+} + HO^- + HO\cdot$$

Once this occurs, the body has not only the damage from hydrogen peroxide to contend with, but also the potentially more severe damage that may result from the hydroxyl radical.

Hydrogen peroxide has been linked to the Epstein-Barr virus, which can be a factor in chronic fatigue syndrome. It has also been implicated in lipid peroxidation and DNA damage.

Other Free Radicals

There are many other kinds of free radicals found in the body. Most are derived from those we have examined above. Many of these other radicals include carbon centered radicals ($R\cdot$), and the peroxyl radical ($ROO\cdot$).

When hydroxyl radicals oxidize various carbon centred molecules (RH) such as protein, carbohydrate, lipid, or nucleic acid molecules, the result is the generation of carbon centered radicals.

These carbon centered free radicals are themselves reactive, and may damage cells on their own. Even more damaging is when these radicals react with oxygen to form the peroxyl radical (ROO·). These latter play a large role in the oxidation of lipids. Since lipids are found in the blood and in cellular fluids, and are a major constituent in the membranes that make up cell walls, there is ample scope for the peroxyl radical's destructive activities.

Nitric oxide (NO·) is another radical that has the capacity to harm the body. We have seen that it serves in ways that are beneficial to the body, even necessary to the body, but it also has the capacity to harm. This is particularly so when it reacts with superoxide ($O_2^{-}\cdot$) to form peroxynitrite (ONOO $^{-}$). Peroxynitrite is a powerful oxidant and has demonstrated an involvement with conditions as varied as neurodegenerative disorders, kidney diseases, and rheumatoid arthritis.

LOCATION, LOCATION, LOCATION

We have all heard how important the location of a business or house is, and how strongly location affects its operation or value. A hot dog stand on a busy seaside boardwalk will do a flourishing business. This same stand on an isolated backroad will likely be abandoned in a month.

For free radicals in the body, location too is crucial as to their effects. Two aspects of location that affect the nature of free radical damage have to do with the part of a cell that a free radical is damaging, and the location and type of cell in the body. We will look briefly at the former factor here, and the latter factors in the section on disease.

Cellular Damage

Cell Wall

Free radicals may inflict damage on various parts of a cell.

The cell wall is one part that is especially susceptible to free radical attack. Through a process known as lipid peroxidation (which we touched on above), the lipid components that make up the cell membranes in a cell wall may come under attack. When this occurs the polyunsaturated fatty acids and phospholipids become degraded through a series of chemical reactions to form hydroperoxides.

The most damaging aspect to lipid peroxidation is that one hit by a free radical can set up a chain reaction, such that each assault by a free radical spawns further radicals bent on attacking still more of the fatty acid components in the cell wall. As this onslaught proceeds, a great many chemical by-products may be generated as well, kicked out into the cytoplasm of the cell. So besides the damage that is inflicted on the cell wall, there is the collateral damage inflicted by radicals and biochemical debris accumulating in the cytoplasm, which may then befoul normal chemical reactions taking place there. The result is that the permeability of the cell may be impeded or plugged, keeping desired nutrients out and unwanted chemicals in, leaving the cell running amok chemically, with the walls eventually leaking out the cytoplasm that is its life.

If you picture the cell as being like a swimming pool, the free radicals might be likened to scuba divers swimming underwater with chisels, knocking chunks out of the pool walls. Some of these shards may blast into other parts of the pool wall, knocking out still more bits. Now, if there are other swimmers in the pool moving in orderly rows doing laps, they may occasionally be struck by errant pieces of debris. As well as being injured themselves, they may begin flailing about, moving erratically out of their own rows, inadvertently striking other swimmers. And being struck, these other swimmers may themselves begin flailing about, causing still more mayhem. Adding to the growing dysfunction, some of the chunks may end up plugging up the inflow vents bringing fresh water into the pool, and they may plug up the outflow drains as well.

Thus, what was originally an orderly movement of desired activity is now a disorderly melee, with shards of the pool wall flying about, swimmers being injured and dislocated from their patterns, drains being plugged, and the water growing cloudy with sediment. Taking this scene to its end point, we would see water leaking out through holes in the pool walls, with dirt and other foreign matter leaking in.

And that is just from the walls being attacked.

Besides attacking the fatty acids in cell walls, free radicals may also attack fatty acids elsewhere in the cell and in the body. Where they oxidize lipids in the blood, they transform them into a substance that tends to agglutinate, which then attaches to the walls of arteries, adding to plaque. Where the plaque buildup becomes extensive enough a hardening of the arteries – or atherosclerosis – occurs, which may then lead to heart attack or stroke.

Also, it is the oxidation of fats that makes them spoil or become rancid. When fats become rancid they also become toxic. Where this occurs to fatty acids in the blood it means that the immune system and the liver will have more work to do in cleaning up these toxins.

And because the oxidification of lipids is susceptible to chain reaction, the damage described above can all begin with a single free radical.

Mitochondria

Nearly 4 billion years ago the atmosphere on our planet contained little oxygen and cells were anaerobic (needing no oxygen). In fact oxygen was toxic and many of these cells have failed to survive to our present 20% oxygen air. An early aerobic bacterial cell called a peroxisome was incorporated into other cells by phagocytosis (digestion by engulfing as a whole) and that this peroxisome helped rid the cell of its dangerous oxygen by turning it into H_2O_2 and this was turned into water by the enzyme catalase. These peroxisomes gave

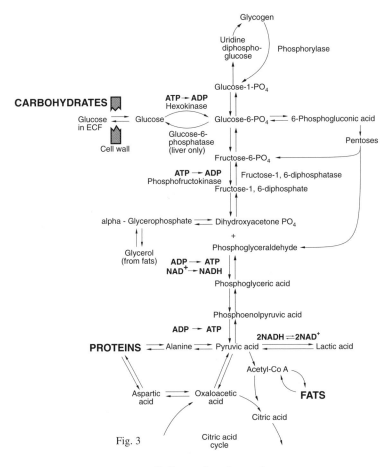

Fig. 3

Cell production of energy

up some DNA and also took on other responsibilities in the cell that they joined (symbiosis). They produced an energy rich Adenosine Tri-Phosphate (ATP) which the cell in the richer oxygen environment began to utilize for energy. These incorporated simple cells are now known as mitochondria. The mother cell nucleus incorporated some of the mitochondrial DNA to make mitochondrial proteins necessary for function. They were likely taken into our eukaryotic cells (possessing a nucleus) 3.5 billion years ago, not long after the earth cooled. Cumulatively, their energy becomes the energy used by the body in carrying out its multitude of daily tasks. Our liver cells may have 800 but our sperm cells may only have 20 of these mitochondria or powerhouses. The number of mitochondria per differentiated cell is fixed and so once lost in a cell, we have no way yet to replace them. Protect your mitochondria.

The mitochondria are like miniature furnaces that "burn" sugar, except that they do not burn sugar in the way wood is burned in a normal furnace. When wood is burned it mainly involves a single reaction. The wood is oxidized directly in one step, with the immediate release of its chemical energy, which we detect as heat and flames.

The oxidation of sugar carried out in the mitochondria is a slower, stepwise process. The simple sugar, glucose, is oxidized through a series of reactions, ultimately producing a substance called adenosine triphosphate, or ATP. The body can then use the energy stored in ATP for its various tasks.

In this stepwise process, as the glucose molecules undergo oxidation, there is an accompanying transfer of electrons that takes place. In the complexities of these reactions and electron transfers, it is not uncommon for an occasional electron to go astray. You might compare it to a person who is dealing cards around a table and tries to go too fast, with the outcome being that once in a while a card goes astray, sailing off the table and onto the floor.

When an electron is tossed out of the reactions involved in sugar metabolism, it will almost immediately attach itself to whatever is nearby. All too often it is an oxygen molecule

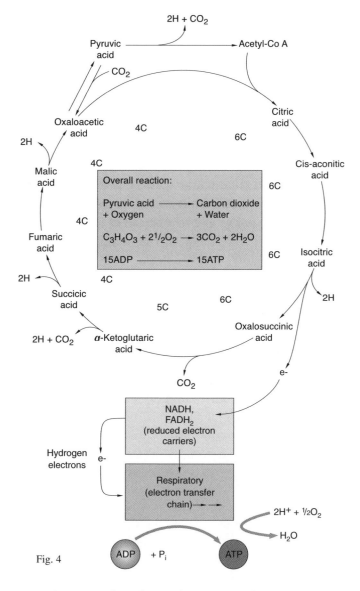

Citric acid cycle producing ATP for energy in the mitochondria

that the electron attaches itself to. This brings about the formation of a superoxide radical (O_2^-), which then goes on its rampage of destruction in the mitochondrion. There is another possible outcome in that the superoxide radical may give rise to a hydroxyl radical, which is even more reactive and destructive. It too will inflict its damage on the mitochondria.

Over time, where the mitochondria are sufficiently damaged, and where there are a sufficient number of cells operating at less than full capacity, the body will have less energy with which to function.

All too often we will see these diminishing energy levels manifesting themselves in people as they go through middle age and beyond. And we will observe these energy levels in people drop even more markedly as this damage continues to accumulate with a further passing of the years. Eventually, we will see these same individuals take on the slow moving gait of old age. Why do our parents end up in the easy chair earlier each evening?

And finally we will see these same changes in ourselves.

DNA

DNA is like the cell's memory bank, the cell's blueprint. It is composed of genes that are arranged on larger, longer units called chromosomes. The chemical composition of the many thousands of genes in humans, and their arrangement on the 46 human chromosomes, make up a blueprint complete with sufficient directions to bring about the development of a fertilized egg cell into a fully formed, human infant. This same genetic information will then continue to direct the operations of each cell throughout its lifetime, and the lifetime of the person in whom it is a constituent part. This blueprint, in directing the production of muscle, bone, enzymes and the like, will also determine things like height, hair color, eye color, and maybe even the death genes on chromosome 4.

Much of this development and growth in the body will depend on cell division or cell replication. These cell divisions, in turn, will involve the replication of each chromosome (with all the genes of which it is composed) into an exact copy. This allows the daughter cells to have the same memory, the same correct blueprint, so that they will be in harmony with each other and with the other cells in the body, as they continue directing the biochemical reactions necessary to the normal functioning of the body as a whole.

When this genetic material becomes altered or damaged, the proper physiological functioning of the cell becomes compromised. Even worse is what occurs when future cell divisions are sent into chaos, with the cell dividing out of control. For, it is such out-of-control cell divisions that give rise to various cancers.

Obviously, then, when the destructive effects of free radicals are brought to bear on the nucleus of a cell – and its genetic material within – the results can be catastrophic. Equally catastrophic are cases where such damage occurs in the reproductive cells (sperm cells and egg cells), and then leads to deformed or incapacitated newborns.

EXTERNAL EXACERBATIONS

Cave Man, Modern man

Cave men (and women) did not concern themselves about free radicals or antioxidants. They did not trouble themselves with optimizing their body chemistry, with keeping in check the free radicals that were a natural part of their physiology. They allowed the body's natural defences to take care of it.

And on average, they lived to the ripe old age of twenty-something.

To be sure, there were a great many other factors present that may well have tended to shorten a cave dweller's life besides free radicals, things like saber tooth tigers, wolves, and snakes. As Thomas Hobbes put it, life then was "...solitary, poor, nasty, brutish, and short."

We no longer have to worry about tigers and wolves roaming our living spaces, at least in most parts of the world. In general, many of the threats to life and limb faced by our ancestors in the caves have been eliminated. Now we have new ones. And amongst these new ones are some of the conditions that tend to promote and increase free radical activity in the body. These are the external exacerbations that are upon modern man and modern woman in the world of today.

Pollution

The word "pollution" is not a pretty word, and in the decades to come it will become even less pretty. The very derivation of the word implies dirt and defilement, and in modern parlance it has almost become synonymous with the word "poison".

The sources of pollution around us are many.

Frequently, the first source that comes to mind is the pollution from automobile exhaust. We have all seen dirty brown smog hanging over our cities at evening. And even smaller communities are not immune. Auto exhaust afflicts almost every urban community, because cars are virtually everywhere. Even when the concentration of auto exhaust has not reached the point where it is visible, it is still harming our bodies. Carbon monoxide, nitric oxide, ozone – just a few of the poisons spewed out by the automobile. Very recently a study was published from St. Paul's hospital in

British Columbia, Canada showing that urban vehicle smog was just as dangerous and carcinogenic (cancer producing) as second hand cigarette smoke.

Once wind and weather have cleared the air over a city we may feel that this is the end of the smog, at least for the moment. But that is not the case. These poisons, although now diluted in the atmosphere, remain there until they come down in rain or snow.

Industry is another source of pollution. We are a bright, inventive species, and we have learned to make thousands of different substances. In so doing, however, we also produce thousands of harmful new products. Many of these products find their way up smokestacks into the atmosphere, and into our lungs

Again, a large measure of these smokestack emissions will come back to earth in snow and rain, which has brought about the coining of another odious phrase: acid rain.

Many of these industrial wastes are also flushed away as liquids or slurries, finding their way into rivers, lakes, and streams – and sometimes even into our drinking water and our food.

Some of the poisons we find around us derive from our use of herbicides and pesticides. We sprinkle and spray them on our lawns, we apply them liberally and in quantity in our agriculture. Again, through leaching and dissolution, these poisons find their way into our waterways and beyond. And, as with the chemicals carried to earth in snow and rain, some dissolve down into our aquifers, and thence to our drinking water.

Many of our cosmetics have harmful ingredients and are absorbed through our largest organ, the skin. Dr. Samuel Epstein gives us an insight into the dangerous world of free radicals and carcinogens that are plaguing our industries in his warnings to the consumer.

Other Sources

Nor are our foodstuffs without taint. Our fruits and vegetables, even after washing and preparation for market, may carry residues of herbicides and pesticides. Our meats, as well, bring unwanted substances to the table. Cattle, swine, poultry – almost all our livestock are injected with or fed hormones and antibiotics, administered to speed and ensure growth to maturity. Afterwards, from abattoir to supermarket, they may take on bacterial and other contaminants. "Hamburger disease" is yet one more phrase that has recently entered the lexicon. (Not to be confused with Dr. Victor Hamburger who died in 2001 at age 100 years, he proved that the nervous system develops in part by selective cell death in the embryo)

Processing, too, adversely affects our foodstuffs, often robbing foods of their inherent nutrients, or adding things like preservatives, dyes, or other alleged helpful ingredients.

Stress, as well, is another, less obvious, external exacerbant. To be sure, much of how we deal with external stimuli depends on ourselves. But there is no denying that there is an abundance of harmful stimuli coming at us these days, sometimes to an almost overwhelming degree. And there is no denying that it is taking a toll. In the early 90s, the top three selling drugs in America were all designed to counter effects brought on by stress. In the interim, the stresses have only become worse.

Again, words recently coined tell the story: stress leave, strung out, burnout, karoshi. (The latter is a Japanese word that applies to the instance of a worker virtually working him or herself to death.)

On the other hand, stress can be a good thing, and it can even save your life in certain circumstances. If a bear or a mountain lion comes charging at you, stress triggers the

flight or fight reaction, and sets in motion a physiology suited to that moment: the heart beats faster, and blood flow is
shut down to the internal organs and is directed to the skeletal muscles; the digestive processes stall; the adrenal glands
release adrenalin; endorphin levels rise (and we wish for a
Winchester). The many physiological changes that occur
under stress allow us to fight harder, run faster, and feel less
pain, which is of immense value in our encounters in Canada
with bears and cougars.

But it is unlikely that our cave ancestors faced bear
attacks in frequent succession, and certainly not day after
day. Consequently, our fight or flight physiology is not
designed for frequent and repeated use in the body. And yet
modern living often inflicts one stress after another upon us
in any given day. And often for many days in a row. Which
means that our fight or flight physiology is elicited many
times a day, and many days in the week.

However, since the body is not designed for these frequent physiological reactions or for continuous use, it can
"burn out." Like an overused electrical circuit, it can blow a
switch from being turned off and on so many times, maybe it
will get stuck on or stay shut off.

As for stress related drugs, they are just the tip of the ice-
berg. There is a plethora of drugs being used today. And very
few of them do not have some side effects – side effects that
are indicative of a disrupted and besieged physiology. And
these are the legal drugs. The illegal drugs may be more
harmful still.

For smokers there is the self-inflicted beleaguerment of
a normal physiology brought on by cigarette smoke.
Cigarette smoke has over four thousand chemical entities –
most of them poisonous, few, if any, good. All of these toxins tax the normal body chemistry, all force it into battle
when it should be on standown.

The same can be said for too much alcohol. A couple glasses of wine or beer per day will do most people no particular harm, and for many, may actually be beneficial. But extend this to four, five, six drinks a day and once more we impose work loads on the normal body chemistry that are harmful.

Some think another source of possible harm lies in the miles of electrical wiring that surround most of us through most of our days – in the walls around us, in transmission lines above ground, under ground, as well as electrical appliances, TVs, computer terminals – all creating electromagnetic fields that may be damaging if in close proximity to the body and overused like electric blankets and cell phones??

And then there is the ozone layer. At least, for the time being. In decades to come people may well be saying: There goes the ozone layer. And that will be because the ozone layer that lies high over the earth is diminishing, at the north and south poles. Each of these ozone "clouds" have holes in their centers, like holes in donuts, and the holes keep growing larger, while the total quantity of ozone is depleting. Given that this ozone layer screens out considerable amounts of ultraviolet radiation, its depletion means that we are losing much of our earth's protective shield. Which means that we will be exposed to more and more of these harmful rays of the sun in years and decades to come.

And when you add them all up, these external exacerbations are certainly taking their toll.

The Toll

The toll taken on the body by these external exacerbants is substantial. They either introduce a jacked-up load of free radicals into the body directly, or they induce the generation of greater quantities of free radicals than the body would have produced in its everyday biochemical processes. In addition, these poisons from the outside attack and weaken the body via their own toxic biochemical pathways, leaving it that much more susceptible to free radical damage.

Thus, heavy metals from auto exhaust (some parts of the world still use leaded gasoline), and from smokestack emissions, are extremely conducive to free radical production in the body. It is embarrassing to note that the countries that comprise NAFTA (North American Free Trade Agreement; Canada, Mexico and the U.S.) contribute 28% of the world's current annual 8 billion tons of carbon emissions. Ozone (O_3), while beneficial to us in the upper atmosphere, is harmful to us at ground level, where it constitutes yet another component found in the pollution around us. Ozone is very hard on the lungs, and strives immediately to rid itself of the third oxygen atom, creating additional free radicals with which the body must contend.

Cigarette smoke, amongst its multitude of noxious chemicals, contains huge numbers of free radicals which it introduces directly into the lungs.

Increased levels of free radicals also result when the skin is bombarded with the stronger UV radiation reaching earth through its depleting ozone layer.

Perhaps worst of all is that the thousands of artificial substances that come at us from the outside all have their own toxic pathways in the body. Each inflicts its own kind of biochemical damage on the body. For example, mercury, in its effect on the brain and nervous system, has given rise to Minimata's disease, first described in Japan.

Many of these toxins are carcinogens (cancer producing), and may affect the lungs, liver, and kidneys. Often, the immune system is dragged into the fray, frequently inducing it to produce still more free radicals, and weakening it in the process.

Whatever their specific actions, the result of these toxins inevitably means they will introduce more free radicals into the body; or they will induce the body to produce more free radicals; or they will damage various tissues and organs at the cellular level – leaving them that much more vulnerable to free radical damage.

Our ancestors from the caves did not have to contend with any of these external exacerbants, but we do. Fortunately, as we will soon see, we can counteract much of the harm these modern toxins would inflict on us by means of a very simple and inexpensive expedient.

The Toll of a Different Kind

In his famous poem John Donne wrote:

"...never send to know for whom the bell tolls;
It tolls for thee."

These external exacerbants are also like the tolling of a bell, and they, too, "toll for thee." Each molecule of toxic waste that enters the body, each free radical that it elicits, and each free radical "hit" – each of these is like a tolling of a bell that portends the laying down of the body and the ending of our days. And every one of them "tolls for thee." For none of us can escape them. Because there is no escape from these poisons, not totally. Each cell in our body may get about 10,000 hits by free radicals per day.

There may be some lucky few – living a distant, rustic existence – who may be able to minimize these toxins from without. They, like our cave ancestors, may escape a considerable amount of their effects. But most of us are not so lucky. Most of us, in making a living (or for other reasons), have to reside in urban settings – which offer all that these settings entail by way of auto exhaust, industrial emissions, background electromagnetic radiation, second hand smoke and not so fresh organic foods.

"The rain falls on the just and the unjust alike." And that includes acid rain. For most of us, there simply is no escape. We are today, as Marshall McLuhan suggested, the inhabitants of a "global village". A near meltdown in Chernobyl does not affect just the inhabitants of Chernobyl – it affects the countryside beyond, the nations beyond, and even the continents beyond.

We may reduce the degree to which we are subjected to the pollution and radiation around us. We may refrain from smoking and from eating junk food. But the fact is, in the modern world we cannot avoid an increased load of free radicals. However, there is one simple way to counteract the free radicals occurring inside ourselves – both the free radicals brought into being by natural physiological processes and those brought into being by external factors – and the call is easy: ANTIOXIDANTS. It is the only toll-free call but you need to know the number or in this instance the right combination.

Our Cells, Ourselves

Our cells are ourselves – the sum total of our physical selves, at any rate. They are the building blocks out of which the body is composed, and it is in the cells where our body chemistry takes place.

In this brief overview on free radicals, we have looked at – albeit in a cursory fashion – the principal free radicals that damage our cells. We have also looked at ways in which they inflict their damage, and where in the cell they inflict it.

Because of this free radical damage, cells can and do become incapacitated – perhaps only slightly so in our younger days (when the body is more capable of repairing itself), but then more severely as time goes by. As we will see in the immediate pages ahead, it is this incapacitation of our cells, as well as the attendant senescence and death of our cells, that is in large measure responsible for the phenomenon we know as aging. Further, where other causes of aging are thought to be involved, free radical damage will often be seen playing an underlying role as a factor affecting and augmenting their influences as well.

SECTION III

Aging

"You've probably noticed that although people are living longer, too many are plagued by diseases that not only hamper their ability to make the most of those added years, but sometimes even seem to make them a curse."

–Dr. Lester Packer

"Free radicals and aging are strongly linked. These diseases that we doctors still attribute to your age really have little to do with time, but are directly related to the accumulation of free radical damage in cells of your body."

–Dr. James F. Balch

"I'll never make the mistake of bein' seventy again."

–Casey Stengel

"The really frightening thing about middle age is the knowledge that you'll outgrow it."

–Doris Day

"He's so old that when he orders a 3 minute egg, they always ask for the money up front!"

–Milton Berle

Aging

GROWING OLD

"Growing old is not a matter of life and death – it's worse than that!"

So read the inscription on a home made birthday card done up by an acquaintance of ours. And although the words on the card may overstate the case, for many people they do express the antipathy felt for the deterioration that generally accompanies growing old.

We have seen this deterioration take place in grandparents, parents, aunts and uncles – where the encroachment of age on a youthful, robust body brings it eventually to a sorrowful incapacitation: where a sturdy man who could lift a sack of potatoes with ease is now – with the onslaught of the years – barely capable of lifting a serving of potatoes to his plate. We have seen where a grandmother or mother who could clean an entire house with ease (down on hands and knees scrubbing floors and stretching on tiptoes while cleaning the uppermost corners in windows), and is now, after the relentless march of time, barely able to clean her own spectacles. Where a former president of the U.S. is powerless in mind and a princess has lived her way into decline. And yet a queen that lives past 100 years only to suffer the finality with frailty and sadness.

So too it is for flexibility. We have all seen babies and infants who almost seem to be made of rubber, and are able to bend and stretch like Gumby and Pokey dolls. And then decades later, after the sands have flowed through the hour-glass, these same individuals are eventually creaking and cracking as though some of that sand has run directly into their joints – which are now as slow moving as the Wizard of Oz Tin Man, after a rain.

Energy levels, too, are affected. In growing old the body takes a licking but it keeps on ticking. Only now it ticks at a much slower pace. Comedian Tim Conway captured this well on the Carol Burnett Show, where he often portrayed an old man taking baby steps at such a slow pace that it would take him ten minutes to walk across a room – except that one of the other characters would intervene, of course, with some kind of joke. Or Mr. Bean would have the worst time trying to overtake an aged senior blocking a long, winding flight of stairs. But the diminishing energy levels that come with age are no joke. And as these levels become lower and lower it is as though the fire is going out in the body's furnace. And this fading of the fire invariably shows up in the eyes, as they gradually lose their fire, their sparkle for life.

And so it is for most things about growing old. They are, none of them, attractive. None of them desirable. There may be a wisdom that comes at this stage of life – for a time. And then that, too, is gone, slipping off into the haze of forgetfulness and enfeeblement.

Not for nothing that we look with distaste at the approach of our own decline. Not for nothing that our hopes and wishes are such as to will this decline gone, or counteracted, or at least forestalled.

Great strides have been taken in combating aging in the recent past, with greater ones being taken at the present time. And in the future – well, we'll probably see the greatest strides of all.

If the process of aging is looked upon as a problem to be solved, then a good place to begin in seeking a solution lies in examining the nature of the problem, in understanding the underlying aspects of the problem.

In the abstract, aging is a fascinating problem, one that has intrigued human beings from the time we first became human.

Philosophy and Attitude to Aging

Many of our colleagues have debated the benefits of a longer life. Today we have had in our office, patients claiming that they do not want to live past the age of 100 years. They cite the problems of the world today that seem overwhelming such as pollution and overpopulation. Of course we cannot ignore problems of the Third World like starvation and lack of clean drinking water but should that stop our quest for knowledge about aging? No one questioned the introduction of Penicillin by Sir Alexander Fleming that would suddenly allow those with resources to beat an early demise. Many politicians see the benefits of good health in the elderly such that many centenarians will remain as valuable contributors to society especially with all their wisdom and experience. If the diseases of aging can be held off for a few more decades instead of beginning to plague us in our 5th decade, then the benefits must seem obvious to us all. Conservative estimates tell us that by 2050, there will be a million centenarians living in North America. There will be a shift in population demographics such that the elderly will be a majority. The younger crowd will not be able to care for the aging population and thus the aged group had better learn to care for themselves. The Health and Longevity Centre in Kelowna sees that independent patient that has decided to take the next step in healthcare and spend their children's inheritance on a longer, more productive and enjoyable life. There will be a sudden rush for the technology as the rest of the population finds out what their neighbors are doing. Aging is a disease that we are determined to beat, just as we are eventually determined to leave the confines of our original home, earth.

Attitude is so important as we battle aging. We must convince ourselves on every front that we are not decrepit and beyond repair. We all know the power of optimism but of course one has to be careful. We don't want you risking injury because you want to join the youth set with skate boarding or snow boarding. If you have the brain connections (neuronal synapses) that helped you with a sport when you were a child then maybe that is the sport to concentrate on now. An interesting study done by Harvard psychologist Ellen Kager in the 1980's took elderly men (greater than 70 years) to a retreat and allowed only picture I.D. of them 30 years earlier and only news and events from 30 years earlier were allowed to be discussed. Amazingly some of their biological aging parameters reversed after their ordeal. Of course there are many variables that were difficult to control but the concept is interesting for future health resorts. People that are satisfied with their lives generally live longer than those disappointed. Although a recent publication claimed that mildly depressed individuals lived longer than the non-depressed. Less risk taking, less accidents and emotional stability may explain this counterintuitive finding. Dissatisfied men in a Finnish study (American Journal of Epidemiology November 2000) were twice as likely to die over 20 year follow up as the men with satisfaction about their lives. There is a difference between dissatisfaction and depression. One doesn't have to have one to be the other?

Connections

A man named James Burke authored a column titled "Connections" in the journal "Scientific American". He also hosted a TV show of the same name some years back. In these a series of causal events was examined. For example, the show might have begun with an ancient Greek astronomer, then move on through subsequent individuals that the astronomer's thought might have had an affect on, move on further still to the discovery of lodestone and the compass, and then on to the discovery of the astrolabe, the sextant, the light telescope (and Galileo's refinement of it), and on through further centuries and developments, until finally arriving at the modern Hubble telescope which, from its location in space, is able to capture the fascinating images of distant galaxies. (The foregoing sentence might also serve as an example of such connections, with one phrase or clause leading to the next, and so on to the end.)

Making connections is what we will try to do as we look at the various theories of aging that follow, with a strong focus on The Free Radical Theory. We will try to string together certain pieces of evidence entailed by these theories and see how they connect and interconnect. So that in the end we will – hopefully – have some insight into the problem. And more importantly, into its solution.

Theories of Aging

There are a number of theories as to why we grow old, why we age. Most of them look at a particular aspect of the aging process, and therefore, will not encompass the entire picture. But the ones we will examine do offer important insights into the aging process, and they do have strong evidence to support them. All of which suggests, from the outset, that there are a number of factors involved in the aging process.

Some of the theories have to do with the wear and tear on the body that accrues over time. Others deal with how organs or systems in the body develop and deteriorate over time. Still others deal with genetics, and how we may be programmed to die. One of the most important of these theories, dealing with the actual chemical process of aging, in our opinion (given the information currently available), deals with free radicals. And we say this for the following reasons.

First of all, the Free Radical Theory tends to underlie or connect to the other theories in many significant aspects. Secondly, the free radical theory suggests immediate steps we can take in countering the process of aging, steps that we can take immediately, at any stage of life.

It is true that research into hormone replacement therapy has also provided strong anti-aging measures, and will almost certainly add to these measures in the future. And it may be that work in the field of genetics will ultimately bring about a fundamental understanding concerning the nature of life. But all of these are linked with the Free Radical Theory and it is this theory that suggests the simplest and least expensive way of slowing and countering the aging process that we have at present.

Somatic Mutation Theory

Most cells of the body undergo cell division throughout their (and our) existence. This cell division generally brings about identical replication to replace older dysfunctional cells and is directed (as are all cell activities) by the genetic blueprint, DNA. On occasion, however, a mutation in the DNA occurs. The Somatic Mutation Theory postulates that an accumulation of these somatic mutations contribute to the aging process. There are enzymes that are able to effect repairs to the altered or damaged nuclear DNA, but this repair process becomes less effective over time. With their accumulations, these mutations bring about changes that usher in the aging process.

The effects of ionizing radiation, a powerful mutagen, have been shown to shorten the lifespan of experimental animals. This offers a pertinent point of corroboration to the somatic mutation theory. Interestingly, we have seen that ionizing radiation also increases the generation of free radicals, and almost certainly some of the DNA mutation is the result of such oxidative damage.

Error Catastrophe Theory

This theory, building on the Somatic Mutation Theory, suggests that damage to DNA can result in an incorrect synthesis of proteins. This, then, gives rise to proteins that do not have the correct molecular makeup, which therefore renders them less than suitable as chemical messengers or signalers. These abnormal proteins might be likened to misshapen Lego blocks that are not able to fit evenly and securely with others in the construction of a wall, for example.

Although abnormal proteins do accumulate with age, they have not yet been shown to be a major contributing factor to the aging process. But we believe the age of "proteomics" is just beginning and will fundamentally change our understanding of a healthy longevity.

Protein Glycosylation

Glucose, a simple sugar occurring in the blood, has been found to undergo reactions in the body with various proteins, such as enzymes, elastin, and collagen. (It can also undergo reactions with nucleic acids as well.) Protein glycosylation gives rise to compounds called advanced glycosylated end products, or AGEs.

We might think of these glycosylated proteins as being something like brown sugar baked onto a ham. If we were to start cutting this sugared ham down into smaller and smaller pieces (a la Democritus), eventually we would get smaller bits of sugar stuck to protein. When we got down to the molecular level these molecular "bits" would be somewhat akin (in a very general sense) to glycosylated proteins.

AGES = Advanced Glycosylated End Products

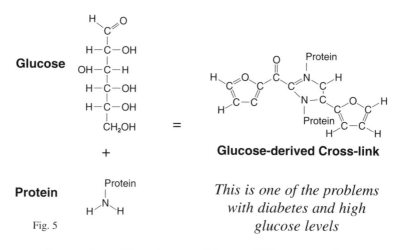

Fig. 5

This is one of the problems with diabetes and high glucose levels

Just as these bits of sugared ham will have a tendency to stick together when they come in contact with one another, so too will glycosylated proteins. And in so doing they will give rise to cross-linked structures. This cross-linkage tends to introduce a stiffening and a rigidity to the tissues in which they occur. If you picture how cooked spaghetti noodles are in a pot after being cooked and the water drained off, you will recall that the noodles are pliable and slip over and about one another with ease. But if they are left in the pot this way overnight, by morning some of them will have congealed together. And in this congealed state they will not slip over one another as they did before, nor will they be as pliable. In fact, the congealed clump will be much more rigid. Although congealed spaghetti noodles are a far cry from the cross link-ages that occurs with glycosylated proteins, this comparison does give us some idea of what cross linkage is about.

When cross-linkages in glycosylated proteins occur in elastin and collagen tissue, for example, we get the brittle skin that so often accompanies aging. Where they occur in organs such as the heart, the stiffness and rigidity these cross links engender are more serious. Here the loss of elasticity may effect an increased resistance to motion – and function.

These glycosylated proteins may also diminish the elasticity and permeability of individual cells, reducing their capacity to take in nutrient or to expel wastes.

Where this process of glycosylation affects genetic material in a cell, further impairment may ensue. The cell's genetic material – its DNA and RNA – are composed such that a multitude of genes are arranged in long strings called chromosomes. It is this arrangement – the makeup of the gene and its location on a particular chromosome – that embodies the information carried by the genetic material. And it is this arrangement that serves as a code, a blueprint which contains the information needed in directing the workings of a cell.

When glycosylation takes place in this genetic material, the information then becomes garbled, incoherent.

You might think of this in terms of wampum beads, or Catholic rosary beads. Both of these strings of beads carry information – the wampum beads as to money, the rosary as to which prayers to recite and in which order. If a dollup of honey were to be plopped onto these strings of beads, such that it stuck them into a clump, it would render them much less capable of conveying their intended information.

The Protein Glycosylation Theory also postulates that products of lipid peroxidation such as malondialdehyde (as well as other aldehydes and ketones) may be involved in other cross-linkages. Some of these cross- links would entail bonds of protein-protein, protein-carbohydrate, protein-DNA, and so on.

(Given the intensity with which free radicals effect lipid

peroxidation, we see an obvious connection here to the glycosylation theory.) What's really interesting with this theory though is its link with Diabetes Mellitus where it has been shown conclusively that the higher your blood sugar is over time the higher the glycosylated end products and the more damage there is.

The Neuroendocrine Theory

This theory postulates that the hypothalamus-pituitary system is programmed from its inception to bring about aging through the evolution of neural and hormonal directives.

The pituitary is the body's master gland. It is through commands issuing from the pituitary in the form of hormones that other hormonal glands and systems in the body are directed. The pituitary works in close conjunction with a part of the brain called the hypothalamus, and the two of them interact through various feedback mechanisms. Together they make up something of a central command post, which directs a great many of the body's functions.

Central to the neuroendocrine theory is the fact that the levels of most hormones in the body do decline as we approach middle age, with some beginning the decline even sooner than that. Evidence has shown that where hormone replacement therapy is initiated in a timely way, many of the parameters of the aging process may be offset or stalled. This is especially so in cases where there is Human Growth Hormone deficiency – inevitable as we age. Beneficial results have also been shown for the sex hormones, and as well for DHEA, melatonin, and others when used in conjunction or "harmony" as anti-aging Doctors postulate.

Although hormonal decline is certainly not the whole story to aging, it does undeniably play a large role, as we have described in our previous book, "Doctors' Secrets: The Road to Longevity".

As for melatonin, produced in the pineal gland, in addition to its role as a hormone, it has been shown to exhibit very strong properties as a free radical scavenger since it moves freely into the cells and body fluids. It is particularly effective in quenching the most destructive free radical – the hydroxyl radical. The implication here is that, in addition to its functioning as a hormone in the body, melatonin will also be acting as an antioxidant, with its effects being most pronounced in the pineal gland, where it is produced.

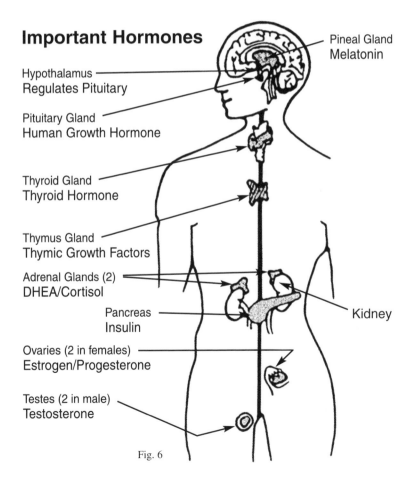

Important Hormones

Pineal Gland
Melatonin

Hypothalamus
Regulates Pituitary

Pituitary Gland
Human Growth Hormone

Thyroid Gland
Thyroid Hormone

Thymus Gland
Thymic Growth Factors

Adrenal Glands (2)
DHEA/Cortisol

Pancreas
Insulin

Kidney

Ovaries (2 in females)
Estrogen/Progesterone

Testes (2 in male)
Testosterone

Fig. 6

With the Neuroendocrine Theory, too, a free radical connection is obvious. Given that free radicals wreak their damage in all cells of the body, this will include the brain and the endocrine glands, and free radical damage is very likely a significant factor in the decline of hormone production in these glands, as we age as we previously pointed out.

Immune System Decline Theory

In our advancing years, the immune system goes into decline, leaving us more vulnerable to a host of microbial and viral predators.

The thymus gland plays a large role in the function and performance of the immune system, and it too declines and deteriorates with age. The decline of the thymus, in contrast with the decline in other glands and organs, enters its onset much earlier – about the time of early adolescence. Around the age of 25, the decline of the thymus is quite apparent through the already diminishing levels of thymic hormones.

Since the thymus plays a large role in the formation and incubation of numerous immune system warriors, such as interleukin-2 and T-cells, this gradual shriveling of the thymus strongly diminishes the effectiveness of the immune system.

A decline in the function of the Kupffer cells in the liver has been postulated by Horan and Fox as a further cause of immune system decline. Here, compounding this decline, are endotoxins found in the digestive tract cell walls. These toxins enter the venous portal system and reach the liver, where they are acted upon by the Kupffer cells and removed from circulation. However, as Kupffer cell function declines with age (and use), it is thought that the untreated endotoxins make their way back into the surrounding circulation, where they then inflict damage on other cells of the immune system that are called upon to do battle with them.

Besides the thymus, other glands of the endocrine system dictate the operation of the immune system and would explain many of the longevity benefits conferred by "Hormone Harmony" when it is finally achieved as mentioned earlier. And all could well play a role in the regulation in the levels of the antioxidant enzyme, superoxide dismutase.

A free radical connection to the immune system, too, is obvious, and we will examine it in more detail toward the end of this section.

Genetic Programming Theory

This theory postulates that all cells are genetically programmed from their inception. Which means that this genetic programming will determine the number of times a cell will divide and over what period of time, and in so doing will determine the growth, maturation, decline, and eventual death of a cell.

An everyday observation that tends to bear this out is found in the fact that people who come from long lived progenitors tend to be long lived themselves. Another indication lies in the fact that a number of diseases appear to have a strong genetic component, which means that – as in the case of diabetes, for example – these diseases will tend to correlate with a diminished life span.

Hayflick Limit

An intriguing piece of the aging puzzle was put in place in 1966 by a scientist named Dr. Leonard Hayflick. Working with another cell biologist, Dr. Moorehead, Hayflick determined that there was a finite limit to how many times most cells could carry out mitotic cell division.

For human fibroblast (cyte) diploid cells, serially cultured in vitro, the limit to the number of times a cell could divide was approximately 50 times. Once a cell reaches that limit it enters a period of senescence, after which it eventually dies. When a sufficient number of cells reach this end point and senescence ensues, the tissues or organs composed of these cells will become weakened. With sufficient weakness the organ fails, and with sufficient organ failure, the organism dies.

There is much evidence to support the thesis that this process is ultimately under genetic control. Some of this evidence we will examine momentarily. As a corollary to the idea of programmed cell senescence, it is not an unreasonable hypothesis that, were we able to bring about the means of conferring an indefinite number of controlled cell divisions, along with cellular detoxification or free radical damage correction the cells would live forever. And then, so would we – except for the incidence of disease, accident, or warfare.

The Telomerase Theory

The mechanisms that most likely give rise to the Hayflick Limit involve telomeres and telomerase.

Telomeres are the structures at the ends of chromosomes that have been compared to the protective plastic tips on the ends of shoelaces. With each cell (and chromosomal) division, these tips shorten a little. Once they have shortened to a certain critical length, the cell stops dividing and goes into senescence.

This shortening of the telomeres is almost certainly governed by the enzyme telomerase, which in turn is controlled through genetic expression. Experiments have shown that human cell senescence can be reversed by transfection with the gene controlling the catalytic component of telomerase. In a sense, this jump starts the cell, presumably by resetting gene expression in the telomere, which in turn, renews the capacity for continued cell division, much the same way cancer cells become immortal.

Obviously, there is great promise in this area for future discoveries, discoveries that may well significantly extend the human lifespan. Geron Corporation continues with research into this field as an avenue to control cancer growth. At this time our best way of expressing telomerase and keeping these telomeres longer is with HGH and hormone replacement.

The Free Radical Theory

As mentioned earlier, the Free Radical Theory was first proposed by Denham Harmon in 1954. The theory postulates that it is damage to cells by oxygen derived free radicals that brings about their eventual senescence: damage to enzymes and other proteins, to unsaturated fatty acids and phospholipids, and as well to DNA and RNA. At the macroscopic level, this free radical damage brings about aging.

Although it took decades for this idea to take hold, it is now known that free radicals are generated in great number in all human and animal cells. Further, free radicals can attack virtually all parts of a cell. When they attack the lipid bilayers of cell walls, they are capable of widespread damage. The reason for this is that they set in motion a chain reaction which is autocatalytic, so that when these polyunsaturated fatty acids and phospholipids are beset by free radicals, products of the reaction are released that are capable of feeding back into the process. This brings about still more of these products, which are themselves capable of entering the fray, inflicting their damage and sustaining the chain reaction.

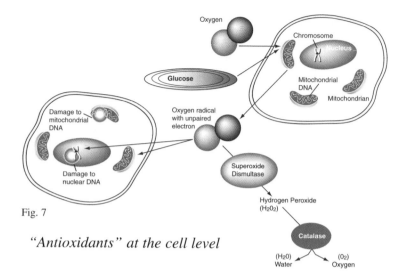

Fig. 7

"Antioxidants" at the cell level

The mitochondria, too, are acutely susceptible to free radical attack. That is because the mitochondria are involved in oxidation-reduction reactions in producing the cell's energy fuel in the form of ATP. Since these reactions entail a complicated series of electron transfers, there is ample opportunity for electrons to escape these reactions. Also, since oxygen is abundant in the mitochondria (they consume approximately 85% of the oxygen used by a cell), there is a high incidence of these errant electrons latching onto an oxygen (or oxygen based) molecule to produce a free radical.

Where anything slows or interferes with this series of electron transfers (things like external exacerbants and toxins), the probability of electrons going astray is increased, which then increases still further the incidence of free radical generation. Thus we see another instance where these external exacerbants bump up the levels of free radical formation. A cascading, amplifying amount of damage to our cells.

With so many free radicals being generated in the mitochondria, this leaves the mitochondrial DNA highly susceptible to free radical damage. The mitochondrial DNA (which is inherited solely from our mothers, so if you have a lively mother, there is a chance that you may inherit this liveliness) is particularly susceptible to attacks on their purine bases, as indicated in a study by Richter. To understand the study it is helpful to know that DNA takes the form of a double helix, the two strands of which are held together by four purine bases: adenine, thymine, guanine, and cytosine. These four bases normally pair up such that adenine joins with thymine, and guanine with cytosine. However, genetic damage may change that. Where hydroxyl radicals convert guanine into 8-hydroxydeoxyguanosine, this latter may – during DNA replication – join with adenine instead. Such DNA abnormalities are highly conducive to mutation. In the Richter study, this circumstance was indicated by a high steady-state concentration of 8-hydroxydeoxyguanosine, indicative of the likely anomalous mispairings between the bases, and potential point mutations. More serious still, free radical damage, where severe and intense, may leave mitochondrial DNA fragmented. This is doubly harmful, since mitochondrial DNA does not have the capacity to repair itself as does nuclear DNA. Such fragmentation may well be indicated by gene deletions and it appears that the circular DNA of mitochondria is more easily damaged (as opposed to our long, stranded, coiled, cell nuclear DNA).

The first known disease involving mitochondrial DNA damage, is that of Leber's hereditary optic neuropathy, and was not identified until 1986. Other diseases now linked to mitochondrial DNA mutation initiated by free radical damage include cancer, diabetes, and heart disease, as well as a number of neurodegenerative disorders.

To add insult to injury, these somatic mitochondrial DNA mutations, as they accumulate, act to interfere with the electron transfer reactions mentioned above. This then creates the possibility, in a roundabout fashion, of yet another cyclical chain reaction: errant electrons bringing about the formation of free radicals, which cause mutations in the mitochondrial DNA, which in turn bring about increased numbers of errant electrons. And on and on.

Wallace has identified free radical induced mitochondrial damage as being responsible for (not surprisingly) diminished energy production, which in turn is a factor in decreased stamina. Such damage has also been linked to memory loss, as well as vision loss, hearing impairment, and chronic fatigue.

Over the past two or three decades there has been a great deal of research done concerning free radicals and antioxidants. Over the next few pages we will look at studies and evidence that further links various aspects of the aging process to free radicals.

Rate of Living and Lifespan

The bigger the organism, the longer it lives. With some exceptions, this idea is indeed borne out by observation. Dogs live longer than mice, horses live longer than dogs, elephants live longer than horses. (Humans, as one of the exceptions, live longer than any of these but more of that later.)

As well, the bigger the organism, the slower its metabolic rate, its rate of living. Again, with some exceptions.

Most interesting is the fact that there is a high positive correlation between metabolic rate and the occurrence of age pigments, lipid peroxidation, and shorter lifespan. What this means is that, in general, smaller animals will have a higher metabolic rate, a higher rate of free radical activity, a higher incidence of age pigments, and a shorter lifespan. Compare the 100,000 free radical "hits" per day on the average rat cell versus the 10,000 "hits" for the average human cell. This in itself is strongly suggestive – albeit indirectly – of a causal link between free radical activity and aging.

Caloric Restriction

In the world around us we have ample everyday evidence that if we don't overeat, we will be healthier. It is not quite as obvious that if we "under eat", while at the same time getting all necessary nutrients, that we will be healthier still, and live longer. Statistically speaking, of course.

This premise was substantiated by a study done in 1935 by McKay et al. In the study young rats were put on a calorie restricted diet, while at the same time given all other necessary nutrients. They lived considerably longer than those who were allowed to eat freely, or ad libitum.

Other studies done using older rats showed similar results, although the differential in life spans was diminished. Further studies done over the years have corroborated these results.

A number of explanations as to how caloric restriction brings about extended lifespans have been put forth. Some of them postulate that improvements in the immune system, or changes in hormones (increasing HGH and DHEA but lowering insulin) are involved, maybe less ingested food toxins or just a lower adjusted metabolic rate also play a role.

One area of thought, involving the role of free radicals and antioxidants, has amassed a substantial body of evidence, evidence supporting the idea that, indeed, free radicals and antioxidants are a large part of the picture.

A study done by Koizumi et al shows that long term caloric restriction in mice brings about selective increases in activity for the enzymic antioxidant, catalase, and an attendant decrease in hepatic lipoproteins.

Other studies have shown that the loss of immunoreactive catalase – a condition that tends to accompany aging – was diminished by means of caloric restriction.

Still other studies have shown caloric restriction to have a positive effect on other enzymes, as well. One of these enzymes, creatine kinase, tends to show decreasing activity with age. Caloric restriction limited these decreases significantly, and in addition, forestalled the age-associated buildup of protein carbonyls, which are also associated with aging, and very likely with free radical activity. A caloric restriction mimic 2DG (2-deoxy-D-glucose) has been tested on rodents but has been proven too risky for humans.

Further Observations

As we age we tend to acquire age spots. These consist mainly of lipofuscin and ceroid lipopigments. These pigments derive from free radical reactions and lipid peroxidation.

It is thought that where partially reduced oxygen species (ROS) interact with the autophagocytic degradation occurring inside lysosomes, the formation of lipofuscin will be one of the resulting products. Thus when hydrogen peroxide generated in the mitochondria eats its way through the lysosomal membrane, it is then free to act with the iron compounds that make up some of the material being degraded in the lysosomes. At this point, reactions of the sort described by Fenton occur, generating hydroxyl radicals. The hydroxyl radicals, in turn, bring about lipid peroxidation, the products of which then engender intermolecular cross-links, and the formation of lipofuscin.

As has already been mentioned, these bodies of lipofuscin introduce an unnatural rigidity and brittleness to the tissues in which they occur. Further, they are indicative of ongoing and excessive lipid peroxidation. Ultimately, they indicate an obvious lack of antioxidant counteraction against this oxidative stress.

Protein Oxidation

Another kind of oxidative stress lies in the instance of postranslational proteins being altered by various ROS. Where this occurs as damage to enzymes, the reactions these enzymes were intended to facilitate will be impeded. Similarly for other proteins: where they have been altered (and usually enlarged) they will be dysfunctional for their intended roles.

In a study done by Starke-Reed and Oliver in 1989, rats ranging in age from 3 to 6 months of age and in which oxidized protein had accumulated, were tested. The tests showed that the accumulated modified protein correlated with a loss of glutamine synthetase, without an accompanying loss of immunological cross-reactivity. Further, in the hepatocytes (liver cells) of the 26 month old rats, the level of alkaline proteases (that degrade oxidized proteins in the liver) was only 20% that of 3 month old rats. This strongly indicates that the accumulation of oxidized protein is due – in part at least – to inoperative or deficient proteases.

In another study done by Sohal and associates (1993), the protein carbonyl content was measured as an indicator of molecular modification in houseflies. These measurements were compared to the physiological age of the flies rather than their chronological age. When the flies were subjected to sublethal hyperoxia (100% oxygen) it was found to irreversibly raise the protein carbonyl levels, and brought about a decrease in their rate of oxygen consumption.

These findings support the general thesis that mitochondrial superoxide and hydrogen peroxide generation tends to increase with age – with the oxidative molecular damage correlating with physiological age rather than the chronological age. (Some people of similar chronological age may differ in physiological age due to hereditary or environmental factors, as well as good versus bad living habits. Hence, although two individuals may be 50 years old, one may look 40 and the other 60, as a result of differing physiological ages.) The oxidative stress also brought about a shortening of the physiological lifespan. Based on data of this sort, it has been proposed that the levels of protein carbonyl may well serve as an indicator of aging.

It has further been suggested (Stadtman) that the quantities of oxidized protein may serve as an indicator of accumulated, unrepaired DNA damage, which also indirectly affects the rates of oxidized protein formation and degradation of oxidized protein.

We have already seen how the extremely destructive free radical, peroxynitrite, is the product of reactions between the nitric oxide free radical and the superoxide free radical. Peroxynitrite is particularly reactive with protein, and shows a strong selectivity towards it. A study by Viner measured the Ca-ATPase in the skeletal muscles of young and aged rats for nitrotyrosine. They found higher levels of nitrotyrosine in the aged rats compared to the levels in young rats, which suggests that protein oxidation does tend to show an increase with age.

Fast Tracks to Aging

There are a number of diseases or syndromes embodying a common element, which is that the people with these syndromes have a considerably diminished lifespan.

It is as though they are on a fast track through life, a fast track through aging, and a fast track to the grave.

Two of these syndromes, Hutchinson-Gilford syndrome (early onset progeria) and Werner's syndrome (adult onset progeria), both take their victims rapidly through the aging process and early to the grave. In both cases various outward and inward premature manifestations of aging occur. As well, these people are then prone to numerous age-related diseases, such as malignant growths and osteoporosis. In addition, both conditions tend to bring about premature atherosclerosis and heart attack.

In the case of Werner's syndrome, levels of Cu-Zn and Mn superoxide dismutase appear to be normal, as are those for catalase and glutathione peroxidase – all of which are some of the most powerful antioxidants produced by the body. Also, normal rates of lipid peroxidation have been reported. In spite of the above data, however, there have been findings of higher levels of oxidatively modified protein, which does suggest the occurrence of oxidative stress from some source, and that free radicals are playing some role here.

Another condition that accelerates aging and death is Down's syndrome. Down's syndrome is caused by the presence of an extra chromosome in addition to the normal forty-six. The mechanisms by which this chromosomal abnormality translates into accelerated aging are as yet unknown.

What is known is that patients with Down's syndrome do exhibit increased levels of lipoperoxides, which are also strong generators of hydroxyl radicals. As well, reports have indicated an increased activity for erythrocyte superoxide dismutase (SOD) and glutathione peroxidase, both of which are strong neutralizers of the above mentioned ROS. These two points of information are highly contradictory. One would have thought that high levels of free radicals would accompany low levels of antioxidants. And vice versa – since antioxidants often become diminished or depleted in neutralizing excessive quantities of free radicals. One explanation that has been offered is that this overexpression of superoxide dismutase, along with the unaccountably high levels of hydrogen peroxide, may in some way embody the mechanism for cerebral toxicity in patients with Down's syndrome.

Too much SOD and only a normal amount of catalase prevents a proper neutralizing of hydroxyl radicals. In other
words the balance or "harmony" of this natural system is lost.

Another experiment may tend to implicate more strongly the action of free radicals here as a primary cause. In this
experiment, cortical neurons taken from fetal Down's syndrome subjects were compared to those of age matched normal brain cells in cell culture. The normal neurons developed
and differentiated normally, and remained viable; the Down's
syndrome neurons tended to degenerate and succumb to
apoptosis (programmed cell death). Further, the Down's syndrome neurons showed three or four time the increase in
intracellular ROS and lipid peroxidation prior to undergoing
apoptosis. Of signal importance, when the Down's syndrome
neurons were treated with catalase or other free radical scavengers, the degeneration that had been observed in the
untreated neurons was prevented.

Altered Genes

Work by Friedman and Johnson in 1988 produced more
evidence that if free radical activity can be controlled and
diminished, chances of a longer lifespan will follow.

In one study, using the nematode Caenorhabditis elegans, they were able to induce mutations that extended the
lifespan of these mutant worms by 40 to 100%. The new
mutant worms showed a resistance to such stressors as free
radicals, ultraviolet light, and temperature. In addition, studies by Larson and Vanfleteren have demonstrated that one
particular mutant form, age-1, had a strong ability to counteract oxidative stress through an increased capacity for neutralizing hydrogen peroxide and paraquat – both of which are
potent generators of hydroxyl radicals.

Another study – this one done by Melov, Lithgow, and

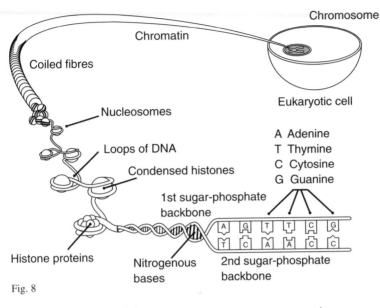

Fig. 8

*Free radical damage may occur to any portion
of the DNA in the nucleus.*

Fischer has shown that these same mutant strains of worm
that have demonstrated an oxidative stress resistance, were
also less susceptible to another age-related problem – they
accumulated fewer mitochondrial genome deletions.

Still other mutant forms of this worm, those which have
an altered gene called the clock gene, have – in a study by
Lakowski and Hekini – been shown to possess a lifespan
nearly five times longer than the lifespan of the normal, wild
worms.

In experiments with the fruit fly, Drosophila
melanogaster, the connection between antioxidants and
increased lifespan is further demonstrated. These transgenic
fruit flies had been altered such that they were carrying three
copies for two of the enzyme antioxidants: superoxide dismutase (SOD), and catalase (Cat). Superoxide dismutase and
catalase are two of the most effective and powerful antioxidants produced in the body. They are especially effective in

neutralizing both the superoxide radical and hydrogen peroxide, the latter also being a natural precursor to the hydroxyl radical.

The overexpression of these two antioxidant enzymes in fruit flies, and the concommitant increased capacity for neutralizing ROS, produced the following results in work done by Orr, Sohal, A. Agarawal and S. Agarawal: a lifespan increase by as much as 33%; an increased mortality rate doubling time; decreased oxidative damage; and a delayed loss of physical activity.

From the above there is one irresistible conclusion to be inferred: The genetic control of free radicals confers both an increased lifespan, and a delayed onset of physical infirmity. As a corollary, one might also conclude that raised antioxidant levels by other means will also provide similar beneficial results.

More Connections

The theories on aging we have examined above all have substantial evidence of their involvement with, and contribution to, our eventual decline and decay.

In general, each theory proposes and circumscribes its own area of involvement, its own set of mechanisms, its own mode of operation – although there are some areas of overlap. Which is to say, between these theories there are a number of connections and inter-connections.

For example, genetics tends to underlie virtually all operations carried out by a cell: protein synthesis, sugar metabolism, and so on. Which means that genetics has a great many causal chains or connections to the mechanisms proposed by the other theories. However, the Free Radical Theory has underpinnings even to genetics, which suggests that the Free Radical Theory has the most connections of all.

Free Radical Connections

In considering the Somatic Mutation Theory, it is virtually certain that damage to DNA by free radicals will tend to increase the probability of mutations. Also, where free radical damage occurs to DNA repair enzymes, there will be an increased incidence of DNA damage going unrepaired. There is also a strong likelihood that some of this unrepaired DNA damage will result in proteins being synthesized incorrectly, leaving them ill-suited to their tasks. This shows an indirect connection, at the least, of free radicals to "protein incorrectness". The beginnings of our understanding of what we have already said will be the biological imperative of the early 21st century, "proteomics".

Another indirect connection occurs between free radicals and protein glycosylation. Since high blood glucose levels tend to generate a higher incidence of glycosylated proteins, free radical damage to enzymes involved in sugar metabolism will then add to these glucose levels and also to insulin resistance by the cells (as in Diabetes Type II). This is especially so where damage to cells and enzymes are involved with insulin production. In this case, free radical damage may ultimately diminish insulin production, which here, too, will give rise to elevated glucose levels in the blood, and again to higher rates of protein glycosylation. In diabetics, where high glucose levels are a problem, there tends to be higher levels of free radicals as well – a double whammy. (One may well be inclined to wonder, then, if an increased incidence of cross-linkage might also be a result.)

A more direct connection occurs where free radicals bring about lipid peroxidation, and the production of substances such as malondialdehyde (as well as other aldehydes and ketones). Where this occurs, a whole variety of cross links may be the undesired result.

As for free radical connections to the neuroendocrine

system, since free radicals are capable of inflicting damage on all cells of the body – including neurons and the constituent cells of the hormone producing endocrine glands – this damage will then play a part in their decline. To be sure, genetic influences will also be playing a part in the diminishing capacity of these glands with age, and their decreasing hormonal secretions. But there can be no doubt of the free radical component as well.

The fact that free radicals can damage the DNA in these cells, as well as all others, includes them automatically as an influence. Also, the levels of free radicals (and their probable indicators) are in an approximate inverse ratio with hormonal levels. Which means that about the time that hormonal levels begin showing significant decreases, the levels of free radicals – where left unchecked – begin showing significant increases. Given the destructive nature of free radicals in the body, the cause and effect relationship here is well nigh incontrovertible.

More speculative is a possible effect of free radicals on the pineal gland. We will recall that the pineal gland is the chief supplier of the hormone melatonin. And although it does not play nearly as large a role in the aging process as human growth hormone, melatonin almost certainly plays some role here. We will also recall that melatonin has shown considerable properties as an antioxidant. Given melatonin's antioxidant properties, it is not too great a stretch to hypothesize that as free radicals come into ascendancy with age, eventually they are able to overcome some portion of the melatonin defenders in the pineal gland, wreaking their typical damage. Which will then result in a diminished melatonin output. In this scenario, there could even be a cyclical effect here: more free radicals causing less melatonin, and less melatonin giving rise to still more free radicals, and on and on. In addition, there is also the harm wrought by the diminished quantities of melatonin left for its regular hormonal operations.

The effects of free radicals on the immune system are also quite direct. Where they harm the thymus gland, they diminish the production and incubation of immune cell warriors. The same may be said for damage in the marrow of long bones. Here, stem cell production may be compromised, meaning fewer T-cells coming off the production line.

The Kupffer cells in the liver, too, will incur free radical damage over time, meaning more endotoxins will be re-entering the blood. Which will entail more work for the immune system, and the likely generation of still more free radicals.

More pervasively, where accumulated free radical damage has been instrumental in damaging or weakening tissues anywhere in the body, these tissues will be that much more susceptible to inflammation and infection. Which will again bring the immune system into play, taxing it further, often inducing the immune cell warriors to employ still more free radicals as part of their weaponry.

The Importance of Free Radicals

Given the ubiquitousness of free radicals in humans and other animals, one would not be surprised if they were one day found even on Mars. (Of course, finding life on Mars would be the main surprise.)

Today, the existence of free radicals – and their destructiveness – is no longer in question. Also, in addition to the destruction they cause on their own, there is the further destruction in which they are complicit: the damage to other proposed mechanisms of aging. Given the damage and destruction caused by free radicals in the body, especially as we get on in years, it is little wonder that the free radical aspect of aging has now come to the fore.

There is no doubt that the fields of genetics and proteomics will eventually provide a greater understanding of the fundamentals of life processes some day. And it may be that hormone replacement therapy already offers huge beneficial results in checking the aging process. But given the pervasiveness and destructiveness of free radicals, and given that there are simple and inexpensive ways of countering them, it would seem folly indeed to ignore this avenue of treatment as well. Which is why we, the authors, feel so strongly in emphasizing the importance of free radicals, and the importance of countering their activity.

In Summary

Scientists like to measure aging in the lab. We measure aging in our offices with a collection of physiological tests (measuring many aging parameters) referred to as an H-scan. This gives us a Biological Age to work with in our antiaging clinics. But for lab tests on tissue to measure aging we have the Biomarkers of Age.

- Protein carbonyls in tissue

- Aging glycation end products (AGE)

- DNA mitochondrial damage

- Beta-galactosidase in skin biopsy

- Lenticular glutathione

- DNA unwinding rate

We do not die from aging. We die from specific diseases – pneumonia, cancer, heart attack, and the like. For those of an advanced age, there are often a number of diseases working together that take them down. Aging is merely the handmaiden – the forerunner – that sets the table for the diseases, and ultimately, death. And handmaiden to the aging process is the free radical.

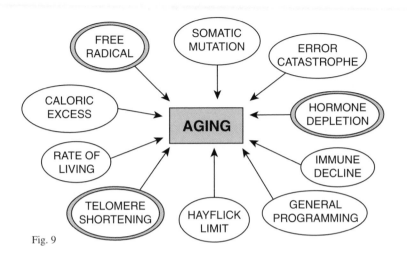

Fig. 9

On this point there is no longer any doubt. Well, there may be a few – hopefully very few – isolated pockets of doubt. But then, there are still people who belong to the "The Flat Earth Society". And even a few who believe that man has never walked on the moon.

In general, the evidence overwhelmingly supports the Free Radical Theory of aging. It also supports the idea that free radicals work to exacerbate other mechanisms of aging as well – by means of DNA damage, mitochondrial damage, and so on. And given the increase in external exacerbants, the harm free radicals do is likely to increase over the years to come.

Ames et al estimate that for every rat cell – even after all natural defenses have been brought into play – there are 100,000 points of attack or "hits" in the cell by free radicals on any given day. For humans, the number of free radical hits per day for each cell is thought to be around the 10,000 mark. This in spite of the fact that the body's natural defenses have been in full operation. One can only guess at what this number would be without the body's defenses battling on our behalf.

Without the battlers in our bodies that do manage to neutralize a large proportion of the vandalizing free radicals, one can hardly imagine the shape we'd be in by day's end. A picture that does come to mind is that of the body melted down into little more than a collapsed pool of protoplasm surrounding a smoking pair of shoes – something like the Wicked Witch of the West (in the Wizard of Oz story) after a pail of water had been poured over her.

Fortunately, we do have free radical battlers in the body, and these battlers are the antioxidants within us. In their variety they do manage to check a great deal of the free radical activity, and the damage that would otherwise assail us. They do manage to keep us whole, to keep us from dissolving (figuratively) into that smoking pool of protoplasm puddled around our shoes.

They are the good guys, the All Star Team. The more we have of them working inside us the better. And the more of them we can introduce into our body chemistry, the better. Because the more antioxidants we have inside us, the better we will be able to ward off and forestall the aging process. And to that end we take the next step along the Antioxidant Miracle pathway.

Preserving The Cell Circle Of Life

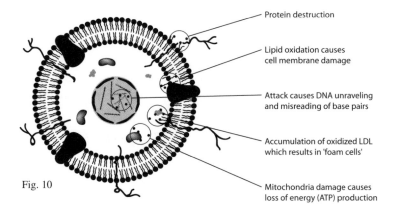

Protein destruction

Lipid oxidation causes cell membrane damage

Attack causes DNA unraveling and misreading of base pairs

Accumulation of oxidized LDL which results in 'foam cells'

Fig. 10

Mitochondria damage causes loss of energy (ATP) production

Notes

SECTION IV

Antioxidants

"By controlling free radicals, antioxidants can make the difference between life and death, as well as influence how fast and how well we age... Antioxidants work together in the body to maintain our health and vigor well into the late decades of life. They do this by protecting us from damage caused by free radicals, which can injure healthy cells and tissues."

–Dr. Lester Packer

"Within a decade antioxidants will be regarded as vitamins are now: necessary for maintaining good health and in preventing disease, and in slowing the aging process as well."

–Dr. Philip A. White M.D.

"Anti-aging medicine helps people die young... as old as possible."

–Dr. Donald M. McLeod M.D.

Antioxidants

THE ALL-STARS

We have seen that the destructive elements in our body chemistry – the free radicals – come in a number of forms. Fortunately, the body's warriors that battle the free radicals come in an even greater assortment of forms. They vary not only in their chemical makeup, but also in how they function. This variance in makeup and function, enables them to counter the varying stratagems employed by the free radicals. But despite their variety, they are all striving for the same objective: to keep us whole; to keep us healthy. And in this regard, no matter how different the antioxidants may be from one another in form and function, they are all working together on our behalf. They are all working as a team, our All-Star Team.

A standard medical textbook that all doctors used in the 1970's said that vitamin and mineral supplementation was largely wasteful and unnecessary and this shaped many prejudices and emotion about the last 30 years of medical treatment. We would like to state that "fighting disease may soon be a term that is relegated to our failures at preventing disease". And you heard it here first.

Enzyme Antioxidants

There are antioxidants that come in the form of enzymes (which are substances that serve as biochemical catalysts for particular reactions). These antioxidant enzymes are arguably the most effective of the antioxidants for the following reasons:

1) In the biochemical scheme of things, they are able to disarm reactive oxygen species before they begin their damage. Just as an all star defensive end in American football can get into the opponent's backfield and break up a play before it gets going, the antioxidant enzymes are able to neutralize free radicals before they get started on their destructive operations.

2) The antioxidant enzymes are especially capable of disarming two of the most insidious players on the free radical team – the superoxide radical and hydrogen peroxide. Thus, like an all-star defensive tackle or guard in football, they are able to take on the most formidable of opponents that may be coming at them.

3) Because the antioxidant enzymes function as catalysts, they may be altered but not used up by the reactions they catalyze. This means they can re-enter the fray time after time but some may need re-energising. In this regard they might be compared to a sturdy all-star footballer or rugby player who is tough enough to make tackle after tackle, and still have the endurance to step up to the line for the next play.

Scavenger Antioxidants

In addition to the enzyme antioxidants, there are also antioxidants which have been categorized as scavengers. This appellation stems, no doubt, from their mode of operation. In contrast to the enzyme antioxidants – which operate in closer conjunction with various physiological processes in the body – the scavenger antioxidants roam at large in the body. They are opportunistic and latch onto free radicals wherever and however they find them. These scavenger antioxidants might be compared to a rover in the defensive backfield, moving about freely depending on the formation of the opposing team's offensive line, and tackling the ball carrier no matter where he may encounter him.

These scavenger antioxidants include certain vitamins, carotenoids, and flavonoids. Also operating as scavengers are a number of other substances produced in the body. These include uric acid, bilirubin and a number of sulfur-containing substances called thiols.

The Lone Eagles

There are two antioxidants that do not fit into any of the other broad categories. They are the unique lone eagles. In the football analogy, they might be compared to the quarter-

Antioxidant Classification

A Antioxidant Enzymes
   Catalase
   Glutathione peroxidase
   Glutathione reductase
   Super oxide dismutase (both Cu-Zn and Mn)

B Metal-Binding Proteins
   Ceruloplasmin
   Ferritin
   Lactoferrin
   Metallotheinein
   Transferrin
   Hemoglobin
   Myoglobin

C Common Antioxidants ("Scavengers")
   Bilirubin
   Carotenoids (beta-carotene, lycopene, etc.)
   Flavonoids (quercetin, rutin, catechin, etc.)
   Uric acid
   Thiols (R-SH)
   Vitamins A, C and E

D Other Antioxidants
   Copper
   Glutathione (GSH)
   Alpha Lipoic acid
   Manganese
   Selenium
   Zinc

back or the place kicker. But because these antioxidants do not fit into the other categories, this in no way connotes a lesser effectiveness on their part. In fact, just the opposite is true. These two antioxidants – glutathione and alpha lipoic acid – are amongst the most versatile and effective of all the antioxidants. They are two of the body's most impressive all-stars.

Antioxidant Metals

A great deal of their effectiveness, as we will presently see, derives from their ability to function as part of the team, working in conjunction with other antioxidants.

Various metals, in their ionic form make up another group of antioxidants. Members of this group – including copper, zinc, selenium, and manganese ions – are generally bound up as constituent parts of some of the antioxidant enzymes. In this regard, then, they too are regarded as members of the antioxidant all-star team.

Metal Binding Proteins

In the human body, metals act as a two-edged sword – they can cut both ways. That is, acting in one fashion they may cause us harm, and yet in other ways they are beneficial to us, even necessary to us (somewhat reminiscent of our findings concerning oxygen). Iron is a good example of this two-edged sword.

Where iron is bound up in hemoglobin, for example, it is then part of a useful substance in erythrocytes – our red blood cells. So constituted, these cells may form a loose bond with oxygen in the capillaries of the lungs. This allows the erythrocytes to transport oxygen to other tissues, where it is needed in "burning sugar" to provide us with energy.

However, where there is too much iron, and it is unbound and moving about freely in its ionic form, this "maverick" iron may bring about the generation of free radicals, as per the Fenton reaction. (We have seen that some of this iron may at times come from lysosomes whose outer membrane has been eaten away by free radical attacks.)

Copper, too, may cause us harm in the right (or wrong) circumstances, as may other heavy metals. There are certain proteins, however, that have an affinity for these maverick metals. They are able to bind with them, tying them up before they can enter into what would be destructive reactions. Many of our patients swear by their copper bracelets for arthritis and perhaps the absorbed copper subdues inflammatory processes via the antioxidant superoxide dismutase.

Included amongst these metal binding proteins are ceruloplasmin, hemoglobin/myoglobin, cytochrome oxidases, lactoferrin, ferritin, metalothionine and transferrin.

Teamwork

We have mentioned some antioxidants as being particularly potent or effective. In so characterizing them, the intent is not to seemingly damn the others with faint praise. They are all worthy to be on this all-star team. Of paramount importance is the fact that, just as it takes all 12 players to make up a complete football team, so too it takes each and every one of the antioxidants to make up a complete antioxidant team. In football, if you can field only nine or ten players, you will not have a full team. More to the point, this incomplete team will not be as effective as a full team. So too it is for antioxidants. Where this one or that one is missing – or is in short supply – this incomplete team of antioxidants will be diminished in its effectiveness.

In American football, where a coach has not managed to

get a player onto the field to replace a player coming off in time for a play, his team will be short one man for that play. This means that the opposing team will be able to "double team" one of his players on the field. Or that with this extra player advantage, the opposing team will have one man who is not covered. If the opposing team with the extra player is on defense when this occurs, it may well use this "uncovered" player to rush in and nail the quarterback for a quarterback sack. This is referred to as the power play when discussing ice hockey.

These analogies, however fanciful, are fairly apt in looking at the team of antioxidants. Where there is a deficiency of a particular antioxidant, the team of free radicals will have an advantage, and may be able to double team some of the other antioxidants. Where the free radicals are able to overwhelm the remaining antioxidants, then some part of the body will take a hit, maybe allowing a score or a goal.

Obviously then, fielding a complete team of antioxidants is of signal importance. In this regard one might be enjoined to recall the old bromide: "For want of a nail the shoe was lost, for want of a shoe the horse was lost..." and on to the point where the battle was lost.

Another key point to be made here is that teamwork amongst the antioxidants is also of crucial importance. They work best when they work together, as a team. When they work together as a team they stand the best chance of winning the game, of defeating the opposing free radicals. Vince Lombardi, hard driving coach of the formidable Green Bay Packers of old, once said "Winning isn't everything. It is the only thing." In sports, this may seem to express a very hard-nosed attitude, and perhaps reflect an extreme stance. In battling the free radicals it is not an extreme stance. It should be everyone's chief battle cry.

The team of antioxidants have different "builds" or

chemical makeup, and therefore will excel at differing functions. For example, some will be better at preemptive strikes, neutralizing free radicals before they launch their attacks. Others will specialize in countering free radicals once an attack is in progress, and then mopping up afterwards. Some antioxidants will be more suited to taking on this or that free radical; others will be more suited to a different quarry altogether. Which is why teamwork is so important.

As we look at the various antioxidants in the pages ahead, not only will we examine their individual strengths and abilities, we will also see how they function as part of their specialty teams. Because very often, it is the way that two or three of them are able to work together as a specialty team that makes them so effective. And it is by this working together, by working in conjunction with one another, that they achieve their strong synergistic effect. Interestingly, some very recent papers published in prestigious medical and scientific journals have failed to show benefits when antioxidants have been used experimentally. We are realizing that a "harmonious combination" in a proper dosage is required for antioxidants to be effective. This may be the key.

SPECIALTY TEAMS

Antioxidant Enzymes

An excellent example of teamwork amongst the members on specialty teams is exemplified in the action of the enzyme antioxidants. These include superoxide dismutase (SOD), glutathione peroxidase (GPx), and catalase. Also playing on this specialty team is the antioxidant, glutathione.

We have seen that superoxide dismutase (SOD) is able to neutralize the superoxide free radical, transforming it to hydrogen peroxide and oxygen, as shown in the following reaction:

$$2O_2^{-\cdot} + 2H + \;\rightarrow\; SOD \text{ (catalyst)} \;\rightarrow\; H_2O_2 + O_2$$

This still leaves us with the moderately destructive hydrogen peroxide. However, hydrogen peroxide does pose a dangerous threat in that it is easily converted (via the Fenton reaction) to produce the formidable and highly destructive hydroxyl radical. And this is where teamwork comes in.

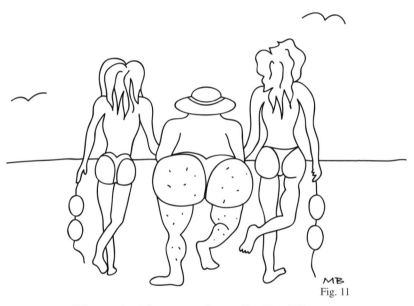

MB
Fig. 11

The antioxidants can be radically different,
but they work well as a team!

Before the hydrogen peroxide can be converted to the hydroxyl radical, two other members of this specialty team are frequently able to intervene. These are glutathione in its reduced or antioxidant form (GSH), which we will discuss in more detail further along, and the antioxidant enzyme glutathione peroxidase (GPx). Together, as shown in the following reaction, these two players double team the hydrogen peroxide and neutralize it. In this reaction, the products are glutathione in its oxidized form (GSSG), and harmless water.

$$2GSH + 2H_2O_2 \;\rightarrow\; GPx \text{ (catalyst)} \rightarrow\; GSSG + 2H_2O$$

(We might interject here that Glutathione peroxidase contains selenium, a mineral antioxidant which we will discuss later as well.)

In a reaction somewhat similar to the one above, the antioxidant enzyme catalase (Cat) is also able to catalyze a reaction that more directly converts hydrogen peroxide to water and oxygen.

$$2H_2O_2 \rightarrow (Catalase) \rightarrow 2H_2O + O_2$$

We might compare these four antioxidants to the front four linemen in football. At the line of scrimmage in football, it is the front four that line up nose to nose with the opposing team's front line. It is their job to nail the opposing team's ball carrier before he makes it past the line of scrimmage, and before he makes any gains. So too for the body's front four antioxidants. It is their job to nail the ROS before they make any gains, to nail them even before they get started.

These antioxidant enzymes occur in virtually all cells of the body. They are an innate physiological component of the body – produced in the body by the body. They are the body's front line of defence. Because they are the body's front four, it is important to maintain a diet that provides us with the necessary building blocks to maintain ideals levels of these – and the other – antioxidants. Because, the best way of cheering on the front four is by beefing them up to the max. Fortunately, this is now becoming possible through supplements that have only recently become available

For a number of antioxidants, the surest way of achieving ideal levels is through the use of high quality supplements. Again, we will discuss more on the aspect of diet and supplements further along in the section on nutrition.

SCAVENGER ANTIOXIDANTS

Antioxidant Vitamins

ACEs

There is another specialty team of antioxidants that takes on the free radical oxidizers inside our bodies. These are the vitamin antioxidants. The prominent ones on this team include vitamins A, C, and E. We might regard them – and remember them – as the body's ACE players.

Like all vitamins, they are necessary to the body in maintaining good health and proper functioning. Most of the vitamins are not produced by humans, and therefore must be supplied to the body either through diet or supplements. And although their role as necessary nutrients has been known for years, it is only more recently that their importance as scavenger antioxidants has come to the fore.

Vitamins A, C, and E are included amongst the scavenger antioxidants in that they roam the body freely, searching out and latching onto free radicals wherever they may find them. Keeping with the football model, a scavenger antioxidant is like a roving defensive back who moves with the play, seeking out the ball carrier wherever he may find him, and then latches onto him and takes him down.

Notwithstanding that we are taking a certain poetic license in our use of a football metaphor, and that we are grossly anthropomorphizing these lifeless chemical entities, this characterizing of their operations is reasonably apt.

Vitamin A

In its role as a vitamin, vitamin A is of major importance in maintaining the health of mucous membranes, skin, hair, and the eyes. It is also involved in the development of healthy bones and teeth. In addition vitamin A assists in the storage of fat in the body, and in protein metabolism. Because vitamin A is necessary for proper functioning of the eyes, without it we become susceptible to impaired vision, and especially, impaired night vision. As well, where severe and prolonged deficiencies occur, there may be impaired growth in the body.

Vitamin A occurs in the form of retinol, and may be derived from beta-carotene. Because it is necessary for healthy skin, it has been used in a number of skin preparations.

Vitamin A is a fat soluble vitamin, which means that by taking too much of it, vitamin A may then accumulate in our fat. As a consequence, it is possible to get too much of it, and for that reason, supplements containing vitamin A should be monitored closely to ensure only the optimal amounts are taken.

Beta-carotene, on the other hand, does not present the problem of excessive usage, and is safe even when taken in large amounts. A simple solution, then, is to take adequate amounts of vitamin A, with additional supplements of beta-carotene. This will allow the body to manufacture more vitamin A from the beta-carotene (when necessary), and as we will see, beta-carotene is a fine antioxidant on its own. Studies such as the CARAT and the ABTC study imply that caution again must be exercised with cigarette smokers showing increased incidence of disease with beta-carotene.

Vitamin A: The Grade A Antioxidant

In its role as an antioxidant, vitamin A is a capable warrior, and might be thought of as a Grade A antioxidant. Because it is fat soluble, vitamin A is able to work quite well in most of the body's fatty mediums.

Since it does much of its work as a vitamin in the mucous membranes, it works as a strong antioxidant in these areas as well. This allows it to scavenge free radicals in the lining of the mouth and lungs. For those who are particularly subject to air pollution, vitamin A is highly recommended to help battle the increased levels of free radical activity engendered by these external exacerbants.

In an experiment involving radiation on rats, it was found that those on a high vitamin A diet showed much less DNA damage, as was indicated by fewer DNA mutations. These rats also showed higher leukocyte levels and much higher levels of vitamin A stored in the liver when compared to the control group. This would tend to indicate that the ingestion of greater amounts of vitamin A prevented its depletion in battling the increased free radical activity induced by radiation, and that its presence was also conducive to maintaining high levels of immune cells. The overall conclusion here is that vitamin A, by means of both its antioxidant properties and its repair capacities, was effective in countering the deleterious effects of radiation on these rats.

With the boost to the immune system that vitamin A offers by assisting in the control of free radicals, it is also effective in helping us counteract infection. Further, vitamin A enhances the receptors on antibodies so that they are better able to latch onto foreign intruders such as bacteria.

Most likely, it is through its antioxidant effects as described above, that vitamin A contributes to the prevention of various cancers.

By means of its antioxidant scavenging, vitamin A is able to counter the oxidative assault by free radicals in the smooth muscle lining of blood vessels, and in so doing assists in preventing damage there. Also, by promoting the health of the endothelial lining of these vessels, and by neutralizing free radicals that would otherwise oxidize low density lipoprotein cholesterol (LDL) in the blood, vitamin A makes a valuable contribution to the prevention of atherosclerosis, and to the promotion of heart health in general.

Through this same antioxidant activity, vitamin A is of great benefit to those subject to extreme oxidative stress. Beside smokers, whom we have already mentioned as members in this category, another group subject to high levels of free radical activity are diabetics. One study has shown that the cells of the pancreas that produce insulin, the islets of Langerhans, doubled their production of insulin when in a medium rich in retinol. So far this result has not shown positive results for application in humans, but one can hope that further research here, and in other areas, will change this. In any event, the fact that vitamin A is an able antioxidant scavenger will always be of benefit to those susceptible to high levels of free radical activity – if they keep their levels up.

Grade A Performance

In its role as an antioxidant, vitamin A may not be as versatile as vitamins C and E, but it is nevertheless a grade A antioxidant. And this should not be taken as disparagement because it is not the intent here to damn with faint praise. Vitamin A performs functions that the others cannot, and it is a necessary member of the team.

By way of illustration, one is reminded of an old Fellini movie called La Strada. In the movie a pitiable waif is lamenting her lack of importance in the general scheme of things. The hero (you can tell it is a European movie because in contradistinction from American movies, the hero dies at the end) – the hero holds up a small stone and tells the waif that even this lowly stone has a place and purpose in the universe. And through his compelling and eloquent appeal is able to cheer the waif and make her feel a sense of her own worth (another tipoff that it is a European movie).

The point being made here is that all that exists has been created for a purpose, and for that reason will always be of importance in the grand scheme of things. In the case of the small stone, for instance, one would soon find it to be of telling importance after walking with it in one's shoe for half an hour. So, although not as highly touted as vitamin C and vitamin E, vitamin A is nevertheless a very important antioxidant, and has a unique and necessary role to play. And this is why we will, throughout this book, stress the importance of all antioxidants, and the teamwork that exists between them. Each has its place in the grand physiological scheme of things, each has a role to play. And by bringing as many antioxidants to bear on the free radicals in the body, the better our chances of forestalling their negative effects.

Vitamin C

The Central Vitamin Antioxidant

Vitamin C is centrally placed in our triumvirate of vitamins A, C, and E. It is also central to our health both as a vitamin, and as an antioxidant. In its role as a vitamin it is central to numerous duties in so many parts of the body. As an antioxidant it not only plays a central role in many parts of the body, it is also of central importance in its role as a member of this specialty team of ACEs (vitamins A, C, and E).

Limeys

We have all heard of people from England referred to as "Limeys". But not all will have heard of the reason for this, and the vitamin C connection.

Centuries back, when Brittania ruled the waves, her sailors would frequently come down with a dreadful disease called scurvy. Because voyages on those old sailing vessels were long, and foodstuffs limited, poor diet eventually became a suspect in the causation of this disease. In the late 1700s, an experiment was carried out by British physician James Lind. His experiments showed that if citrus fruits – including limes – were added to the naval larder and the sea-man's diet, the disease did not occur. Limes and other citrus fruits were thereafter included aboard ships in the British navy, and the incidence of scurvy plummeted. And thereafter as well, the British sailors – and in time all Brits – became known as "Limeys".

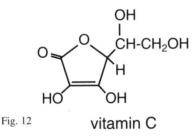

Fig. 12   vitamin C

More than a century later the miracle substance in citrus fruits that produced the remarkable victory over scurvy was identified. It subsequently became known as vitamin C. Since that time vitamin C has been extensively researched, and its many facets and properties recorded. More recently, its role as an antioxidant has been examined, and these prop-erties too have been demonstrated and proclaimed, with still more research continuing at the present time.

The Central Vitamin

Vitamin C plays a central role in the health of the body through its activity in the formation and maintenance of var-ious body tissues.

In the formation of collagen, for example, vitamin C is a necessary player. It is also a crucial player, since collagen is found in so many parts of the body. You might think of collagen as something of a glue, an elastic "bio-glue" that holds much of the body together in that it helps hold cells together. In this regard it strengthens the composition of the body in general, including blood vessels, muscles, and so on.

Collagen is a primary component of connective tissue, and as such provides the supple foundation for a healthy skin. It is also a necessary component of cartilage and bone. Given that collagen is necessary in the formation of tissues, it is equally necessary in hastening the healing of wounds and broken bones. Vitamin C as an ester (ascorbityl palmitate) is an excellent antioxidant skin care product because this form of vitamin C is now lipid soluble and absorbed into the cells of the skin.

Since vitamin C is instrumental in the formation of tissues found throughout the body, its effects are also felt throughout the body. Or more accurately, the shortage of vitamin C is felt throughout the body. In mild deficiencies, bleeding gums and a susceptibility to bruising occurs. And of course, with severe deficiencies, scurvy, where capillaries become so weakened that there is a great deal of internal bleeding, tissues become spongy, teeth fall out – and in the end it leads finally to death.

The numerous health benefits conferred by vitamin C have been studied and recorded over many decades. Only more recent is the discovery that many of these benefits owe their occurrence to the wonderful antioxidant properties of vitamin C.

The Central Antioxidant

Because so many of its health benefits derive from vitamin C's action as an antioxidant, and because these benefits affect so much of the body, calling vitamin C the central antioxidant is not an exaggeration.

The reason vitamin C can bring about its effects in so many areas of the body is that it is water soluble. Since the blood has a high water content, vitamin C may be carried easily in the blood, and may also operate in much of the body's protoplasm. Vitamin C is not fat soluble, however, and for this reason cannot effect its antioxidant action in areas such as the lipid bilayers that make up parts of cell walls. And yet, even in such fatty areas, vitamin C manages to assist – indirectly – in waging war on free radicals there. It does this by "recycling" or restoring vitamin E, which is fat soluble and is able to operate in fatty mediums. All of which means that there are few places where vitamin C is not able to assist in prosecuting the war against free radicals.

Not for nothing that we regard vitamin C as the central antioxidant vitamin.

Immune System Enhancer

By now almost everyone has heard of vitamin C's ability as a cold and flu fighter. Although it may not cure a cold, vitamin C has shown that it can reduce the length and severity of colds in many individuals. And when taken on a regular basis, it can help to reduce the incidence of cold and flu, as well as other infectious diseases.

Although the physiological details of how vitamin C affects these results are not yet known, current thought holds that much of these effects result from vitamin C's ability to strengthen the immune system.

A strong point of evidence for this is that vitamin C has been found in immune cells at levels that are anywhere from 20-100 times those found in the blood. Since many immune cells maintain high concentrations of free radicals as part of their weaponry in battling foreign invaders, the possibility exists that at times the free radicals may get out of hand. Should this happen these immune cells may become over-taxed and weakened. With high levels of vitamin C on hand this unwanted circumstance is averted, and the immune system is bolstered and kept strong.

This hypothesis may help to explain why vitamin C has accumulated much documented evidence showing that it can decrease the incidence of throat and lung infections, such as bronchitis and tonsillitis.

Studies have also shown that vitamin C has the ability to suppress replication in viruses. The rhinovirus, responsible for the stuffy nose during a cold, is one of these viruses so affected by vitamin C. Again, the pathway by which vitamin C achieves these results is unknown. But some studies do suggest that certain antioxidants may block the activation of genes that bring about replication in these viruses.

If these findings are borne out by further studies in the future, and with greater amplification, we should by then have a more detailed explanation as to how vitamin C is so formidable in battling colds, flu, and other infectious diseases.

Vitamin C vs Pollutants

Vitamin C is a superior warrior in battling free radicals generated by pollutants, as well as those generated by other external exacerbants. No matter where the pollutants come from – auto exhaust, cigarette smoke, drinking water – vitamin C is one of the staunchest antioxidants we can send into the fray on our behalf.

Because it is a scavenger, vitamin C neutralizes free radicals wherever it finds them. Because it is water soluble it can get to so many places in the body to do its scavenging.

Because it is water soluble, and because of its very makeup, toxicity for vitamin C is not a factor. As a rule, an excessive amount of vitamin C does not cause any major problems – it merely produces expensive urine, in which the excess is excreted. Since this is the case, one may aim for maximum levels in the body without concerns about a toxic buildup. Finally, as a supplement vitamin C is a very inexpensive vitamin to buy, and as well, it occurs in a number of wonderful fruits and vegetables. High doses of vitamin C may offer some problems though, to smokers. People who smoke will almost chronically have higher levels of free radicals, and these high levels deplete vitamin C more rapidly than in non-smokers but cigarette smoke contains cadmium which can combine with ascorbic acid to form a lethal combination 100 times more deadly to the DNA than the cadmium alone. Dr. Huq of Sydney University in Australia recommends no extraordinary doses of vitamin C for smokers. Please try to end your cigarette smoking as soon as possible.

People exposed to greater quantities of air pollution on a regular basis will also benefit from extra vitamin C supplementation. Ditto for those who are at risk of higher free radical activity generated by any of the external exacerbants.

When considering pollution, we would do well to keep in mind the various chemicals and preservatives added to food. In fact, the authors feel that many of these additives should come under the heading of "food pollution". Most particularly are those additives regarded as carcinogens, and which should be most avoided when considering food pollution – a subject which could fill a book of its own.

Carcinogens such as the nitrosamines, for example, have been linked to cancer of the mouth, stomach, and colon. Fortunately, pollutants such as these are strongly combatted by vitamin C.

Cancer

A number of studies have shown a link between cancer prevention and vitamin C. We have already mentioned that vitamin C can counter agents that almost certainly contribute to the occurrence of stomach and colon cancer. Other studies have shown that vitamin C plays a substantial role in preventing lung cancer as well. Similar conclusions have resulted from studies involving cancer of the prostate and the pancreas.

Since vitamin C is a solid immune system booster, and since vitamin C neutralizes free radicals wherever it encounters them – including those which would otherwise cause DNA damage – it should come as no surprise that vitamin C is a cancer fighter. The correlation between vitamin C and decreased risk of cancer are a natural consequence of its many attributes.

That being said, we would offer a strong cautionary note: It is folly to court carcinogens in the belief that vitamin C will be an absolute and certain shield against cancer. Vitamin therapy should never be used in the place of standard cancer therapies. Although vitamin C confers undeniable benefits in reducing the risk of various cancers, avoidance of carcinogens wherever possible is strongly advised. Because nothing in life is certain, and nobody, except for identical twins or clones can be the same.

Diabetes

Diabetics are particularly prone to high levels of free radical activity. For one thing, there is a loose association between vitamin C and insulin. Vitamin C is sometimes carried by insulin, and both use the same pathway to gain entry into a cell. In this competition to gain entry, insulin usually wins, meaning there will often be a shortage of vitamin C in the cell.

In addition, with the insulin either in short supply, or being inefficiently used, diabetics exhibit high sugar levels. This excess blood sugar may bond with various proteins, or may be oxidized itself. Both of these processes are the result of free radical activity, and both may be conducive to further free radical activity. Because of the unique physiology accompanying diabetes, the cells of a diabetic will generally be under greater oxidative stress than those of a non diabetic.

Research by R. S. Maxwell has shown that such reduced antioxidant activity, and the accompanying increased oxidative stress, leave diabetics fighting a vicious circle. When insulin is low in Type I Diabetes, less vitamin C is carried through the body. And when antioxidant levels drop, the insulin levels are depressed still further in.

Obviously, an increased uptake of vitamin C, and other antioxidant supplements, will help break this cycle and counter the increased free radical activity diabetics must contend with.

We will continue to examine diabetes in greater detail in later chapters.

Cataracts

There has long been the suspicion amongst many clinicians that vitamin C might be a factor in reducing the incidence of cataracts occurring in those of advancing years. And now evidence is accumulating that bears this out.

In one study involving over 300 women ranging in age from 56 to 77 years of age, vitamin C was indeed shown to be a significant factor in reducing cataracts. Of the 165 women who had taken vitamin C as a supplement over the previous ten years, 77% had a lower incidence of lens opacity. As for moderate lens opacity, the decrease in occurrence was 83 percent.

One more reason for keeping up the levels of vitamin C in the body, especially as we approach our later years.

Cardiovascular Disease

Because vitamin C is water soluble, it travels freely in the blood, where it is on a constant search-and-destroy mission against free radicals. One study has shown vitamin C to be particularly effective in reducing the superoxide radicals there, and in so doing, reducing the number of oxidized LDL (low density lipoprotein) molecules there.

The LDL (as opposed to the HDL) are the harmful ones. Where the oxidized LDL find a suitable spot on the inside of an arterial wall (often where oxidative damage has occurred), they may attach themselves there and begin the formation of plaque. With the buildup of plaque, the arteries become narrower, more constricted. This restricts the flow of blood and increases the pressure on the walls, producing high blood pressure. High blood pressure overworks the heart, which over time can be quite dangerous.

When sufficient plaque has formed we get a hardening of the arteries or atherosclerosis. Obviously, neutralizing free radicals before they can oxidize the LDL particles in the blood is of extreme importance to cardiovascular health. And this is exactly what vitamin C has been shown to do. Almost certainly it achieves this effect – at least in part – by working alongside vitamin E, which is particularly effective as an antioxidant in the endothelial lining of the arterial walls. And vitamin C does this by recycling or restoring vitamin E.

Restoring Vitamin E

Remember a scene from the old "I Love Lucy" show, where Lucy and her friend Ethel are working on an assembly line at a chocolate shop. As the chocolates come to Lucy on a conveyor belt she has to wrap them before they get by her, so that they are ready for packaging further along the line. The chocolates are coming down the belt to Lucy far too quickly, however, and Lucy cannot keep up. This leaves her scrambling madly in the attempt, even to the point of cramming many of the chocolates into her mouth, with others falling off the end of the belt onto the floor. (the cramming in the mouth bit might be okay as Penn State University has shown that dark chocolate flavonoids reduce LDL cholesterol)

What we would like to do – with a particular purpose in mind – is to rewrite this scene. Picture this:

Lucy is working at a baked potato factory. She is tending an extremely hot oven which ejects blistering hot potatoes if they are not removed in time. And if these potatoes come in contact with the walls or floor they will burn these surfaces badly.

Since Lucy has very long arms and is wearing long protective mitts, her job is to reach into the oven and remove the potatoes before they eject, and then place them in an appropriate container across the room. However, on her own Lucy cannot keep up, and the potatoes begin to eject, hitting the walls and floor – burning them, scarring them, and even starting small fires here and there – and all the while she dashes about trying to cope with they mayhem. There is ample room for comedy in this scene, but in real life such a situation would not be so funny.

Now add Ethel Mertz and her husband Fred to the scene. They both have short arms and short protective mitts, and cannot reach into the oven as Lucy can. But what they can do is take the potatoes from Lucy as soon as she removes them from the oven, and take them to the appropriate container, and then return for more. This allows Lucy more time to keep up and do what only she can do in this scenario – to reach into the oven and remove the potatoes before they eject and cause harm. (Perhaps the stress reduction here will make up for the lack of chocolate and reduced LDL cholesterol!)

In the scene we have just scripted, the action between the characters bears some resemblance to the interaction between vitamin C and vitamin E, and the way vitamin C can assist vitamin E to do the job that only it can do. Admittedly, this takes a long stretch of the imagination, but if we cast vitamin E in the part Lucy played, and a pair of vitamin Cs as Ethel and Fred, then all we have to do is substitute a lipid bilayer from a cell wall as the oven, and some free radicals as the hot potatoes. And then call: "Action!"

In this scenario, only vitamin E can operate in the fatty medium of the lipid bilayer. Which means that only vitamin E can latch onto or neutralize the free radicals there. Once it has done so, vitamin E then itself becomes a free radical, although a much less harmful free radical, since it is a much larger entity than the original free radical, and the electrical imbalance is spread out over a larger area, and is less intense. (It is a bit like Lucy holding a hot potato between her oven mitts – some of the heat is now impeded, and it is kept away from walls and floors where it can do harm.)

Once vitamin E has latched onto a free radical, it cannot latch onto more. And since the concentration of vitamin E in this part of the body is limited, once it has reduced a free radical it is then hors de combat – out of the war. Further, it is fairly difficult for vitamin E to escape the lipid bilayer and travel through the blood to carry the free radical away. However, if sufficient vitamin C has been supplied to the body, there will be optimal levels of it in the bloodstream.

In this circumstance the vitamin C in the blood is able to come in close contact with the vitamin E in the lipid bilayer, remove the free radical from vitamin E (reduce it), and move off through the blood to dispose of it. This restores vitamin E to its original state, still in place on the battlefield, and ready to take on another free radical in the lipid bilayer.

Thus, although each of the two dramas above has a very different cast of characters, the function of the corresponding members is not all that different. In corroboration of vitamin C's role as depicted above, there are studies that indicate that keeping vitamin C levels high also improves the levels of vitamin E in the body. For one such study done at Tufts University, where subjects were given 220 milligrams of vitamin C daily, it raised their levels of vitamin E by 18 percent. Which suggests strongly that for all of us, keeping vitamin C front and center in the cast of characters in the body can prevent the drama within from becoming a tragedy. People with a glucose-6-dehydrogenase deficiency, kidney stones, kidney failure or with iron overload should discuss with their doctor before taking Vitamin C supplements.

Wound Healing and Scars

When wounds heal, there is a complex sequence of steps that take place to ensure strong, functional tissue is layed down to fill in the voids created by injury. Initially cytokines will cause inflammation then clotting and vasoconstriction followed by prostaglandins and histamines causing vasodilation. Growth factors, lactic acid and vitamin C will stimulate the fibroblasts to produce collagen. It is essential to have an adequate intake of protein and the amino acid, arginine, in doses of 20 grams per day has been shown to improve protein synthesis for wound healing. Some of this may be due to extra HGH production via the arginine although studies show oral arginine alone don't elevate HGH. Elevated blood sugar (glucose) may impair the wound healing by preventing vitamin C transport into fibroblasts and white blood cells, interfering with collagen production and immunity. Vitamin A improves collagen synthesis and counter the effects of steroids on wound healing. Vitamin E orally and on the skin does not appear to help wound healing or prevent scarring in studies done on burn patients. Vitamin K is necessary to promote clotting. Zinc deficiency must be corrected and supplements of 30 mg per day have been recommended especially for the elderly. Serum ceruloplasmin levels should be checked or else copper supplemented at 3 mg per day will ensure that adequate copper is available to act as a cofactor for crosslinking of collagen and elastin via lysyl oxidase. Iron is necessary for hemoglobin carrying oxygen to the wound and also for hydroxylation of amino acids, lysine and proline for collagen synthesis. Of course fats are required. Linoleic acid (omega-6 from vegetable oils, corn, soybean and safflower) will lead to arachidonic acid and inflammatory, immunosuppressive prostaglandins. Linolenic acid (omega-3 from fish oils, flaxseed and canola oils) will lead to vasodilation, anti-inflammatory and immune enhancing prostaglandins. Interferons have been used to reduce scar formation by inhibiting Type I collagen messenger RNA and histamine production. Transforming growth factor beta (TGF-beta) is a cytokine that can enhance scar formation as a topical cream and used in combination with interferon alpha 2b (IFN-alpha 2b) cream (which decreases scarring) at various stages of skin wound healing, the ultimate minimal scarring wound may be attained.

Vitamin E

We would not be amiss in stating that the "E" in vitamin E might well stand for "Excellent". Vitamin E serves as an excellent vitamin, conferring numerous benefits on the body in this capacity. And with the above foreshadowing of vitamin E as a team player with vitamin C, we might easily guess that in its role as an antioxidant it might even be graded "Most Excellent".

As A Vitamin

Vitamin E was discovered in 1922 by researchers Herbert Evans and Katherine Bishop. They found that an unknown substance in green lettuce was instrumental in preventing miscarriage in rats. In 1936 this unknown substance was finally isolated and identified. It subsequently became known as vitamin E. Over the decades more and more has been discovered about vitamin E as a necessary ingredient in our diet, an ingredient without which we would fall into failing health.

Various Types of Vitamin E

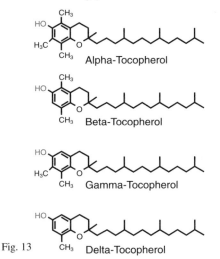

Alpha-Tocopherol

Beta-Tocopherol

Gamma-Tocopherol

Fig. 13   Delta-Tocopherol

In general, vitamin E is necessary in preventing pronounced muscle weakness and wasting. Concomitant with that, vitamin E is also, then, conducive to the healing and repairing of damaged tissues; to the reduction of scarring from such damage; to the effective clotting of blood at the site of a wound; and to the lowering of blood pressure.

In addition to building and repairing healthy muscle, vitamin E has also been associated with maintaining healthy nerves, skin, and hair. As well, vitamin E has been linked to preventing cataracts, to relieving symptoms of PMS, and to relaxing leg cramps.

With the mountain of evidence attesting to the necessity and the benefits of vitamin E, it is unlikely therefore that the scoffers of the past would, themselves, undertake an experiment today in which they were to be deprived of it.

As An Antioxidant

If vitamin E is an excellent vitamin, it is then a most excellent antioxidant. There are a number of reasons for this, and underpinning most of them is the fact that vitamin E is fat soluble.

To get some importance of this, picture a bottle of liquid Italian salad dressing that you have just taken out of the fridge. You can see that if it has not been shaken recently it will have separated into two different layers – layers largely composed of oil and water. Since oil and water are mutually insoluble, their molecules will not intimately intermingle, as for example, will those of vinegar and water. Which is why we have to shake these kinds of dressings immediately before using to get a mixture of the two onto the salad.

Further observation has shown that if a substance is fairly soluble in water, then it will be less so in oil. And vice-versa. Thus, although vitamin E is not particularly water soluble, it is fat soluble. And it is this property that allows its molecules into places in the body such as the fat based lipid bilayers that make up part of the cell wall.

Because vitamin E can enter fatty mediums and move about in them, and can do so better than any other scavenger antioxidant, it assumes a signal importance here. We have seen that where free radicals are permitted to attack these areas willy nilly, not only do they bring about isolated incidences of lipid peroxidation – they almost certainly set in motion a chain reaction: one produces two; two produce four; four produce eight; and so on. Not unlike the chain reaction in uranium 235, or plutonium – only with free radicals it is the cell that can be destroyed. And after that, another, and another....

Although vitamin E is present in cell membranes in very low concentrations when compared to the lipid molecules (perhaps 1:1000 or 1:2000), it does a powerful job in preventing lipid peroxidation. No doubt a great deal of its ability to take on such odds rests with its ability to curtail the attendant chain reactions before they get started. But when vitamin E is allowed to drop below the optimal level – that is when the free radicals begin to win. And one end result is an accelerated aging process. Another is the fast track to heart disease.

Cardiovascular Disease

It had been known for quite some time after its discovery that vitamin E possessed antioxidant properties, and was able to prevent the oxidation of polyunsaturated fats – that is, to keep them from going rancid. But it was only in 1954 that A. L. Tappel, a biochemist at the University of California at Davis, was able to prove that vitamin E could also prevent the same kind of oxidation from occurring to fats in the blood.

Since vitamin E is not water soluble, it cannot travel easily in the blood, which is largely water based. It gets around this in a rather ingenious fashion. It hitchhikes through the blood on particles of lipoprotein. These lipoproteins are manufactured in the liver and serve as transport units for cholesterol. The low density lipoproteins (LDL) carry cholesterol to the tissues to be used in the construction and maintenance of cells. The high density lipoproteins (HDL) carry cholesterol to the liver where it can be excreted in the bile.

Where these lipoproteins – especially the LDL – undergo oxidation as the result of free radical attack, they become transformed at their molecular level. In this oxidized state they are now able to activate receptor sites on macrophages, which are part of the body's defense system against foreign invaders. The macrophages "engulf" the oxidized lipoproteins much as an amoeba engulfs a food particle. This bloats and distorts the macrophages into what have come to be known as foam cells. In this state the bloated foam cells take on an affinity for the endothelial lining of the inner artery walls. Where they are able to secure purchase there they attach themselves, sort of like molecular barnacles.

Exacerbating the situation still further are instances of oxidative damage to the endothelial linings of the arterial walls which initiates the process of inflammation. It is amazing to think that until about 5 years ago only fat accumulation was considered to be the cause of atherosclerosis, not the inflammation that we now know as the major driver of problems leading to stroke and heart attacks. We have seen that free radicals are especially destructive in these areas, partly from their ability to set in motion ruinous chain reactions. Once this damage has occurred it makes it that much easier for foam cells to attach and proliferate there. This might be compared to the way a new coat of varathane will adhere better to a previous coat if it has been sanded and scuffed a little. The damaged area on the artery wall allows a better adhesion for the foam cells.

So here we have the oxidative (leading to inflammation) process slamming us with a double whammy: it is indirectly responsible for the existence of foam cells, and it damages artery walls to provide a better sticking spot. One is reminded of contact cement: apply it to two different surfaces, then later press them together and presto! Sticks elephants to ceilings. Only with the lipoproteins and the artery walls, the contact cement is free radical oxidation.

Where there is a sufficient buildup of these foam cells, packed onto the sides of arterial walls, you eventually get a more rigid accretion called plaque; and where there is sufficient plaque you get a hardening of the arteries; and where you get a hardening of the arteries you can get high blood pressure; and where the coronary or carotid arteries are affected you can get a heart attack, or stroke. And you know on which side of the sod that can get you.

All from a loathsome little free radical and its oxygen!

Now picture the above series of events running backward, like a movie being shown in reverse, and stop it at the point where the free radical is about to strike the lipoprotein. Only now let your ears hark to the clarion call of a trumpet sounding out the first notes of the William Tell Overture (aka the Lone Ranger's theme)! And now picture a vitamin E astride its steed of another lipoprotein molecule, riding down on the nefarious free radical and disarming it. Just in the nick of time, of course.

And, of course, we are being just a little more than fanciful here. But the above histrionics – notwithstanding the fancy – is a rough approximation of what takes place in the blood within your arterial walls – and the damage that can be prevented – if you have maintained sufficient levels of vitamin E in your body. Which you will have if you have been wise in your choice of diet and supplements. Again prevention is the key since there is more evidence to demonstrate prevention of progression than there is to show easy reversal of hardening of the arteries.

Heart Health

That vitamin E is an effective agent in promoting heart health is supported by an ever growing body of evidence.

One of the earliest studies on vitamin E was conducted

by two Canadian cardiologists, Wilfred and Evan Shute. After treating over 30,000 patients with vitamin E, they reported achieving strong positive results, detailed in their book "Vitamin E for Healthy and Ailing Hearts", published in 1972.

More recently Lester Packer has shown equally positive results in his studies on vitamin E, particularly in its use in preventing heart disease.

Numerous studies continue to confirm the benefits of vitamin E in the prevention of heart disease. Two Harvard-based studies in particular, involving over 87,000 female nurses and 29,000 male health professionals, demonstrated clearly the boost to heart health conferred by vitamin E. The two groups showed a 41% and a 37% decreased risk of heart disease respectively.

Even for those with heart disease, beginning a program of vitamin E supplementation can be of tremendous benefit. In a double blind study known as the Cambridge Heart Antioxidant Study, dramatic results were obtained. In this study, which involved 2002 patients with serious heart disease, 1035 were given either 400 I.U. or 800 I.U. of vitamin E daily. The remaining 967 patients were given a placebo. After 510 days the study was discontinued – not because vitamin E was not working, but because it was working so well. Those receiving vitamin E had 77% fewer heart attacks compared to those on the placebo. The reason the study was discontinued is that it was decided to put all the patients on vitamin E so as not to deprive them of its benefits.

Obviously, where vitamin E can demonstrate such amazing results for diseased hearts, there can be little doubt that it will show equally fine results in preventing heart trouble in the first place.

Although there has been considerable skepticism shown vitamin E over the past few decades, the tide has now turned.

The mechanisms by which vitamin E works are ever more widely being elucidated upon in the wake of research going on throughout the world. And the results continue to corroborate earlier positive findings that support vitamin E as a promoter of heart health, and in other areas as well. We will discuss further the results of the Heart Protection Study.

Cancer

Vitamin E, as an active scavenger and quencher of free radicals, also prevents DNA damage, which is often a harbinger of cancer. Besides fighting cancer in this way, vitamin E has also shown an involvement in signaling pathways that turn on and off genes, and that also affect cell growth.

Researcher Angelo Azzi in Switzerland has shown that vitamin E inhibits the activity of protein kinase C, which activates enzymes that stimulate growth in tumors.

Another study, this one conducted by Katalin G. Losonczy, a researcher with the National Institute on Aging, also supports vitamin E as a cancer fighter. Her results, involving a study on over 11,000 people whose ages ranged from 65 to 105, were dramatic. Those taking daily supplements of vitamin E exhibited a 41% less chance of dying from cancer. Not surprisingly, the results were also favorable with respect to heart disease, where those in the study had a 40% decreased likelihood of dying from this cause.

Longevity

In view of the foregoing results, a skeptic might wonder: although vitamin E may well have demonstrated a reduced risk of dying from cancer or heart disease, does it in fact actually promote longevity? So far, this appears to be the case. Vitamin E can increase the likelihood of an increased lifespan. As well, vitamin E – especially in conjunction with other antioxidants – appears eminently capable of improving the quality of a person's life in those later years.

One study, conducted by David Deamer at the University of California at Davis, involved the culturing of human cells, and the production of lipofuscin by these cells. Lipofuscin, we will recall, is an age pigment that shows up in the skin as age spots. It also shows up in other tissues and organs. The incidence and accumulation of lipofuscin tends to increase with age, particularly in nerve tissue and heart muscle.

In the Deamer experiment, young cells were grown in a medium of 10% serum, in which they developed and grew normally. The did not begin showing accumulations of lipofuscin until they were well along their span of cell divisions – that is, until they had grown old. The same kinds of cells were then grown in a medium low in serum, subjecting them to a nutrient-poor existence. Early on, these cells demonstrated difficulties in dividing properly and repairing themselves. These same cells accumulated large amounts of lipofuscin early in their lifespan. They had aged prematurely.

However, when cells such as these were grown in this same nutrient-poor medium – with the exception of 100 micrograms of vitamin E being added – the cells did not exhibit this early formation of lipofuscin, as had those without the vitamin E. They did not exhibit this signal of premature aging. And the sole difference was vitamin E!

In another experiment, vitamin E was actually able to extend the lifespan of cultured human cells. In this experiment, cells which had a normal lifespan of 50 divisions (before reaching their Hayflick Limit) were grown in a vitamin E enriched medium. In this vitamin E enriched environment the cells reached an astounding 100 cell divisions. In this case, vitamin E had doubled their lifespan!

Granted, as humans we do not live our lives as isolated cells in petri dishes or in test tubes, dividing our lonely way to the Hayflick Limit. But we are composed of groups of cells, and these cells do undergo cell division and they do eventually reach the Hayflick Limit. So experiments of this sort are of great merit in suggesting what may be going on at the cellular level, and therefore, in the entire human animal.

In the area of longevity, much of the evidence concerning vitamin E is indirect evidence of the sort considered above. A major reason is that in America, humans today have a projected lifespan of almost 80 years. However, since much of the vitamin E research was only begun in the last decade or two, direct studies on humans with respect to longevity will not bear fruit for some time to come. This being said, the following point must be emphasized: those studies that do exist strongly indicate that vitamin E is an important factor in attaining an increased lifespan. Just as important, vitamin E also improves the quality of life in those years by improving an individual's health, allowing us the bonus of a healthy lifespan.

Other Benefits

Vitamin E has also been shown to exert a positive influence on other diseases to which we humans are susceptible, especially as we get older – which is another way in which this vitamin can help extend the human lifespan.

As was the case for vitamin C, vitamin E also helps in the prevention of cataracts. Since the formation of cataracts is thought to come about from lipid and protein oxidation – particularly of the crystallins of which the lens is largely composed – it is not surprising that vitamin E has shown the ability to prevent cataracts.

Arthritis is another condition in which vitamin E has

demonstrated an ameliorating effect. A number of studies have indicated that through vitamin E supplementation, the severity of the stiffness and pain – and the attendant reduced mobility – can be significantly curtailed.

Perhaps most encouraging is that vitamin E has shown positive results in preventing, delaying, or diminishing the severity of Alzheimer's disease. Since this cruel disease occurs as the result of a deterioration in the brain, and that some of this deterioration is very likely the result of oxidative damage to nerve tissue, the action of vitamin E as an antioxidant is surely one way in which it has been able to effect its positive results. And although the ultimate cause of this disease is still presently unknown – much less a complete cure looming on the immediate horizon – until such is the case, vitamin E can at least offer the potential for valuable help here.

Whether as a preventive or palliative, vitamin E offers a simple and effective solution – albeit only partial – in diminishing the severity of Alzheimer's disease. For this disease especially, unless one has experienced the sorrow it causes (not only for those afflicted but also for the loved ones in attendance), it may be difficult to fully comprehend the stark reality that half a loaf here is so much better than none.

Natural vs Synthetic

Over the past few years there has been a running debate as to the benefits of natural vitamin E versus synthetic vitamin E. To best evaluate the two, a number of salient points should first be considered.

To begin with, vitamin E – as it occurs in nature – is not a single chemical entity. Rather, vitamin E comes in two similar molecular forms, tocopherols and tocotrienols. Each of these in turn, have four isomeric forms: alpha, beta, delta, and gamma. Thus you can have alpha, beta, delta, or gamma tocopherols, as well as the four corresponding tocotrienols. If names such as alpha tocotrienol seem a bit abstruse or technical, they are hardly so in comparison to their actual chemical names. Which, unless you have PhDs in biochemistry, you really do not want to know.

Of these eight vitamin E forms, alpha tocopherol is the most active in the body, and the one most available in foodstuffs throughout the world. It is also the one that is preferentially selected by the liver to be set up as a "hitchhiker" on a lipoprotein. As a consequence, alpha tocopherol (listed as d-alpha tocopherol) is the form most commonly found in natural source vitamin E supplements today.

So what form, then, does synthetic vitamin E take? Synthetic vitamin E, most commonly produced from petrochemicals, takes the form of stereoisomers of the natural vitamins. This means that they are similarly composed but have a slightly different geometrical arrangement in space. Thus, they too may assume 8 slightly different guises.

Studies comparing the two – natural and synthetic – are quite recent and still not in total agreement. The preponderance of evidence so far suggests that the natural form of vitamin E brings about higher levels in the body and is used more efficiently by the body. That is, it has a greater bioavailability. So, as you can see with matters biochemical and biological, nothing is ever as simple as they seem but we can work through the complexities.

In essence, this means that natural vitamin E is selected by the liver and processed for use by the body more readily than the synthetic versions. Some of the most recent studies indicate that natural vitamin E, in the form of alpha tocopherol derived primarily from wheat germ oil, confers about double the effectiveness of synthetic vitamin E. However, by increasing the dosage of synthetic vitamin E, up to a point, the differential can be reduced substantially.

As a guide to consumers, the natural vitamin E will be listed under the ingredients as d-alpha tocopherol, while synthetic vitamin E will be listed as dl-alpha tocopherol.

Gamma Tocopherol

Adding to the vitamin E confusion are some of the other forms in which this vitamin occurs, such as gamma tocopherol. Gamma tocopherol is the prevalent form that occurs in soy beans and corn, and in their oils. In North America it was at one time the form of vitamin E that most commonly found its way into the average American's diet. But over the decades that has changed.

Nowadays, gamma tocopherol is generally removed from these oils, and used for other purposes, including (ironically) the production of natural sourced vitamin E, in the form of alpha tocopherol. As a consequence, for most North Americans, alpha tocopherol predominates both in the diet and in supplements. Notwithstanding that the body uses alpha tocopherol more efficiently, gamma tocopherol has its own special functions, and its widespread removal from the diet is not an ideal tradeoff.

Current research so far indicates that gamma tocopherol can do some things better than other forms of vitamin E. It is remarkable, for instance, in its ability to protect people from lung cancer, especially smokers. A study conducted in the South Pacific indicated this property most emphatically.

In this study, two distinct populations with similar smoking habits were involved, those in Fiji and those in the Cook Islands. The gamma tocohperol levels were determined for the two groups and then compared to their respective rates of lung cancer. The Fijians, whose diet supplies greater quantities of gamma tocopherol, were found to have twice the serum levels of gamma tocopherol than the Cook Islanders. Even more telling is this: although the smoking habits for both were similar, the rate of lung cancer for the Fijians was about a tenth of that for the Cook Islanders.

Although research on the subject is preliminary, one explanation of how gamma tocopherol guards against lung cancer may lie in the following: nitrogen dioxide is a significant component of tobacco smoke and is easily converted into a potential carcinogen. Gamma tocopherol, however, is able to interact with nitrogen dioxide and deflect it down a different biochemical pathway, thereby reducing the number of carcinogens produced, and the risk of cancer.

Gamma tocopherol has also shown an unmistakable ability in reducing heart disease. One mechanism proposed to explain this derives from the fact that the body produces a diuretic called LLU alpha, which is concerned with the elimination of water from the body, and less directly, in the regulation of mineral levels in the body. It turns out that gamma tocopherol is a key player in the production of LLU alpha, and where gamma tocopherol is lacking, LLU alpha may then be lacking as well. This in turn may throw the body's water and mineral balance off the mark, and in so doing, contribute to the occurrence of high blood pressure. Which in turn increases the risk of heart attack and stroke.

There is a fly in the ointment as concerns gamma tocopherol, however. It stems from the fact that preliminary research suggests that alpha tocopherol may tend to block the uptake of gamma tocopherol in the body. For those (such as smokers) who are particularly at risk for developing lung cancer, or those who already have high blood pressure, one suggestion might be for these individuals use vitamin E supplements now available that consist solely of gamma tocopherol, in addition to their regular vitamin E supplements.

Tocotrienols

The tocotrienols, too, have demonstrated a specialized function in the body. And as ever, function follows form. In the case of the tocotrienols, it is their form – their molecular configuration – that confers this special function, this special ability.

The vitamin E molecules take the approximate form of a dragon head with a long tail, with bits of chemical ornamentation here and there, particularly at the ends. In the case of the tocotrienols, the tail is so configured as to allow it to move about more freely in the fatty membranes of the body than is possible for their tocopherol siblings. The fact that their molecular form more closely resembles the molecules that make up the matrix of the lipid membranes is a large factor in this mobility. With this mobility, the tocotrienols are then able to spread out through in the membranes of arteries, for example, to distribute and disperse themselves more readily and more evenly than the tocopherols, which tend to occur in clusters. This makes the tocotrienols that much more efficient as scavenger antioxidants in these tissues.

The tocotrienols possess another big plus in their antioxidant activity. There is research to suggest that, of the various forms of vitamin E, the tocotrienols are the most easily restored to their original state by vitamin C, after they have neutralized a free radical. Part of this may be due to their mobility. Since they are able to move to the edge of the fatty membrane more readily than the tocopherols, they may be restored more quickly, and brought back to fighting trim. That is, they may more quickly hand off the electrical imbalance they have taken on in neutralizing a free radical to a vitamin C molecule, and then with their mobility, return more quickly to the fray.

No doubt it is by possessing these properties that the tocotrienols are especially adept in preventing atherosclerosis, and in preventing high cholesterol levels. More impressive still, they have quite recently shown that they can be of immense value in treating these conditions after they have already come into being.

Areas of particular concern involving the buildup of plaque are the carotid arteries, which supply blood to the brain. Where this buildup is sufficient to constrict the flow of blood to the brain, we have an instance of carotid stenosis. Eventually such plaque deposits may cut off blood supply to the brain – causing a stroke. Or bits of the plaque may come loose, and, finding their way to the brain, may in this way cause a stroke.

Until recently, one way of preventing this dire consequence required an operation in which the carotid arteries were cut open and scraped, clearing away the plaque and opening up the arteries once more. This is a dangerous operation, however, in that bits of the plaque may escape the area and end up in the brain anyway, bringing about the unwanted stroke that the operation was intending to prevent. Which illustrates the adage that desperate measures require desperate means.

But that adage may no longer apply here.

Recently a study was conducted by Dr. Marvin Bierenbaum of the Kenneth L. Jordan Heart Foundation on patients with carotid stenosis due to the buildup of plaque. The patients were divided into two groups, with one group receiving tocotrienol supplementation over a four year period, and the other group receiving a placebo. Both groups were given ultrasound scans after periods of six months, twelve months, and then yearly after that.

Of those receiving tocotrienol supplements, 94% either improved or remained the same. Of the control (placebo) group, none improved and over half grew worse.

Perhaps just as remarkable are results Dr. Bierenbaum obtained in another study, this one looking at tocotrienol's ability to improve cholesterol levels. In this experiment patients had been placed for a time on a regime of palm derived tocotrienols, during which some patients had seen little improvement in their cholesterol levels. Three years into the study the patients were then switched to tocotrienols derived from rice bran, which also included the rice bran phytochemicals. (Phytochemicals are substances such as flavonoids, carotenoids, tocopherols, and phenolic acids, which occur along with other nutrients and vitamins in fruits and vegetables, and which appear to confer an enhancing effect on the performance of these vitamins. Also, many phytochemicals serve as antioxidants as well.)

Those patients whose cholesterol levels had remained unchanged under the palm derived tocotrienols, afterwards improved while using the bran derived tocotrienols, which included their accompanying phytochemicals. Obviously here, the whole is more than the sum of the parts, and certainly, more than some of the parts. Not only was the bad cholesterol (LDL) reduced, but the good cholesterol (HDL) was increased, bringing about an improvement in the entire blood profile.

The tocotrienols have also demonstrated a positive effect as agents in countering breast cancer. To better understand their effects in this area is important first to distinguish between two types of breast cancers, estrogen receptor positive and estrogen receptor negative. In estrogen receptor positive cancers, most often found in post-menopausal women, estrogen is conducive to tumor growth. In estrogen receptor negative cancers, estrogen has no effect on tumor growth. At the crux of the matter is an anti-cancer drug called tamoxifen. Tamoxifen is effective in preventing and treating estrogen positive cancers, but not against estrogen negative cancers. More damning, it also has serious side effects, such as carrying an increased risk for uterine cancer.

In a study conducted in laboratories at the University of Western Ontario, the effects of tamoxifen and tocotrienols on both types of cancer was compared. This in vitro experiment showed that the tocotrienols inhibited the development of both types of cancer. To be sure, these are preliminary findings, obtained from laboratory experiments. Undoubtedly field trials will follow, but similar positive results are expected.

In addition to working on the inside of the body, particularly in the membranes of artery walls, the tocotrienols are also effective much closer to the surface. They tend to gravitate to the skin as well. Here again, in their role as powerful antioxidants, the tocotrienols play a large part in how vitamin E is able to counter free radical activity in this outer covering of the body. Because it is in the skin that free radical activity is especially increased by ozone and ultraviolet rays. Which is why vitamin E has so often been part of the various preparations designed to keep the skin healthy and smooth, and forestall the effects of aging.

A Brief Guide

There has been controversy concerning vitamin E in the past, much of which has been put to rest with the host of recent research. But with this same research comes a welter of information about vitamin E, and its numerous guises. Much of it can be simplified but we must keep in mind some of the complexity mentioned earlier and remember that vitamin E, as part of the larger antioxidant team, is itself a team, with its various constituent players offering varying benefits between them. This team concept is often ignored in many of the trials and experiments reported in the publications we review. And with that in mind, the following points will have a greater contextual backdrop upon which to anchor them.

1. Vitamin E, as the most effective of the fat soluble antioxidants, is of great benefit in countering the effects of aging, and in reducing the risk of many serious diseases, including heart disease, stroke, and cancer.

2. Whether in natural or synthetic form, vitamin E is a valuable supplement, with the natural form working more efficiently in the body. Given that much of the North American diet has been stripped of the vitamin E previously found in certain oils and foodstuffs, most people will benefit from vitamin E supplements.

3.With new information surfacing almost daily, one may expect a large variety of vitamin E preparations in the near future. Already gamma tocopherol is available, and the tocotrienols will soon be available as well. This variety will allow those at particular risk, or those with particular needs, to obtain the combinations of vitamin E that are of most benefit to them.

4.Although it may be difficult to obtain all necessary vitamin E from foodstuffs, this is the desired objective at which to aim. And then, according to need, use additional appropriate supplements as...supplements.

THE CAROTENOIDS

The carotenoids make up another specialty team operating as antioxidant scavengers. They occur as natural pigments in fruits and vegetables, frequently giving them their orange, red, and yellow colors. As well, they occur in green, leafy vegetables, but the colors there are masked by the green of the chlorophyll.

Although over 700 carotenoids have been identified, only about 60 are found in food. Of these, only a half dozen or so have been studied in any detail for their antioxidant properties. Preeminent amongst these are alpha-carotene, beta-carotene, and lycopene, with cryptoxanthin, lutein, and zeaxanthin also currently being researched.

In general, the carotenoids excel in reducing the risk of heart disease, and most particularly in reducing the risk of cancer.

In one study, for example, the carotenoid levels in over 2000 individuals was monitored over a 13 year period. During that time, those with the highest carotenoid levels had 40% fewer heart attacks. Similar statistical studies have shown that high levels of carotenoids correlate well with a reduced risk of cancer.

Other studies have also been conducted over the past decade or so on the individual carotenoids. In these studies many of their specialized functions – their areas of particular benefit – have been identified.

From these studies a familiar theme emerges: The carotenoids do indeed have their own areas of specialized function. However they also tend to have a pronounced synergistic effect on one another – that is, they most often work best as a team. Interesting how this theme runs through the whole arena of cellular chemistry.

As we look at the individual carotenoids we will, as we have with the other antioxidants, be considering the experiments and studies that support the claims made for them. It is true that there are a great many numbers and statistics set forth in these studies. And although the use of these numbers and statistics are necessary in measuring or assessing certain factors or properties, it may at times seem like a boring numbers game. But that is the point: it is a numbers game. We are gathering the "odds" from the various scientific "bookmakers" as to how the various antioxidants will win, place, or show. And then we use these odds – these numbers – in

selecting our various lifestyle components in order to optimize the life in our days, and the days in our lives.

There is an old Black spiritual that says: "I wanna be in
that number, when the saints go marchin' in." We might
wanna be in that number, but we don't wanna be in that number any sooner than necessary.

Beta-Carotene

Probably the best known of the carotenoids is beta-
carotene. For many years its main claim to fame was as a precursor to vitamin A. Since it does not show toxicity when
taken in large amounts, beta-carotene is a safe way to augment vitamin A levels in the body. Which allows it to promote many of the benefits associated with vitamin A.

However, beta-carotene has its own areas of specialized
function. For example, beta-carotene has demonstrated itself
to be a more formidable cancer fighter than vitamin A.

The conclusions from a number of experiments, and a
chain of reasoned thought, show how beta-carotene may – at
least in part – achieve its ability to reduce the risk of cancer.

To begin with, studies have shown that beta-carotene is
particularly good at neutralizing singlet oxygen. Now
although singlet oxygen is not itself a free radical, we have
generally regarded it as such since it does readily give rise to
free radicals. Other studies have shown that the free radicals
generated are then able to wreak damage on most parts of the
cell, including the DNA. And where you have damaged
DNA, you will likely have cells dividing improperly, and
sometimes out of control – giving rise to tumors and the like.
In other words, cancer. But where oxidative damage is curtailed by antioxidants such as beta-carotene, studies have
shown that the risk of cancer drops except with smokers.

By way of example, one very interesting study (B.L. Pool-Zobel, R. Bub, H. Mueller et al) had the participants follow a normal diet, with one glaring omission – it was low in carotenoids. During this phase of the experiment the DNA damage was assessed by measuring strands of DNA breaks due to oxidation. After this phase, the subjects were then placed on a high carotenoid diet, which was then followed by further DNA damage assessment. The experiment showed that the diet rich in carotenoids (carrots, tomatoes, spinach) did indeed bring about reduced oxidative damage to the DNA. Of the carotenoids tested, the alpha and beta-carotene, and lycopene (in tomatoes) were shown to effect the greatest reduction in DNA damage.

Two Further Mechanisms

There are other ways in which beta-carotene battles cancer, ways in which other mechanisms appear to be at work.

One of these mechanisms involves the concept of cellular communication. (And we are not talking about telephones here.) In ways still unknown to researchers, it appears that cells in close proximity are able to communicate with one another by means of what are called gap junctions. Undoubtedly this communication will not be on a par with the Socratic dialogues of Plato, but it does allow the cells to divide in a reliable and organized manner. However where a diminished gap junction was found between cells, it was also accompanied by an increased probability of cancer.

In an experiment conducted by G. Wolfe in the early 1990s, it was shown that beta-carotene was able to enhance the communication – or gap junction – between cells. The compelling conclusion, then, is that one mechanism by which beta-carotene is able to reduce the risk of cancer is by enhancing this necessary communication between cells, thereby making cell division more reliable.

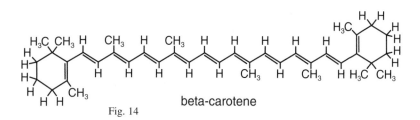

Fig. 14   beta-carotene

Since various components of the immune system are warriors against foreign invaders and rogue cancer cells, another way in which beta-carotene may reduce the risk of cancer lies in its ability to enhance the immune system. Some white blood cells of the immune system have the means of identifying foreign invaders. These white blood cells carry a protein on their outer surfaces called MHC2. This protein, in a little understood fashion, is able to identify foreign invaders and alert the immune cell, directing the cell into its attack and destroy mission.

In the late 1990s, Dr. David Hughs, working at the Institute of Food Research in England, found that beta-carotene played an intrinsic role in the above process. He found that beta-carotene (and possibly other carotenoids) increased the quantity of MHC2 proteins available. Here the obvious conclusion is that beta-carotene promotes the supply of MHC2 proteins, and when in full supply these proteins will be able to fortify the white blood cells and maintain them at full strength. Which will then enable them to optimally protect the body from foreign invaders – and against fifth columnists such as cancer cells.

In addition, Dr. Hughes has found that elevated beta-carotene levels were instrumental in enhancing another cancer fighter in the body called tumor necrosis factor alpha.

Other research has shown that beta-carotene is also capable of enhancing other members of the "immune emergency response team", such as T-cell and B-cell lymphocytes, and the aptly named "natural killer cells".

Because of its potent antioxidant properties, beta-carotene – like many of the other antioxidants – has demonstrated (Journal of Arteriosclerosis, Thrombosis, and Vascular Biology, June 1995) an ability to inhibit the oxidation of polyunsaturated fatty acids and lipoproteins in the blood. We have already seen how the oxidation of these molecules is conducive to the buildup of plaque on arterial walls, thereby increasing the risk of heart attack. A study bearing this out was conducted by J.M. Gazeiano, where male physicians taking beta-carotene on alternate days, showed a 40% reduced risk of heart attack.

Some years back a study was done which did not bear out the fine results for beta-carotene that were normally obtained. However, it is felt by many researchers that the study in question involved smokers and former smokers, many of whom had been exposed to asbestos on the job. And because of this the sampling was atypical, and produced skewed results.

One explanation that has been put forth for this out-of-step result is that once smokers (or those with lung damage due to the inhalation of asbestos particles for much of their lives) reach an advanced age – and an advanced stage of serious deterioration – then even beta-carotene may not be effective checking or reversing this deterioration.

Most studies, however, indicate that most people will benefit from optimal levels of beta-carotene. There is simply so much information out there that is favorable to the benefits of beta-carotene. To ignore it is to throw out the baby with the bathwater.

And, although your mother may not have been familiar with all of the scientific information validating beta-carotene, she was right as usual when she told you to "Eat your carrots!" and today she would add "Take your vitamins."

Alpha-Carotene

Although alpha comes before beta, it is only recently that alpha-carotene has come to the fore. And that is because it is only recently that scientists have begun looking at alpha-carotene in earnest.

In Japan, researcher Michiaki Murakoshi is of the opinion that future research may prove alpha-carotene to be an even better cancer battler than beta-carotene. Leading a team of biochemists at the Kyoto Prefectural University of Medicine, Murakoshi made an important discovery using a type of cancer cell called neuroblastoma cells (NCI Cancer Weekly). These neuroblastoma cells contain a gene called N-myc, that codes for cell growth and can contribute to cancer development. In his work, Murakoshi coated these cancer cells with carotenoids to see whether the carotenoids would have any inhibitory effects on this gene. Not surprisingly, they did show just such an inhibitory effect. What was surprising, though, was the fact that alpha-carotene showed approximately 10 time the inhibitory effect than that exhibited by beta-carotene.

Other studies on animals have shown that alpha-carotene was especially effective in preventing carcinogen-induced cancers.

Although much of the research on alpha-carotene has consisted of in vitro laboratory studies, or have used animals rather than people, the results have been very positive. Ensuing research will no doubt involve human studies, and researchers in the field anticipate that alpha-carotene, in its role as a vital antioxidant, will continue to shine.

Cryptoxanthin

Cryptoxanthin, along with alpha and beta-carotene, make up the three carotenoids commonly found in the diet that serve as precursors to vitamin A.

As with many studies on the carotenoids, cryptoxanthin has more often been researched in conjunction with other carotenoids, rather than on its own. That is because many of these studies have used actual fruits and vegetables, rather than isolated carotenes in a preparation. Invariably these fruits and vegetables will have any number of carotenoids present, with a certain few predominating. And very often, these predominant carotenoids will tend to work together, conferring a synergistic effect.

Such is the case for cryptoxanthin in conjunction with alpha-carotene. In one study, the two of them together produced a significant reduction for the risk of developing cervical cancer.

In another study conducted in 1993, high levels of cryptoxanthin correlated well with a reduced incidence of cancer.

Although cryptoxanthin may never achieve the prominence of alpha or beta-carotene, in conjunction with the others it will almost always be contributing to a synergistic effect.

Lutein and Zeaxanthin

Lutein and zeaxanthin are two more of the lesser known carotenoids that have been studied in combination, both with each other and occasionally with other carotenoids as well.

In one study, supplements of lutein, zeaxanthin, and beta-carotene were used along with foods high in vitamin A. This combination was shown to be effective in reducing the risk of premenopausal breast cancer. The results were even more impressive for women especially at risk for the disease, due to a history of cancer or alcohol consumption.

Lutein, zeaxanthin, and alpha-carotene were teamed up in another study, and in this combination were shown to bring about a reduced risk of lung cancer.

The role of carotenoids in the prevention of macular degeneration was examined in the United States in 1994. (Macular degeneration is a disease of the macula, the spot where light focuses on the retina. It is the principal cause of blindness in the U.S. today.) About a thousand patients and controls were involved in this experiment, and the results showed that lutein and zeaxanthin were the carotenoids that offered the most protection in preventing macular degeneration. More recent studies have shown that with zinc, these antioxidants can reduce the risk of macular degeneration by 25% (commonest cause of blindness in Americans over 50 years).

Once more in this case, as in so many others where the carotenoids are at work, the value of teamwork presents itself.

Lycopene

We now come to the all-star of the carotenoid antioxidants – lycopene. Not only is lycopene one of the more potent antioxidants, it comes in a tasty and attractive package – the tomato. And not only are the benefits of lycopene to be had from fresh tomatoes, they are even more pronounced in cooked and processed tomatoes. A rarity in the case of fruits and vegetables.

So in moments of gustatory pleasure, when we are enjoying a toasted tomato sandwich, or a slice of juicy tomato with an omelet, or chunks of tangy tomato in a crisp green salad, we may also take pleasure in the fact that we are filling up the physiological tank with lycopene. And when we are savoring the rich tomato sauce in a lasagna, or on pizza, or with spaghetti, we are filling the tank even fuller.

We are better able to absorb lycopene from processed tomatoes than from fresh ones since the tomato cell walls are destroyed releasing the lycopene. In fact, we can do so about two and a half times better. It is thought that in processed forms such as tomato paste, pizza sauce, and the like, that the lycopene is more concentrated. Also, there are usually small quantities of fats in these products, or in dishes or recipes where tomatoes are called for, and this bit of fat may also add to the absorbability of lycopene. Pinch yourself if you think you are dreaming, but all of this is true!

However this comes to be understood, there are few who don't enjoy a savory tomato-based feast in at least a few of its many delicious dishes and entrees. And few there are in the field of research whose experiments will not attest to the benefits conferred by the lycopene to be found in such dishes.

The Benefits

To restate the obvious, lycopene is a powerful antioxidant, and many of its benefits derive from this property directly. The data is now flooding in and is well nigh incontrovertible.

Perhaps one of the most significant findings is that, just as lutein tends to concentrate in the retina, lycopene in men tends to concentrate in the prostate. Which is, no doubt, why it has shown a pronounced ability to reduce the risk of prostate cancer.

A study conducted at Harvard University on 48,000 men showed that consuming tomato products 10 times per week produced a 35% reduced risk of prostate cancer, when compared to those consuming less than 1.5 servings per week.

(One might safely assume that if all the men in America were reading this book on the same day, and were to arrive at the above passage all at the same moment, the collective sigh of relief would set all anemometers at weather stations into a dizzying spin, and that the following stampede out the door for a pizza would leave most of the world's seismographs ajar.)

But the good news is not reserved for men only. Research in breast cancer, lung cancer, and endometrial cancer that was done at Ben Gurion University and Soroka Medical Center in Israel, has shown that lycopene is even more effective than alpha and beta-carotene in battling these cancers. It does this by somehow causing a delay in the cell cycle progression from one growth phase to the next. Other findings, as well, are tending to support this study, in that they too show links between high lycopene levels and protection from breast cancer.

Another study involving women has shown that the 75% who ate the least amount of tomatoes had a risk factor between 3.5 and 4.7 times higher than for those who ate the most tomatoes, the risk factor here pertaining to a condition known as intraepithelial neoplasia, which entails precancerous changes of the cervix.

Similar kinds of statistics have resulted for the risk of cancer of the gastrointestinal tract, and for heart disease.

For gastrointestinal tract cancer, the 25% who had the greatest intake of tomatoes showed a 30-60% reduced risk for this disease.

In Great Britain, research conducted by Dr. George Truscott of Keele University shows that lycopene has double the capacity of beta-carotene in reducing oxidative damage. Further studies in Israel indicate that lycopenes in a tomato product reduces the oxidation of the harmful cholesterol, which we will recall is instrumental in starting atherosclerosis. Given findings of this sort, it is not surprising to find research steadily accumulating that supports the conclusion that lycopene is a powerful antidote to heart disease.

A major study conducted in Europe, for instance, showed that men who consumed large quantities of lycopene-rich foods were 50% less likely to have a heart attack when compared to men who consumed little. In this experiment, nonsmokers experienced the greatest benefit.

All of this from the red pigment in a tomato!

That lycopene is a superior scavenger antioxidant is now beyond question. Undoubtedly, research in the future will corroborate and refine what we know about lycopene today. Ways of concentrating it, of making it still more effective are being researched at the present time. The list of its marvels and applications can only grow longer.

Given the benefits from lycopene in the various tomato products and tomato dishes, we anticipate there will be a considerable upsurge in those seeking the gustatory pleasures of Mediterranean cuisine. For those who are allergic to tomatoes, or who do not like them in any form, there will be supplements on the market. For the rest, who would rather sit down to a candle-lit meal, with spaghetti and meatballs before us, a Caesar salad on the side, and a glass of red wine glowing in the candlelight, we can only say: Buono Appetito!

And for those who are ready to reshape their intake of foodstuffs and supplements so as to recharge their antioxidant supply, we would prefer to quote the inimitable and flamboyant chef, Emeril Lagasse, and say: BAM !

The Flavonoids

In 1535 French explorer Jacques Cartier and his crew became ice-bound along the St. Lawrence River in this region of Quebec, Canada. They had little by way of fruits and vegetables through that brutal winter, and the men became afflicted with bleeding gums, inflamed body sores, a pervasive weakness, and erratic behavior. It was scurvy. The entire crew were in the throes of desperation, and in the first part of that winter 25 men died.

What saved the others was an act of kindness by the Indians that inhabited the area. They showed the explorers how to brew up a tea using the bark of a tree that grew there, the maritime pine. In his journal Cartier recorded details of the event, and of how the crew miraculously recovered and regained their health within a week or two after drinking this pine bark concoction.

Centuries later in the 1960s, a Canadian scientist, Dr. Jacques Masquelier, came across Cartier's journal and read about the curative powers of the pine bark infusion. Dr. Masquelier was nonplussed at Cartier's account. He knew that the pine bark (and the pine needles) contained little by way of vitamin C. So what had brought about the incredible cure?

Since the 1930s it had been known that a family of compounds called flavonoids were able to enhance the effects of vitamin C. Dr. Mesquelier began research on the pine bark infusion and found that they did indeed contain a rich mixture of flavonoids, with a group known as proanthocyanidins in ample supply. After further research and development, Dr. Mesquelier came up with a potent formulation based on the pine bark infusion that he called Pycnogenol. It is now recognized as one of the more potent antioxidant preparations available today. We are tempted to consider the term "Pineys" for those French settlers that corrected the same deficiency as the "Limeys".

Variety: The Spice of Life, The Device of Life

Where the carotenoids number in the hundreds, the flavonoids number in the thousands – over 4,000 and counting. This number is less daunting when we see that there are well under a hundred that we tend to commonly encounter. And that these fall into less than a dozen different groups. It is less daunting still when we see that there are a limited number of foodstuffs and formulations in which the flavonoids are found.

Like the carotenoids, the flavonoids occur in various plants – in the bark, berries, roots, shoots, leaves, or flowers. Like the carotenoids as well, the flavonoids tend to occur in mixtures, so that one plant or plant part will have mixtures of flavonoids from more than one group or type. Most of the time, however, one group or type will tend to predominate.

Although flavonoids number in the thousands, only about 50 occur in foodstuffs that humans eat. Sometimes flavonoids come to the table in the form of fruits and berries, sometimes in the form of spices, teas, or wines.

Whatever their source and whatever their makeup, one thing is certain – the flavonoids are superb antioxidants. And like the carotenoids, it is in their mixtures that the flavonoids are most effective. If variety is the spice of life, variety is also the device of life.

Over and over again we find Mother Nature playing out this theme, and so it is too in the case of the flavonoids. The combined members in a group are invariably more effective than just a single one, and the groups themselves when found in combination exercise a strong synergistic effect upon one another. Teamwork. Again.

To be sure, the various flavonoid groups possess the general properties of all antioxidants. But each group also has its own areas of special function, of particular effectiveness.

And when we ingest foods or formulations that contain a number of the flavonoid groups or types, it is then that we get the maximum benefit. For then we are able to reduce free radical activity that much more effectively, thereby forestalling the aging process and extending our youthful years.

Truly, variety is the device of life.

History

Flavonoids have been in use by humans for over five thousand years, employed over the centuries by tribal healers such as shamans and medicine men. And although these early practitioners held no medical degrees, nor knew the details of human physiology, they were knowledgeable about flavonoids in a hands-on kind of way. And they were able to use flavonoid potions in treating a number of afflictions, including inflammatory problems, skin conditions, and so on.

One of the oldest uses of flavonoids consisted of those obtained from the ginkgo biloba tree. The early use of ginkgo biloba (or ginkgo for short) goes back thousands of years to ancient China. China was the last bastion of the ginkgo tree, since it had been wiped out in other parts of the earth during the ice ages.

The ginkgo tree is not only an ancient tree, it is a long lived tree, with some of them attaining the age of a thousand years or more. Perhaps it was this quality that set early medicine men experimenting with it for curative properties. And we have already seen how the North American Indians were able to cure Cartier and his men, who, unknowledgeable about scurvy or a cure for it, were dropping like flies from the disease. Since this knowledge was familiar to the Indians hundreds of years back, it is not overly presumptuous to think that their knowledge went back much further still, into the mists of time.

There is an obvious irony in the fact that many of the so called "primitive" peoples had a greater understanding in this area than did the "advanced" explorers.

Notwithstanding that the flavonoids have been in use for thousands of years, the modern "discovery" of them goes back to the 1930s. It was then that Albert Szent-Gyorgyi, the man who first isolated vitamin C, was able to isolate and identify the flavonoids in biochemical terms. He not only identified the flavonoids, he also described their ability to boost the effectiveness of vitamin C.

One way in which this enhancing effect manifested itself lay in the following. Prior to Szent-Gyorgyi's work, attempts had been made to remedy a condition that was characterized by a weakness and vulnerability in the capillary walls. A weakness of this sort would often give rise to leakage from the capillaries, producing edema or swelling in parts of the body. Such weakened capillaries might also buckle in and obstruct the flow of blood. Where vitamin C had been tried on its own as a remedy, it had not been able to effect an improvement. However, Szent-Gyorgyi found than when flavonoids were used along with vitamin C, the condition was remedied. Szent-Gyorgyi referred to these substances – the flavonoids – as vitamin P.

Decades later, the modern research efforts of Lester Packer and others have since demonstrated the signal importance of flavonoids. But the mainstream medical community has been slow in acknowledging the benefits of these marvelous quasi-vitamin antioxidants, and governmental bodies have yet to set a daily recommended allowance (RDA) for them. We see a touch of irony here, not unlike that which has underscored the history of antioxidants in general. All of which tends to stir recollections of Galileo after he was forced to recant his views and state that the earth did not move around the sun – and the words he is said to have muttered a moment afterwards – while still on his knees: "And still it moves!"

It seems that some ideas just take time in finding acceptance.

Antioxidant Activity

The flavonoids are amongst the most powerful of the antioxidant scavengers. For one thing, they tend to occur in a mixed variety, where each confers its synergistic effect upon the other, heightening the potency of all. And although some flavonoid groups or families may appear to be more potent than others, it is in concert where they truly shine. It is the most effective of the flavonoids that we will be examining, for it is these that have come to be used in various foodstuffs or formulations. And it is these that we will recommend for inclusion in the diet, or by way of supplementation.

The flavonoids are most capable of quenching or neutralizing a broad gamut of the reactive oxygen species (ROS), including singlet oxygen and the hydroxyl and superoxide radicals. But where it is first among equals is in taking on the insidious nitric oxide radical, and its pernicious progeny, peroxynitrite.

If the hydroxyl radical is the most destructive free radical, nitric oxide is the most insidious – insidious because it bears a treachery within it.

Our Favorite Mistake

We have seen that as a friend, nitric oxide assists in regulating the flow of blood by controlling the constriction or relaxation of muscles in blood vessels. In a similar way it affects muscles in the digestive tract, thereby aiding in digestion. It also serves as a signaler in turning genes on and off, and as a neurotransmitter, where it plays a part in brain cell communication.

As well, nitric oxide also plays a significant role in the immune system. As part of their weaponry, some of the immune cells produce nitric oxide with which to destroy invading bacteria, or rogue cancer cells. Nitric oxide, generated by the action of nitric oxide synthase (NOS), is produced in other parts of the body as well, including the endothelium (lining artery walls), in central and peripheral nerve cells, in skeletal muscles, and in the epithelial cells lining the bronchi, uterus, and stomach.

Yet for all the good that nitric oxide does, it is also capable of doing us huge harm. It is because nitric oxide masquerades as a friend in one instant and then beats us up in the next that we regard it as insidious. It is like a treacherous turncoat. No doubt if the cells of the body could sing, when singing about nitric oxide they would invariably do a few lines from the Cheryl Crowe song "My Favorite Mistake".

Too Much of a Good Thing

The problem with nitric oxide derives from excess. In just the right amount nitric oxide serves us well. But under the stress of an infectious invasion, for example, or as the result of inflammation, many cells of the body – but especially the immune warriors – increase the production of nitric oxide. When this happens, an interesting and harmful sequence of events ensues.

As a backdrop, we will recall that the antioxidant enzyme called superoxide dismutase (SOD) is in a continuous process of neutralizing the superoxide radical. However, when inflammation or infection induces the body to produce an excess of nitric oxide, this excess of nitric oxide tends to crowd the SOD out of the way and "swarm" the superoxide radicals, combining with them to produce peroxynitrite. Peroxynitrite is extremely reactive, and may attack proteins, lipids, DNA – almost any tissue in the body. It is particularly vicious in that it is so capable of attacking the fatty structures of the body and setting off chain reactions, with free radicals blasting away in all directions – like neutrons in an atomic bomb.

So now, instead of having the weaker nitric oxide radicals in balance, (for the most part benefiting us), and the superoxide radicals under control through the neutralizing effect of SOD, we instead have the production of peroxynitrite coming on stream. And the chain reactions, and the destruction, and the accelerated aging.

Fortunately, the flavonoids are eminently capable of taking on the nitric oxide marauders. The arbitrary Hardwick Limit restricting the total number of sexual encounters for a male may not be important if antioxidants are available to prevent the damage done by NO (nitric oxide).

Restoring Vitamin C: A Triple Treat

Not only do the flavonoids serve wonderfully well in combating the worst of the free radicals, and not only do they work wonderfully well in synergism with one another, they also boost the performance of another team player that we have already met – vitamin C. We saw this in the work of Szent-Gyorgyi, and it has been confirmed in modern times.

The flavonoids, besides filling their own role as antioxidants, help to sustain the levels of vitamin C in the body, and extend these levels over time. They do this much in the way that vitamin C is able to restore vitamin E. And in so doing the flavonoids produce a cascading effect: they not only maintain the levels of vitamin C over an extended period of time, but this then allows vitamin C to maintain higher levels of vitamin E over an extended period of time as well. A triple treat!

PROANTHOCYANADINS: THE PROS

The flavonoids are members of a larger chemical family called polyphenols, which – as the name suggests – have a number of phenolic rings in their molecular structure. In the case of the flavonoids, there are also hydroxyl groups present in their molecular structure. Early research so far indicates that the more hydroxyl groups present in its makeup, the more potent a flavonoid will be as an antioxidant.

To illustrate, one subclass of the flavonoids, the cate-chins, usually have five hydroxyl groups attached, and occasionally six. This confers upon them an excellent antioxidant ability. There is another flavonoid group, however, that has ten hydroxyl groups attached, and it has demonstrated a most superb antioxidant ability. It is this group of flavonoids that tends to predominate in some of the most potent antioxidant preparations available today. They are known as oligomeric proanthocyanidins.

The name is a bit of a tongue twister. However, we can simplify matters by referring to them simply as proantho-cyanidins. And simplify further still by recalling that in sports, the best players are the professionals, or the pros. And we might think of the proanthocyanidins in this regard also – as the pros. For the proanthocyanidins are quite possibly the best of the flavonoid antioxidants, a distinction they owe to their ten hydroxyl groups.

The proanthocyanidins, or the pros, are the flavonoids that are dominant in such excellent antioxidant preparations as gingko biloba, Pycnogenol, and grape seed extract. They are also found in grapes, and give rise to closely related flavonoids found in wines, especially red wines. We drink red wine! Not copiously but sufficiently to provide the benefits that we describe.

Although there are other flavonoid groups to be found in these formulations, all doing their own special jobs and adding their synergistic effect as well, the major effect in these formulations is to be had from the proanthocyanidins, the pros.

Ginkgo Biloba

One of the most potent flavonoid preparations is ginkgo biloba, or ginkgo. Derived from the leaves of the ginkgo tree, ginkgo biloba has shown an ability to benefit the body above the belt and below – everything from brain function and memory to sexual function in men.

Ginkgo's medicinal properties go back thousands of years, where it has helped countless people over the centuries. But it is only recently that it has become more widely known and used.

The proanthocyanidins, which are found in abundance in ginkgo, are likely a major source of ginkgo's powers. But there are other flavonoids as well, such as flavones, flavonols, and bioflavones. And although the proanthocyanidins may be the major players, it is the full synergist mix that always works best.

On the point of synergism, one might be given to a flight of speculative fancy. In so many instances, but especially for the carotenoids and the flavonoids, the various antioxidant components occur in plants in considerable variety, and it is in these combinations that they are of most benefit to humans. And one wonders, did we evolve over the eons in such a way as to most benefit from the mix of antioxidants as they occurred in nature? Or was it merely a happy touch of serendipity bequeathed by the hand of the Creator?

Whatever the cause, the theme of variety and synergism plays out once more in the case of the flavonoids, and particularly for ginkgo.

Blood Circulation

In its action as an antioxidant ginkgo is able to prevent the oxidation of LDLs. This in turn helps prevent the formation of plaque on the artery walls.

Also, ginkgo, through its ability to modulate the effects of nitric oxide, is able to regulate the relaxation and constriction of blood vessels. Which in turn allows it to exert a positive effect on blood pressure. And although the effect produced is significant, it is not huge, and should not be regarded as a cure for hypertension. That being said, it would nonetheless seem that if ginkgo can show positive effects on blood pressure after it has become a problem, then it would likely have a positive effect in preventing or diminishing the severity of hypertension as well. One word of caution: for those on blood thinning agents such as warfarin, there may be an interaction with ginkgo, as well as other antioxidants, so individuals in this circumstance are well advised to check with their physician prior to embarking on a program of antioxidants.

In the Packer Laboratory, at the University of California at Berkeley, a great deal of research into antioxidants has been carried out under the auspices of Dr. Lester Packer. In one experiment ginkgo was shown to hasten recovery after a heart attack. In the experiment, a simulated heart attack was induced in a Langendorff beating heart model, where the heart was flushed with a solution containing no oxygen. After forty minutes the solution was changed to one that did contain oxygen. Under these conditions only about 20-25% of the hearts recover, with the rest sustaining serious damage to the heart muscle. And in the end these hearts soon die. However, when ginkgo was added to the solution, 65% of the hearts recovered, and the damage to the heart muscle was greatly reduced.

With its positive effects on heart health, blood pressure, and circulation, ginkgo is definitely a candidate for the medicine cabinet.

Brain Booster

Brain power requires a lot of energy, and this is delivered to the brain via blood flow. Given the excellent effects ginkgo has on blood circulation, it is not surprising that it has been used as a brain booster. In Europe, particularly in France and Germany, ginkgo has been used for years to enhance mental ability.

Recent experiments in stroke and Alzheimer's patients have also produced positive results. Here again, although the results were significant, they were still a long way from a cure. Nevertheless, these and other studies, suggest that ginkgo would lend itself well as an adjunctive therapy, along with vitamin E, in slowing and diminishing the ravages of Alzheimer's disease.

Sexual Function

Sexual function is extremely important to men. And to women, for that matter. And since men do not concern themselves with health matters often to the same degree that women do, we might direct these words even more so to the distaff side of the readership. Because it often takes a woman's influence to steer a man in the right direction.

Where sexual function is concerned, one cannot regard

it as a command performance – it is not commanded or achieved in the manner in which one might raise one's arm. And sometimes, even when the spirit is willing the system fails. That is, in about 75% of the cases of sexual dysfunction, the cause is thought to be physical.

Where erectile function is concerned, there are two factors to consider. One factor involves our two-faced friend, nitric oxide. Part of the biochemistry that produces swelling and engorgement for both men and women, entails a hormone that activates the production of nitric oxide. This hormone, oxytocin, is released during breast feeding and explains why some women derive pleasure from breast feeding. And although a bit more complicated than covered in our treatment here, the upshot is that with proper quantities of nitric oxide produced, the muscles in the arteries become relaxed, allowing them to fill with blood, which brings about the desired swelling and stiffness. Since ginkgo helps keep nitric oxide in balance, it provides a definite assist on this front.

Ginkgo also assists on another front. The flavonoids are marvelous at preventing the oxidation of LDL cholesterol, and ginkgo is one of the best in this regard. It also excels at preventing free radical damage to the endothelial lining of arterial walls. Taken together, this prevents the buildup of plaque on artery walls. Where such plaque occurs, it restricts the easy flow of blood to the penis. And it is the unobstructed blood flow that is so necessary for proper intercourse. The buildup of plaque in these arteries has been implicated in about half the cases of sexual dysfunction.

In one study, 50 troubled men were put on a regime of ginkgo supplementation. After only six weeks about half of them experienced an improvement in sexual function. After six months these men had all regained full and normal function.

Since ginkgo improves mental function and especially

memory, and since it may improve sexual performance as well, one happy conclusion is that we will all remember what it is for.

Pycnogenol

Since Pycnogenol has been around a long time – perhaps the longest of the modern day antioxidant formulations – there is probably more data on it than for the others. Like ginkgo, Pycnogenol has a preponderance of the pros, or proanthocyanidins, in its makeup, but it contains other flavonoids as well – such as flavonols and flavanonols. In total there are over 40 different antioxidants in Pycnogenol. Both the scope and the value of the results obtained with Pycnogenol are testimony to the quantity and variety of the flavonoids found in it. And the mutually beneficial effect they have on one another.

The Capillary Cadenza

A great deal of the research on Pycnogenol has also been done at the Packer Lab in California. This research has shown that Pycnogenol is a superlative antioxidant, and excels at neutralizing the superoxide and the hydroxyl radicals, and in controlling nitric oxide as well. It is also superb at restoring vitamin C.

We have seen that nitric oxide can be extremely injurious to the membranes lining the blood vessels. We have also seen that vitamin C is a necessary component in the formation of collagen, which is the connective tissue that holds the body together – a sort of bioglue. This bioglue is particularly important in the structure of the capillaries. Where there is poor collagen formation, the capillaries may rupture and leak, or cave in and obstruct blood flow. Either way, the result may be a tendency to bruise easily, or the incidence of edema.

Pycnogenol prevents this by setting in motion a series of events, each following upon the heels of the one before, like the flurry of notes in a musical cadenza. We might think of this flurry of events as the Capillary Cadenza: Pycnogenol holds nitric oxide (and peroxynitrite) at bay, thereby helping maintain the integrity of the capillaries against free radical attack; it neutralizes other free radicals in the blood as well, preventing LDL oxidation and further damage to capillaries; it restores vitamin C and reinforces the levels of vitamin C; which means that blood vessels – especially the capillaries can be built up and appropriately maintained, without weakness and vulnerability; and this means there will be no tendency toward bruising, no edema, no swelling. All from Pycnogenol, and its Capillary Cadenza.

Platelet Aggregation

There is another way in which Pycnogenol promotes cardiovascular health. It protects against platelet aggregation.

Platelets are cells in the blood that are instrumental in bringing about the clotting of blood at an open wound. This helps staunch the blood flow, closes the wound to outside contamination, and eventually hardens into a scab under which the wound heals. However, smoking – and other causes – may predispose platelets to clumping together without the presence of an open wound. These clumps (as was the case for bits of plaque that came loose into the bloodstream) may lead to heart attack or stroke.

Where aspirin is used to "thin" the blood, there is frequently the possibility of serious side effects: gastrointestinal bleeding, ulceration of the stomach lining, stomach upset, and so on. But as Dr. Packer points out: "Pycnogenol works even better than aspirin in terms of platelet aggregation, but without the unwanted side effects associated with aspirin."

Immune Function

Another area where Pycnogenol has demonstrated strong positive effects is on the immune system. Obviously, where Pycnogenol is able to restore vitamin C and reinforce its levels in the body – and improve the performance of vitamin E and glutathione – we would expect that this would show an improvement in immune function. And it does.

One way that Pycnogenol is able to fortify the immune system is by helping protect macrophages against free radical attack. It does this by regulating nitric oxide production.

We will recall that certain immune cells, including macrophages, use free radicals such as nitric oxide as weapons in attacking invading bacteria. However, where too much nitric oxide is produced, the immune cells may then become endangered as well.

Experiments that demonstrated the moderating effect of Pycnogenol on nitric oxide levels were recently carried out, with the following results. Macrophages in cell culture were subjected to bacterial toxins so as to induce the production of nitric oxide. As expected, a point was reached where the nitric oxide concentration began killing off the macrophages as well. But when Pycnogenol was added to the fray, the production of nitric oxide was moderated, and the macrophages were left intact, able to continue in the battle.

As indicated above, this was an in vitro experiment. But the circumstances of the experiment are sufficiently straightforward as to permit at least a tentative conclusion: that Pycnogenol will have a similar moderating effect on nitric oxide in the body.

Another experiment – this one closer to the human model – was conducted at the University of Arizona, where mice were used. The mice used were those whose immune systems had been compromised by either of two conditions:

an HIV-like infection, or alcoholism.

It was found in these immune deficient mice, that Pycnogenol improved immune function by increasing the production of interleukin-2, which in turn brought about an increased activity in T-cells and lymphocytes.

Further, in healthy mice, Pycnogenol heightened the performance of NK (natural killer) cells. NK cells are instrumental in battling cancer by detecting cellular growth of an abnormal nature and attacking the cells involved.

Again, this was not an experiment involving humans. But although the gross morphology of mice may differ vastly from that of humans, the physiology of mammals has an area of huge commonality. In fact the cellular chemistry of all living things has a consistent similarity and the differences are in the details. And since this is an exciting area of research, we may well anticipate human trials in the future that will expand upon and corroborate these findings.

Chronic Fatigue Syndrome, Fibromyalgia & Arthritis

Chronic fatigue syndrome (CFS) and allied disorders are mysterious afflictions that leave their victims with barely the energy to get out of bed some days. This acute lethargy is often accompanied by joint and muscle pain, as well as headaches, swollen glands, and depression. Some of the symptoms appear similar to those of arthritis, and some resemble symptoms of allergic reactions. The theories of the "Yuppie Flus" are slowly getting sorted out and we know four important points about these disorders today:

1) There is overgrowth of bowel bacteria

2) The bowel leaks toxins causing inflammation

3) Toxins and free radicals overwhelm the liver

4) Oxidative stress produces cytokines and mitochondrial damage leading to more inflammation

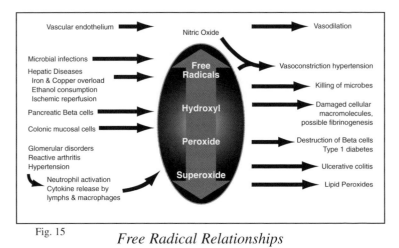

Fig. 15 *Free Radical Relationships*

Once this pathogenesis is accepted, the treatment plan becomes obvious with a resultant improvement in energy (ATP) production as the end result.

Current opinion holds that much of the pain and swelling that accompanies rheumatoid arthritis – and the progression of this disease over time – is caused by free radical damage and cytokine release, at least in part. Pycnogenol, along with vitamins C and E, have been used with success to moderate these symptoms.

Since CFS and fibromyalgia (FM) present some of the symptoms of arthritis, Pycnogenol has recently been used in the treatment of these conditions. The results so far have been favorable.

Dr. Anthony Martin, who presented a paper on the subject in May of 1997, suggests that the positive results obtained in using Pycnogenol to treat CFS may be explained as follows. Since Pycnogenol assists in optimal maintenance of the capillaries, it will improve circulation in joints and muscles, and thereby relieve some of the pain. Also, with its antioxidant activity, Pycnogenol will be relieving a great deal of the inflammation, which is also a probable cause of the discomfort experienced by chronic fatigue and fibromyalgia patients.

Given the limitations CFS and FM impose upon those suffering from them, Pycnogenol is certainly a candidate at the top of the list for those seeking relief.

Slowing The Aging Process

Another experiment carried out at the Packer Lab at Berkeley offers exciting evidence that the antioxidants in Pycnogenol do slow the aging process. Central to the experiment is the concept of apoptosis, which states that cells are programmed to die off after going through their normal life span.

In this experiment brain cells were grown in culture where they were exposed to high levels of glutamate. Glutamate is an amino acid produced in the body and which serves as a neurotransmitter by brain cells. As was the case for nitric oxide, the crux of the matter lies in having just the right amount. Where glutamate occurs at overly high levels, it can destroy glutathione, and bring on the death of brain cells. People with Alzheimer's disease, brain damage, AIDS, and cancer, for example, all show high levels of glutamate present in the brain.

The cultured brain cells, grown in the lab, were exposed to high levels of glutamate, and as expected, began to die off. However, when Pycnogenol was added to the mix, the brain cells did not die off. In fact, they continued to function normally.

To be sure, this experiment was an in vitro experiment carried out in a lab, not on human beings. Nevertheless, the results are impressive and exciting, for they suggest an avenue of fruitful research on humans in the future, and they indicate that similar results may well be obtained in humans. Also, these results add one more piece of evidence to an already growing body of evidence – all of which attests to the anti-aging effects of antioxidants.

Grape Seed Extract

Another stellar member of the pro team, loaded with a high proanthocyanidin content, is grape seed extract. Here again, as with Pycnogenol, Jacques Masquelier has played a central role.

A Potent Alternative

Since the production of Pycnogenol requires the death of the pine tree in obtaining its bark, Masquelier sought an alternate source for the antioxidants it contained. And the alternative he found turned out to be grape seed extract.

There are a number of advantages to grape seed extract when compared to Pycnogenol. For one thing, grape plants mature much faster than pine trees. For another, harvesting the seeds does not require the destruction of the plant. For a third, the grape seeds are to be had as a by-product of an already established industry – wine production, which means that they are more readily available than pine bark. (The maritime pine is found only in limited parts of eastern Canada, and France.)

No doubt the greatest advantage of grape seed extract over Pycnogenol lies in the concentration of proanthocyanidins found in grape seed extract and the content of ellagic acid. Since the proanthocyanidins, themselves, are almost identical, their potency mainly depends upon their concentration in a given source. The proanthocyanidins found in the seeds from green and white grapes have shown the greatest concentrations of all, with many preparations from these grape seeds showing higher concentrations than those found in Pycnogenol – by about 10 percent!

As regards the potency of grape seed extract while it is working in the body, operating as an antioxidant scavenger, its performance is truly amazing. Its potency has been shown to be as much as 50 times greater than that of vitamin E, and 20 times more potent than vitamin C. In addition, the proanthocyanidins in grape seed extract are able to restore vitamin C and sustain its levels in the body, thereby sustaining the levels of vitamin E as well. Another triple treat! It allows vitamin C into the cells.

Benefits of Grape Seed Extract

Since grape seed extract has not been available for nearly as long as Pycnogenol, it has not been as thoroughly researched. However, since it has shown concentrations of proanthocyanidins that are consistently higher than those in Pycnogenol, one would expect it to show a higher effectiveness as well. Mutatis mutandis – change for change. And in fact, early research is showing grape seed extract to be an extremely strong and valuable performer helping in some studies with allergy and viral upper respiratory infections.

In allergic reactions, allergens such as spores or pollen trigger an enzyme in the body to bring about the production of histamines. As the histamines attach to other cells (see Quercetin), they then bring on the varied symptoms of an allergic reaction: nasal congestion, watery eyes, and so on.

Because grape seed extract has the ability to block the enzyme responsible for histamine production, it short-circuits the process, possibly reducing the unwanted symptoms.

It is because of its formidable concentration of proanthocyanidins that grape seed extract is also so effective at countering free radical activity as it affects the cardiovascular system, much in the manner of Pycnogenol. In the case of Pycnogenol, we referred to the related effects of the antioxidants as they prevented the oxidation of LDL, and prevented blood vessel damage due to free radical attacks, and sustained vitamin C in its job of fortifying the matrix of collagen in maintaining strong capillaries – and we referred to all of this as the Capillary Cadenza. In the case of grape seed extract, we might refer to its similar effects in this regard as the Arterial Arpeggio.

Hence, Dr. Michael Murray, author of "The Healing Power of Herbs", recommends the use of grape seed extract in slowing atherosclerosis and in maintaining healthy capillaries and in hastening the healing of wounds. Where the proanthocyanidins promote the building of strong, healthy capillaries, the capillaries will provide a better blood supply to wounds, and speed healing.

Dr. Murray also suggests grape seed extract in preventing retinopathy, both macular degeneration – where the carotenoids were very effective – and diabetic retinopathy.

Because of its anti-inflammatory properties, grape seed extract has also shown itself to be somewhat effective in the treatment of arthritis.

Just as it blocked the enzyme that produced histamines, so too it has shown an ability to inhibit the production of another kind of enzyme – the proteases, which are involved in the breakdown of protein.

Some of the most encouraging news about grape seed extract comes from a study done by Dr. Liviero L. Puglisi. In this study, proanthocyanidins from grape seeds of the plant Vita vinifera were tested for their antimutagenic properties. The results of this study demonstrated that the proanthocyanidins from grape seed extract were "strong agents in counteracting spontaneous mutation, both at the mitochondrial and nuclear level of the cell. This effect, at least in part, is due to the antioxidant properties of proanthocyanidins and could be a rational basis for their potential use in chemo prevention of several pathologic situations (i.e. cancer)."

More data on this front is eagerly anticipated.

With its high concentration of proanthocyanidins, it is expected that in the near future grape seed extract will find itself at the forefront of antioxidant formulations. In fact, in a few years it might even become known as "great seed extract".

Wine

The French Paradox

There can hardly be a wine connoisseur anywhere who has not by now heard that wine is actually good for you.

The clue to wine's healthful effect first surfaced in France, where the inhabitants are renowned for their high-fat diet , replete with creamy sauces and rich cheeses. And where there is also some of the heaviest cigarette smoking on earth. One would certainly be justified in thinking the French would have shorter lives and experience more heart trouble than are found in other lands. And yet – as was observed by French cardiologist Serge Renaud – the rate of cardiovascular problems in France were no higher than in other countries. And in many cases they were lower.

Knowing that the French are also regular wine drinkers, Renaud began investigating this angle to see if there was a relationship between the two.

In Vino Veritas, In VinoVitas

In his initial investigations Renaud found that there was indeed a connection between the consumption of wine in France and the fact that, in spite of their high-fat diet and cigarette smoking, the French had as long a life expectancy as people elsewhere.

There is an expression: In vino veritas – in wine there is truth. With Renaud's findings this expression might be expanded to add: In vino vita – in wine there is life!

In further studies Renaud has since shown that two or three glasses of wine per day – especially red wine – has a salutary effect on the cardiovascular system. In one study Renaud reported a 30% decrease in death rates from all causes associated with moderate wine consumption. For cardiovascular disease there was a 35% reduction. And a 24% reduction for cancer.

All from two glasses of red wine per day. Caution to the alcoholics, any alcohol is harmful and contraindicated since their quantity of consumption is impossible to self control.

Heard it on the Grapevine

Here again one of the chief protagonists turns out to be the pros, the proanthocyanidins. Plentiful in grapes – both in the skins of red grapes as well as the seeds of all grapes – the proanthocyanidins offer us their antioxidant powers in yet another form, and this one so very appealing. For who has not enjoyed crunching a firm juicy grape between the teeth for the explosion of flavor that's in it. And then another, and another...But remember, the proanthocyanidins are in the skins, so avoid Mae West's line and never say: "Peel me a grape". Or if you do, ask for the peel.

Plus Ca Change...

When the grapes are made into wine, many of the proanthocyanidins are converted into anthocyanidins in the acid environment of fermentation. However, the change is slight, and it simply means that we exchange one fine antioxidant for another. Which is in line with the French adage: Plus ca change, plus la meme chose (The more things change, the more they stay the same).

One important point to bear in mind is the limit of 2-3 glasses of wine per day. When this limit is exceeded the benefits are then outweighed by the drawbacks, and then we reap harm rather than health. Otherwise, wine is probably one of the more appealing ways in which to augment our supply of antioxidants (for adults).

Sante!

Quercetin

Quercetin is another important flavonoid and is a member of the flavonol group. It is found in onions, garlic, green tea, and cayenne pepper. Quercetin has the general properties of an antioxidant, but of these, its most important strengths lie in combating circulatory problems, and in preventing cancers of the intestinal tract. In addition, quercetin is likely an even better performer than grape seed extract in countering allergies.

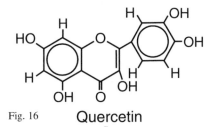

Fig. 16   Quercetin

One study, conducted by M.G.L. Herzog in the Netherlands, showed strong results for quercetin in promoting heart health. In the study, referred to as the Zutpheten Elderly Study, quercetin was one of the chief flavonoids in the diets of 805 elderly men. Their diets included a high intake of tea, onions, and apples. After five years the results showed a 51-68% decreased risk of heart attack or death from heart attack. As well, there was a decrease in the incidence of a first heart attack. Further, the risk of stroke was reduced by as much as a third.

Another study conducted jointly in seven countries, including the United States, also linked quercetin with a pronounced decrease in the risk of heart attack.

These studies are consistent with other reports in which quercetin was associated with similar reductions in heart disease.

Quercetin has shown an ability to counter excesses of iron, and to diminish the occurrence of platelet cells sticking together. Preventing the aggregation of these cells almost certainly contributes to quercetin's positive effects on heart and circulatory health. For we have seen that this tendency toward excessive clotting by platelet cells in the blood is associated with atherosclerosis, and atherosclerosis is an obvious precursor to heart attack or stroke.

Quercetin's ability to quell allergies is another one of its strong points.

An allergic reaction occurs when a stimulus – an allergen – enters the bloodstream and combines with a group of substances called immunoglobulins, which are produced by our immune system. Immunoglobulins are located on what are called mast cells. In response to the allergens, the mast cells release histamines, which are the substances that bring on nasal congestion, watery eyes, itching, and so on. Histamines can also be released from white blood cells called basophils when they are triggered by allergens, again bringing about the allergic reactions.

Where antihistamines work by preventing the binding of the allergens to mast cells, quercetin works by blocking histamines at the site of release – by stabilizing mast cells and basophils. Quercetin also has an inhibitory effect on the inflammatory enzymes, and has been shown to decrease their numbers in the blood.

As for colds and flu, garlic and onions (two fine sources of quercetin) have been used by people for years in "strengthening" the blood against these two banes of winter. Garlic in particular is prized in this regard, and adding to its efficacy are other antioxidants it contains – vitamins A and C, as well as the minerals selenium, germanium, zinc, and manganese.

Undoubtedly further research on quercetin will expand upon its antioxidant benefits in the future. Meanwhile, with the use of onions and garlic in our daily cooking, we will bring to the table a pungency and flavor that is unmatched by any other foodstuff.

Isoflavones

We find another excellent source of flavonoids in soy bean products, especially tofu. Soy products contain genistein and diadzein, which are members of a group called the isoflavones. Of these two isoflavones, genistein is the more prominent and more important.

Although soy products have entered the American diet in a tentative way over the past two or three decades, their use is not commonplace. In Japan soy products have been in the diet for centuries. So it is not surprising to find that much of the initial data about soy and the isoflavones has a strong Japanese connection.

Genistein is the principal isoflavone in soy products. Front and center amongst genistein's effects as an antioxidant is both its cancer fighting ability and its positive influence in promoting heart health. And although both are important, it is as a cancer fighter that genistein initially captures our interest.

Since genistein is found only in soy products – which is prominent in the Japanese diet – and since soy has been little used in America, we have a natural laboratory situation readily at hand. In science, researchers frequently attempt to isolate a single variable and test for its effects. To some extent this has occurred by way of the differences between the Japanese diet and the western or American diet. And although there are other differences as well, one of the most significant lies in the difference in soy consumption.

Accompanying this difference in diet, with the Japanese consuming a great deal of soy products and westerners little, researchers have found corresponding health differences as well. For example, the Japanese have longer life spans in comparison with almost all other peoples on earth. They also have one of the lowest rates for heart disease and cancer.

Two cancers which readily underscore the striking contrast between east and west are found in the rates of prostate cancer and breast cancer. These two cancers, which are common in America, are far less common in Japan. The death rate from breast cancer for women in America is four times higher than the rate for women in Japan. For prostate cancer in men, the death rate in America is five times higher.

Much of genistein's anti-cancer effects derive from its molecular structure. Genistein is easily converted into a molecule that resembles estrogen, but with a much weaker effect. This allows genistein to occupy sites where estrogen molecules would normally attach, sites from which estrogen could begin working its effects conducive to cancer. Since breast cancer and prostate cancer are both strongly affected by hormones, and are said to be hormone dependent, having the weaker genistein-based molecule attach to the activity site is much preferred. Being in place there and blocking estrogen from attaching at these activity sites, genistein thereby blocks estrogen's cancer inducing influence.

In prostate cancer, researchers believe that the isoflavones – and genistein in particular – are able to block the actual development of the cancer.

Autopsies on Japanese men show that they have almost the same incidence of prostate cancer as do American men, but in the Japanese men the cancer had not developed. In many cases it had not progressed to where it had even produced clinical symptoms. A strong indicator that genistein was a significant factor in blocking the development of this cancer lies the fact that the levels of isoflavones in Japanese men were about one hundred times higher than for those found in American men. Also estrogen receptor alpha in the prostate gland cancers may be blocked by phytoestrogens from Japanese soy diets or the soy may be stimulating estrogen receptor beta in these men.

As for heart health, soy bean products such as tofu have shown they can lower cholesterol levels when they are incorporated into the diet. And since the isoflavones in foods such as tofu and miso also prevent the oxidation of LDLs in the blood, we then see why the Japanese have the lowest rate of heart disease in the world despite the high incidence of smoking.

To obtain the benefits of genistein and diadzein, keep in mind that the preferred product is tofu. In contrast, soy sauce has little to offer by way of isoflavones, and is very high in sodium.

For those who have tried tofu and found it wanting in flavor, look upon that as a plus. For one thing, at least it is not offensive. For another, the blandness of tofu allows it to take up other flavors – be they spices, vegetables, or sauces. It beckons to the creative soul in you to give it zest, to give it a flavor worthy of its striking antioxidant benefits. So be brave and give tofu a try. Incorporating soy products like tofu into your diet will soon have your body telling you "Arigato!"

Milk Thistle

In milk thistle is found silymarin, which contains flavonoids of the flavonolignan group. Silymarin has been used with notable success in treating liver impairment and gall bladder problems. Most of its antioxidant effects are largely confined to the liver, where it also appears to inhibit the depletion of glutathione, (whose importance we will be investigating some pages hence).

Those suffering from cirrhosis, hepatitis, or jaundice, will almost certainly benefit from the use of silymarin, as will those suffering liver impairment from alcohol or drug abuse especially in combination with alpha lipoic acid.

Huckleberry or Bilberry

Although this plant has many names (huckleberry in the U.S., whortleberry by the Lord Lyon of Scotland for the official McLeod crest) botanists have agreed to call it bilberry. Shakespeare wrote: "A rose by any other name would smell as sweet..." We might paraphrase this and say "A huckleberry by any other name will provide the same antioxidant benefits." Because no matter what name is used, these plants all serve as a source of another flavonoid family, the anthocyanosides. Not only that, huckleberries are an excellent source of these flavonoids because they carry such a high concentration of them. About 10% of their leaves are made up of polyphenols, which is the large chemical family in which the flavonoids are found.

The anthocyanosides are closely related to the antho-cyanidins found in wine. With that molecular similarity comes a similarity in effect. The anthocyanosides in huckleberry exert their strongest antioxidant action on the circulatory system.

Because the eyes are so highly vascularised, these flavonoids are most beneficial in guarding against conditions such as cataracts, macular degeneration, pigmentary retinitis, and diabetic retinopathy.

These flavonoids were used in the form of jams by Royal Air Force pilots to improve their night vision for combat and bombing missions during World War II.

Because they improve the circulatory system, huckleberry or bilberry have demonstrated strengthening of the capillaries, improving wound healing and lowering blood pressure.

Hawthorn

Hawthorn contains a flavonoid group called the procyanidins. It has been used in herbal preparations for centuries.

The procyanidins in hawthorn appear to be most effective as an adjunctive treatment for heart problems. Hawthorn is thought to improve circulation by bringing about peripheral vasodilation (opening blood vessels in outer areas of the body), and by dilating the coronary arteries. In the case of the latter – improving circulation in the heart – this will improve the transport of oxygen to the heart muscle, which will add to the improved health and efficiency in this vital organ.

In providing yet another source of antioxidant protection, hawthorn is one more arrow in the quiver.

THE LONE EAGLES

When Charles Lindberg flew across the Atlantic in 1927, he became the first person to do so alone. Because he made the flight alone, and because it was such a stellar achievement, he was often referred to as The Lone Eagle. He was in a class by himself. I think he would be amazed today to see Dr. White flying himself to work and meetings with relative ease (as Dr. McLeod struggles with inconvenient, time consuming highway travel).

And now we come to the two antioxidants that we have referred to as lone eagles – alpha lipoic acid and glutathione. Like Lindberg, each of these antioxidants is a stellar performer, and each is in a class by itself.

Alpha Lipoic Acid

Alpha lipoic acid (ALA) – which we will refer to simply as lipoic acid – is an exceptional antioxidant and sometimes referred to as the master nutrient. Unlike the vitamins, which have been identified and studied for decades, lipoic acid has only been seriously investigated in the laboratory over the last decade or so. Because lipoic acid is produced by the body it is not classed as a vitamin. However, it occurs in very small quantities in the body, and these quantities diminish as we age, when our need for lipoic acid is greatest. The news of its properties and benefits is hot off the presses, and with the flurry of research going forward with lipoic acid, we can expect much more information on this remarkable lone eagle in the near future.

Mushroom Poisoning

In 1977, a man and woman were brought into a New Mexico hospital with severe nausea, as well as abdominal cramping and diarrhea. They were diagnosed as having a viral infection, treated, and sent home. Back at home their condition worsened and they became violently ill. At that point their son, a paramedic, drove them back to the hospital, where they continued to decline.

That evening the son recalled an article he had recently read about mushroom poisoning. Upon checking with his parents and finding that they had indeed eaten wild mushrooms, he contacted the doctor who had been mentioned in the article, Dr. Burt Berkson. After speaking with Dr. Berkson on the phone he then drove his parents to the hospital where Dr. Berkson was a medical resident. By now the ailing couple had been nearly given up for dead.

It turns out that Dr. Berkson was familiar with European cases in which lipoic acid had been successful in treating severe liver damage. He contacted Dr. Fredrick Barter who at that time was head of endocrinology at the National Institutes of Health in Washington, D.C. Dr. Barton had some lipoic acid on hand and had it rushed out the same day to Dr. Berkson. Against hospital directives (lipoic acid was not on a list of medications that had been approved of by the hospital), Dr. Berkson administered lipoic acid to the desperately ill couple.

Their improvement was dramatic. Within a week they were feeling much better. Even more encouraging, liver function in each of them had almost returned to normal.

History

Alpha lipoic acid, thioctic acid or lipoic acid as it is more commonly called, is an amino acid that is produced by the body, but in very small amounts. Compounding this is the fact that as we age the body produces even less lipoic acid, just at the time when we would most benefit from it.

Lipoic acid was identified as a necessary but unknown substance in potato extract that allowed bacteria to grow in culture. Little further was determined about lipoic acid until it was isolated in 1951 by Lester Reed, a biochemist who also mapped out its molecular structure. Because lipoic acid does not occur in high concentration in animals (as is the case for humans), it took ten tons of beef hearts to obtain only thirty milligrams of lipoic acid.

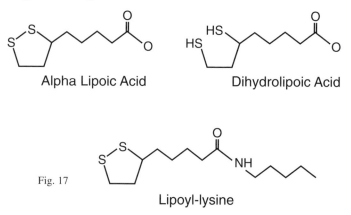

Alpha Lipoic Acid   Dihydrolipoic Acid

Fig. 17

Lipoyl-lysine

Over the decades following its chemical identification there was no great rush to investigate lipoic acid, and it was not until 1989 that the antioxidant properties of lipoic acid came to be recognized. And it is only in recent years that its unique qualities are finally being fully investigated.

The "lipoic" part of the name derives from the fact that lipoic acid is fat soluble. However, lipoic acid is also water soluble, which is another feature of its exceptional nature, and is a major factor as to why lipoic acid is often referred to as the universal antioxidant.

The Universal Antioxidant

Because lipoic acid is hydrophylic it is soluble in a water based environment like the blood, as is the case for vitamin C. But lipoic acid is also lipophylic, which means that it can also operate in a fatty environment like the lipid bilayer of a cell wall, as was the case for vitamin E. This unique characteristic enables it to work its antioxidant magic in virtually all parts of the body. Which is another reason why lipoic acid is so deserving of the term "universal".

Lipoic acid is even able to cross the blood/brain barrier, which as we will see, makes it very effective in stroke situations.

Much of the research on lipoic acid – as was the case for numerous other antioxidants – has been conducted at the Packer Lab under the direction of Dr. Lester Packer. There, and elsewhere, scientists have found lipoic acid to be an amazing performer, and an amazing team player.

A Restoration Masterpiece

Another reason why lipoic acid might be regarded as the universal antioxidant is because it is able to restore or recycle so many other antioxidants.

We have seen that vitamin C can restore vitamin E, and that the flavonoids can restore and fortify vitamin C. But lipoic acid has a scope much broader than that. Lipoic acid is able to restore or recycle no less than the following: vitamin C, vitamin E, CoQ-10, and most importantly, glutathione. Lipoic acid can even restore itself. That lipoic acid can do so is important with respect to all of these antioxidants, but it is especially so for glutathione. As we will presently see, glutathione is one of the most important players in the chemistry of the body. And with the exception of silymarin's inhibitory effects on the depletion of glutathione, lipoic acid is probably the best antioxidant to restore glutathione.

There are a number of prescription drugs that are able to boost the levels of glutathione, but they are somewhat inefficient and often show spotty results. Since depleted glutathione levels are associated with a number of diseases, the fact that lipoic acid is able to help maintain glutathione levels in the body is of signal importance.

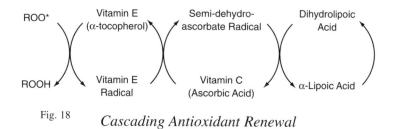

Fig. 18   *Cascading Antioxidant Renewal*

In restoring these antioxidants, it is actually a reduced form of lipoic acid that is involved in the process. This reduced form, called dihydrolipoic acid (DHLA), reduces the oxidized vitamins, as well as glutathione and Co Q-10, back to their original state, ready for action. This converts dihydrolipoic acid back to lipoic acid. Which the body, through other pathways, is able once more to turn into dihydrolipoic acid. With this ability to oxidize and reduce back and forth, lipoic acid – and its alter ego dihydrolipoic acid – are able to serve the body in a unique fashion. For the sake of simplicity we will continue to refer to the two simply as "lipoic acid".

The important thing to remember is that lipoic acid, regardless of terminology, is without equal in restoring other members on the antioxidant team. Because lipoic acid is able to recharge and restore all of these powerful antioxidants, it might well be regarded as a restoration masterpiece.

Cataracts

It is thought that anywhere from 60-80% of our sensory input comes from our sense of sight. To imagine this marvellous sense becoming less sharp, less distinct, and then clouding over forever – that is disquieting. To have it happen for real is tragic.

And yet, with the action of UV rays over time, and the intensified free radical assaults on the lens of the eye that accompany these rays, the result for many people is the development of cataracts. And without appropriate surgery and a favorable outcome, one possibility is the extinction of vision.

It was through work on cataracts that scientists at the Packer Lab first came to see the versatility of lipoic acid. The experiment showing lipoic acid's effect on cataracts is based on a very interesting circumstance: where humans cannot produce vitamin C in the body, many animals can. Rats, for instance, are able to produce vitamin C, except as newborns in their first few weeks of life. During this period they must depend on glutathione for their primary protection against free radical damage. Interestingly, glutathione production is inhibited by a substance called butathione sulfoxamine (BSO).

As further background in the matter, earlier experiments had shown that when newborn rats were given BSO it would inhibit glutathione production in them, with the result that when these rats opened their eyes for the first time at about six weeks of age, they had already developed cataracts.

A subsequent experiment repeated the above experiment, with the rats divided into two groups. Both groups were given BSO, with the second group also given lipoic acid along with the BSO. The first group, as expected, developed cataracts. The second group, however, was almost cataract-free. In addition, when the glutathione levels in the eye lenses were measured for both groups, those for the second group were found to be much higher.

Remarkably, lipoic acid had shown that it could stimulate glutathione production – even in the presence of BSO.

Substitute Player

It is always a plus for a team if one player is able to substitute for another. Such is the case for lipoic acid.

Lipoic acid is not only able to restore vitamin E, it is able to fill in for it, to substitute for it when vitamin E levels are low. This ability to pinch hit for vitamin E is likely due to its being fat soluble. Whatever the mechanism, lipoic acid has shown that it can stand in for – and perform many of the functions – that vitamin E would otherwise carry out, when this vitamin is in short supply.

In an experiment demonstrating this, mice were divided into three groups. The first group was put on a normal diet; the second group was put on a vitamin E deficient diet; and the third group was put on a vitamin E deficient diet with one added feature – the inclusion of lipoic acid to the diet.

As expected, the first group developed normally, while the second group deteriorated – they lost weight, lost muscle mass, and grew weak and scrawny. In short, they aged before their time.

The surprise was with the third group. The mice here continued to grow and develop normally. Obviously, lipoic acid – at least in some circumstances – has shown that it is able to pinch hit for vitamin E. This result also suggests that lipoic acid, like vitamin E, is instrumental in helping forestall the aging process. Dr. Ames of the University of California at Berkley found that ALA and acetyl-L-carnitine combinations caused great improvements in rat's cognition and energy. Hopefully the anti-aging benefits for rats will translate into human benefits and prove fruitful for all the patents that Dr. Ames has initiated for these antioxidants.

Genes

Our genes serve as a blueprint and determine a great deal about how any of us grows and develops. Our physical makeup – our hair color, eye color, etc. – is determined by this blueprint. But this is not the full story, for it is not quite as simple as that. Our environment, and in particular the foodstuffs included in our daily diet, can effect the way in which the blueprint is read and carried out. Which in the main, is a good thing.

If our environment, for instance, is such that we have a nutritionally sound diet in our growing years, we will reach the full potential for height as directed by our genetic blueprint. For a child raised in a poverty-ridden ghetto, on the other hand, where proper nutrition is a hit and miss affair, reaching this potential for full height as set forth in the genetic blueprint will not likely be achieved. However, the encouraging aspect to this is that we can change the environment in many regards. We can improve it such that we permit the full genetic potential to be reached, at least for the "good" genes. Even as adults we can strive to keep our full genetic potential unfolding as it should.

We also carry "bad" genes – genes that would bring about unwanted conditions in ourselves. And there are genes that are defective, or that can be made defective by things like free radicals and carcinogens. Complicating matters further, is the fact that for many "bad" genes, such as those that bring about colon cancer, their function is not that cut and dried. For these genes to express themselves and bring on the disease, it is often the case that certain conditions must be met.

Some of these conditions have to do with signalers in the body, signalers that turn a gene on so that its blueprint can be read. It is a bit like a classical pianist who has a page turner who turns the pages of music for him, which allows the pianist to read the music and play it. If the page turner did not turn the page, the pianist would not be able to go on playing – and the music on the page would not be expressed.

Free radicals often act as "page turners" for bad genes, and activate them to turn on and express themselves. We see an example of this in smokers, who introduce huge numbers of free radicals and other chemicals into their bodies, and who have higher rates of lung cancer as a consequence. With the high concentration of free radicals and carcinogens, the smokers turn on bad genes, those which are conducive to cancer development.

There is a certain natural "page turner" or gene activator in the body called Nuclear Factor Kappa B (NF Kappa B). It is a protein that can bind to DNA and affect the way it is expressed. Where NF Kappa B is working properly, all is well. If it becomes too much of a page turner, things go awry. This causes problems such as inhibiting immune function, or increasing the probability of heart disease, and so on.

Fortunately, antioxidants in general – and lipoic acid in particular – are able to help regulate NF Kappa B by keeping it under control. Fortunately as well, we have a choice in the matter. We have the option of choosing lifestyles that do not promote free radical damage, and we can strive to optimize our levels of lipoic acid and other antioxidants. And in so doing, we can minimize the debit side of the ledger, where free radicals are working to set gene activators out of control. In this way we can keep this page turner under control.

Data of this sort described above is coming from many laboratories around the world today. Antioxidant research - including that concerning lipoic acid – is at the forefront of much of this present day research. As further data arrives concerning antioxidants such as lipoic acid, and their effects on genetic potentiation, we will undoubtedly have even more choices – and more control over disease in the future.

Chelating Agent

A chelating agent is a substance that is able to bind with heavy metals and toxins. There are various metals, such as iron, that are a necessary part of the body's physiology. In fact, hemoglobin is a chelate of iron, and is crucial in oxygen transport throughout the body. For metals such as iron or copper, the right amount in the right place is everything. It is when there is a surfeit of metals such as these, in their ionic form, that we have problems. (We have seen how excess iron can bring about the generation of hydroxyl radicals in the Fenton reaction.)

Some metals, such as lead, arsenic, or mercury, are harmful in even small amounts, and generate an increased toxicity as their concentrations increase. This also brings about increased free radical activity.

Where a chelating agent is able to bind with harmful metals – or those that are in excess – they are then able to neutralize these metals, to prevent them from going along biochemical pathways that are harmful to us. Which – in extreme cases – can even kill us.

You might picture these harmful metal ions as lone, clumsy dancers on a dance floor, gyrating and twisting madly, crashing into other dancers or smacking them with their flailing limbs. When a good dancer embraces a wild one, however, the good dancer brings a settling effect to the wild one like a chelating agent preventing harm from metals. As a chelating agent (and a good dancer), lipoic acid has shown itself to be something of a Fred Astaire.

It has been demonstrated that lipoic acid can chelate high levels of mercury, for example. This highly toxic metal can then be carried away in a relatively harmless state, to where it ultimately reaches the gall bladder and from which it is then excreted.

Arsenic, which finds its way into our environment via industrial and manufacturing processes, also finds its way into many municipal water systems. Arsenic also comes to us via cigarette smoke, pesticides, and smokestack emissions. In addition to murder mystery novels set in foggy London of a century ago, arsenic also finds its way into modern day smog.

Experiments on dogs have shown that lipoic acid is effective at chelating arsenic and removing it from the blood and tissues in these animals. Human trials will likely show its effectiveness here as well.

The toxic metals that lipoic acid has been shown to chelate include excesses of iron and calcium, as well as copper, cadmium, zinc, and lead. Chelation was first demonstrated for lead removal from the body by J. Julian Chisholm who died at age 79 years in June 2001.

Mitochondria

Just as the human body is made up of many different kinds of cells, so too the cell contains within it a number of different structures called organelles. These organelles, one of which is the mitochondrion, all perform their own particular functions which are necessary to the cell's normal operations. And necessary, then, to keeping the body healthy and working well.

Current thought holds that long ago, perhaps 3 billion years or so, primitive cells without nuclei existed, some of which resembled mitochondria. These cells, like mitochondria, excelled at energy production. As the various kinds of early cells evolved, some of them eventually developed a nucleus. Although they had other advanced features, many of these nucleated or eukaryotic cells were sluggish in the area of energy production. One way around this was for the eukaryotic cells to engulf the primitive cells. Over time this practice evolved to where the primitive cells became part of the nucleated cells – they lived inside the nucleated cells in a symbiotic relationship: the primitive cells provided high levels of energy, and the nucleated cell provided a protective home. As time passed the high energy cells became just another part of the nucleated cell, which today we recognize as the mitochondria.

A vague comparison might lie in the way our cave ancestors brought fire into the cave to provide for their energy needs or Tom Hanks created fire for his sojourn on the beach. A somewhat more accurate comparison might be found in the furnace in a modern day house. The furnace provides heat (energy) and the house provides a sheltered environment.

In the case of the present day mitochondrion, energy production is still its principal task. The mitochondrion contains within it chemical "production lines" where sugar is converted into a substance called ATP (adenosine triphosphate). Where energy needs are high, such as in heart muscle, the liver, or the brain, mitochondrial organelles are abundant.

Essential in the mitochondrial energy production, and in this capacity serving as a coenzyme, is lipoic acid. Lipoic acid assists along the production line by facilitating particular reactions in a whole series of reactions. It also serves by assisting in the passage of glucose molecules across the membrane into the mitochondria.

In energy production, we will recall, oxidation-reduction reactions are proceeding apace, with electrons being shunted this way and that, and occasionally going astray. When this happens and the electrons latch onto an oxygen molecule (oxygen is also present in these reactions), we have the formation of the superoxide radical.

Fortunately, lipoic acid is on hand doing its work along

the energy production line, and is capable of wearing many hats. Putting on the white hat, that of a superb antioxidant, it is able to ride herd on the black hats – the superoxide radicals, and other free radicals as well. Which in turn prevents mitochondrial damage.

One in vitro study (Balijepalli S, et al. Neuropharmacology 1999, April) provided evidence of lipoic acid's ability in this regard. Slices of mouse brain treated with a drug called haloperidol brought about reduced levels of glutathione and a decreased ability to counter oxidative processes. When these brain sections were pretreated with lipoic acid and glutathione, they reduced this vulnerability and prevented much of the oxidative damage.

In an in vivo study, a woman suffering from mitochondrial damage was assessed prior to, and after lipoic acid treatment, by the use of phosphorous magnetic resonance spectroscopy (31P-MRS). One of the correlates to this mitochondrial damage in brain cells was a decrease in a substance called phosphocreatine. After only one month of lipoic acid treatment, the patient showed a 55% increase of brain phosphocreatine. There was also impressive improvement in mitochondrial function and skeletal muscle performance, as indicated by assessments done on the calf muscle. By way of subjective corroboration, the patient also reported an improvement in her general condition, and her muscle performance in particular.

There have also been high positive correlations shown for liver impairment and mitochondrial damage. In the case of mushroom poisoning, and the resulting liver impairment, we have seen lipoic acid's dramatic effect in restoring liver function. And we are not amiss in thinking that much of this effect had to do with improved mitochondrial performance.

Dr. Mark Lazarovich of the National Sinus Research Center in Berlin, Vermont has found that a treatment with minimal side effects for migraine type headaches would include a non-sedating antihistamine, an intranasal steroid and Riboflavin (B2). B2 has been shown to correct a mitochondrial metabolism defect that Belgian researchers found in migraine sufferers. He also uses 2-3 liters of water and prophylactic migraine therapies.

A February 2002 report from the "Proceedings of the National Academy of Sciences" has shown the remakable extension in lifespan of rats after administration of alpha lipoic acid with acetyl-L-carnitine. The alpha lipoic acid controls free radical production and the acetyl-L-carnitine helps increase energy production from the mitochondria. Professor Bruce Ames is patenting some of these supplement combinations at the University of California at Berkeley, predicting that these results will apply to humans.

The Liver

The dramatic recovery of the couple who had eaten poisonous mushrooms mirrored results that had been obtained with the use of lipoic acid in Europe. There, doctors had been using lipoic acid for some years in the treatment of liver problems. And now lipoic acid is finally seeing a wider use in America in this regard.

Dr. Berkson, who treated the couple with mushroom poisoning, is at the forefront of lipoic acid use in a clinical setting, and is regarded as one of the leading authorities in its use. In his book "The Alpha Lipoic Acid Breakthrough" he has stated: "I have worked with ALA [lipoic acid] on the FDA investigative drug permit since the late 1970s and believe that it is an excellent therapeutic agent for many types of liver disease, as well as for several other serious medical conditions....Over the past few years numerous scientific papers have been published on the substance. I think that prior to any serious consideration of liver transplant surgery, a doctor should prescribe a course of alpha lipoic acid."

Your liver is your life. And although most of the major organs of the body are all necessary for life, few perform as many complex and varied tasks as does the liver. It maintains and recycles red blood cells; it screens poisons and bacteria from the blood; it stores vitamins and minerals; it produces proteins necessary in maintaining proper blood pressure; it is involved with bile production and digestion; it plays a large role in regulating cholesterol levels. And the list goes on. If the liver had a dozen PhDs in biochemistry it could not do more. And lipoic acid provides it with a marvelous assist.

The liver is like the toxic waste site in the body. Much of the physiological refuse ends up there. That includes many of the poisons that come to us from the modern environment and find their way into the body. Where there is a sudden influx of poison, as in the case of mushroom poisoning, the liver can become overwhelmed. And it is at such times that lipoic acid is invaluable.

Lipoic acid, besides restoring numerous other antioxidants, is an extremely effective antioxidant in its own right. It has two thiol (sulfur) groups in its molecular makeup, and it is these thiol groups that play a large part in reducing free radicals. With two thiol groups, lipoic acid is like a boxer that can deliver a knockout punch with either hand. And it delivers these punches in protecting the liver by neutralizing free radicals and other poisonous substances before they can wreak their damage on the liver.

Diabetics, AIDS patients, people suffering from radiation poisoning – all have extremely high levels of free radicals. In such cases – and others – lipoic acid has demonstrated that with its one-two punch it can greatly improve their circumstances – partly by relieving the strain on the liver. In his book "Lipoic Acid: The Metabolic Antioxidant" Dr. Passwater states: "Lipoic acid has also been used for decades to protect the liver and to detoxify the body of heavy metals such as excessive iron and copper and toxic metals such as cadmium, lead and mercury." He then goes on to say: "One of the most exciting developments is that lipoic acid appears to help slow the progression of HIV infection to clinical AIDS."

Lipoic acid also protects the liver in another fashion. Much in the way that genistein occupied an activity site that estrogen might otherwise have occupied and used to promote cancer, lipoic acid is able to occupy certain protein carriers. Where these protein carriers are unoccupied, various poisons may occupy them and hitch a ride to the liver. As Dr. Berkson describes it: "Some scientists believe ALA reverses poisoning by competing for binding sites on the carrier proteins that bring the toxins to the liver. Carrier proteins are analogous to a passenger train going to the liver, with only a specific number of seats (binding sites). Large passengers (poison molecules) start crowding their way onto the train (carrier protein), but the smaller, swifter passengers (ALA molecules) slip in under the large passengers and take their seats (binding sites) on the train (carrier protein). Consequently the toxins cannot take the train to the liver, and the liver is saved from being poisoned." In the case of many poisons which the liver does not process, they may be passed along in the bile, or to the kidneys, where they are passed off in the urine.

Like many of the antioxidants that have particular areas of the body where they are most effective, that too is the case for lipoic acid. And although lipoic acid is found in virtually every cell in the body, and counters free radical activity in virtually every cell in the body, it does some of its most impressive work in the liver. A great deal of Dr. Berkson's work over the past two decades has helped many patients with liver impairment through the use of lipoic acid.

Since silymarin shows some of its strongest effects in

the liver, Dr. Berkson has also used it in conjunction with lipoic acid. He has also used selenium in this fashion as well. Some of these applications have involved patients with hepatitis, and have produced dramatic effects: "Symptomatic hepatitis C patients with elevated transaminases were placed on a triple antioxidant therapy comprising alpha lipoic acid, selenium, and Silymarin (milk thistle) and all were spared hepatic transplantation, showed improved laboratory indices, and returned to normal working life." (Berkson B M, Med Klin. 1999 Oct) The conclusion summing up the results of this work: "Multiple antioxidant therapy combining alpha lipoic acid with other antioxidant agents such as selenium and the herb milk thistle is synergistic in Hepatitis C therapy and may provide a cost-effective alternative approach, even in cases with a poor prognosis."

Lipoic acid, through its activity in the mitochondria where energy is produced, also appears to benefit the liver indirectly. Researchers have found through autopsies done on people who have died from liver disease, that invariably there was accompanying mitochondrial damage present as well. Since lipoic acid offers excellent protection to the mitochondria, its effect in this regard also helps the liver. This has been borne out in Europe, where patients with liver impairment have been treated with lipoic acid, and have shown very positive results.

Almost always, research is initiated to solve a problem. This is certainly the case for liver disease – and its treatment with lipoic acid. And this research has produced striking results as to the benefits of lipoic acid. However, a further conclusion presenting itself is that if lipoic acid can show such striking effects in combatting liver impairment – even to the point of forestalling or preventing liver transplants – then its day-to-day effects would have to be equally beneficial. So, although most of us do not have the severe levels of poisons in our system as might accompany mushroom poisoning, most of us will have low grade levels of poisons from the world around us – and the associated free radical activity. Through the use of lipoic acid we have a one-two punch to counter these poisons and the ensuing free radical activity.

Cardio–Connection

Many years back one of the authors had a teenaged neighbor living down the road. The young man had an old beater that had been running reasonably well – until its water pump gave out. While replacing the water pump the young man broke a bolt off that was supposed to hold the water pump tight to the block, which left it leaking water. Thereafter, as he raced back from downtown he would arrive at home with the engine spewing water and steam. This cloud of steam and water under the hood eventually ruined the generator, and soon took its toll on the battery as well. Which left the young man in need of the neighborhood kids to push it to get it going, and which on one occasion sent the car out of control and into a tree, taking out a headlight and pushing in a fender. Which for a time rubbed on a tire. The dilapidation continued to take its toll, until finally the old beater was put out of its misery when the motor seized up, and it was unceremoniously towed off to the scrap yard.

This progression of decay in the old car is not that unlike the way things tend to unfold in the aging body. Many of the body parts have interconnections, so if one part becomes somewhat impaired, other parts too may be affected. Just as mitochondrial function has an impact on the liver (and all else in the body), so too an organ like the liver may affect other aspects of our health. Not unlike one part failing in the old car, which then led to other failings as well. Bringing on the untimely end.

For example, if poisons in the environment are generating increased free radical activity in the body, over time an organ like the liver may become overworked. There will be an excess of heavy metals and poisons that the liver cannot process and discharge. And since the liver function has an effect on blood pressure, an overworked liver may produce unwanted consequences in this area too. And since the liver also plays a prominent role in cholesterol levels, where it is failing on this front we may end up with elevated cholesterol readings, meaning more unprocessed LDLs left unattended in the blood – until they are attended to and oxidized by free radicals.

A failing liver may be remiss in properly carrying out another of its duties – that of converting excess blood sugar into glycogen, and storing it there. Leaving more glucose in the blood will then bump up the levels of the AGEs – those pernicious accelerated glycation end products. These "sugared proteins" aid in the formation of cross links in collagen, and where they result in damage in the collagenous matrix of the arteries, the stage is set for further problems. Because now, along with additional damage due to oxidative stress, these damaged spots will be the equivalent of the artery laying out a welcome mat for the oxidized LDLs, gobbled up by the foam cells in the arterial wall with the subsequent formation of plaque.

Atherosclerosis

We see how the conditions described above are conducive to the formation of plaque on the arterial walls – which in turn will readily give rise to atherosclerosis.

Because lipoic acid operates very efficiently as a scavenger antioxidant, it is a strong ally in countering free radical activity throughout the body, including the cardiovascular system. In so doing it offers solid prevention against cardiovascular disease.

But it is probably in its role of restoring vitamins E and C, as well as glutathione and CoQ-10, that lipoic acid achieves its most formidable effects in protecting against cardiovascular disease. Although lipoic acid can get into fatty areas of the body and do its antioxidant work there, vitamin E is unmatched in this regard. Because of its molecular structure, vitamin E has a nimble mobility in places like the matrix of the lipid bilayers. It is almost as though it can chase down free radicals there, and disarm them. So vitamin E is the battler you most want in these front trenches. With vitamin C on hand to restore it. And most of all, you will want lipoic acid present at levels where it can restore both.

In a war situation (and as regards free radicals it is a war situation) you might think of the free radicals as enemy soldiers coming at you and your troops armed with live grenades. Because you (as vitamin E) excel at hand-to-hand combat, you are in the front rank, along with others like you, where you can disarm these enemy soldiers and take away their live grenades. But if you cannot get rid of the grenade, it will get rid of you, removing you from the battle. Fortunately you have backup soldiers (vitamin C) who have the ability to take the grenade from you and dispense with it behind the battle lines. Most fortunate of all, however, is where you have sufficient soldiers of a third kind (lipoic acid), who are able to relieve both yourself and your immediate backup (vitamin C) of your grenades, and dispose of them.

By being able to relieve both vitamins E and C of their deadly burden, lipoic acid serves as a bulwark in preventing atherosclerosis. And where this prevention keeps the arteries clear and open, it helps prevent heart attack and stroke.

Heart

Preventing lipid peroxidation in the lining of the arteries

is of great importance, and with respect to the coronary arteries that supply the heart, it is a matter of life and death. Cardiovascular disease is the leading cause of death in America today, and a large part of this fact derives from heart trouble and heart attack.

Through its antioxidant action, lipoic acid has demonstrated an inhibitory effect on lipid peroxidation. It has also shown that it can interfere with and halt the adhesion of macrophages to the artery walls. Lipoic acid is also thought to prevent damage to the endothelial lining in another way – through its ability to inhibit the effects of the transcription factor NF Kappa B. This inhibitory effect manifests itself in the endothelial cells lining the arteries by protecting against oxidative injury and inflammatory damage and there. "Exogenous alpha-lipoic acid is reduced intracellularly by at least two and possibly three enzymes, and through the actions of its reduced form, it influences a number of cell processes. These include direct radical scavenging, recycling of other antioxidants, accelerating GSH [glutathione] synthesis, and modulating transcription factor activity, especially that of NF-kappa B. These mechanisms may account for the sometimes dramatic effects of alpha-lipoic acid in oxidative stress conditions (e.g., brain ischemia-reperfusion), and point the way to its therapeutic use." (Drug Metabol. Review, 1998 May).

One experiment conducted at the Packer Lab used the Langendorff beating heart model, which consists of a procedure that allows a living, beating heart to be studied outside of the animal. In the experiment a heart attack was simulated by perfusing the beating hearts from rats with a solution that contained no oxygen. The solution was changed to one that contained oxygen after forty minutes had elapsed. Normally, only 20 – 25% of the hearts recover and continue beating normally, while the rest sustain severe damage. However, when lipoic acid was added to the reperfusion solution, the recovery rate jumped to a striking 60 %, almost double the rate for those without lipoic acid, similar to the benefits of Ginkgo.

The old song says "You gotta have heart...." In the future it may be "You gotta have lipoic acid...." Well, it doesn't quite have the same ring to it, so maybe not. But you still gotta have lipoic acid!

Stroke

When blood, and its necessary cargo of oxygen, is interrupted in its flow to the brain, we have an incidence of stroke. In the case a major stroke where death does not occur, physical and mental impairment usually does.

The time to take action is not in our aging years, when the carotid artery that feeds the brain is clogged with plaque, but in our younger years. And especially as we approach middle age, before we begin to deteriorate. An ounce of prevention is worth a pound of cure. And in guarding against stroke, lipoic acid is a formidable ounce of prevention.

An experiment carried out at the Packer Lab graphically illustrates lipoic acid's efficacy in guarding against stroke. In the experiment, stroke in rats was induced by blocking the carotid artery. Blood flow was restored after thirty minutes. We have seen in this situation that with the onrush of blood that comes once its flow is restored, there is usually some reperfusion injury in attendance, brought on by the accompanying burst of free radical activity. In this experiment, the explosion of free radical activity overwhelmed the rats' antioxidant defences, and within 24 hours 80% of them died.

When the experiment was repeated, there were two important differences. First, the rats were injected with lipoic acid just prior to the restoration of blood flow through the carotid artery. Second, within 24 hours only 25% of the rats died! Even more impressive, the survivors recovered completely and showed no sign of impairment.

Other experiments involving induced stroke showed equally impressive results. It was found that injections of lipoic acid were able to reduce free radical damage to various parts of the rats' brains. Further investigation has shown that lipoic acid was able to bring about this reduction of free radical damage in part because of its ability to cross the blood/brain barrier.

An additional result – equally impressive – lay in the fact that lipoic acid was able to boost the levels of the other lone eagle, glutathione. This is significant because, in the animals that were not administered lipoic acid, their levels of glutathione plummeted after the induced stroke – an additional indication that their antioxidant defenses had been vanquished. Obviously, lipoic acid stimulates glutathione production when we need it the most – when the body is under duress.

Diabetes

Diabetes is another area where lipoic acid has provided strong positive results.

This terrible disease, which occurs principally in two forms – Type I and Type II – is the result of impaired sugar metabolism. Not enough of the glucose in the blood can get into the body's cells where it is needed for energy production.

In Type I diabetes, also referred to as juvenile or insulin dependent diabetes, there is not enough insulin produced in the pancreas to facilitate the proper uptake of sugar by the cells.

Type II, or adult onset diabetes, results from an insulin resistance. The body still produces enough insulin, but it no longer works as effectively at "escorting" sugar molecules into the cells, where they can be metabolized.

Type II

It is Type II diabetes which has become one of the fastest growing diseases in North America today. And although genetics plays a large role in the development of this form of diabetes, so does lifestyle – particularly as to diet and exercise.

People who are overweight and sedentary are more at risk for this form of the disease than those who are active and lean.

Age, too, plays a role, with the risk of developing the disease rising steadily over the years. This is borne out by the fact that 85% of Type II occurs in people over thirty-five.

Accompanying this disease are inordinate levels of free radicals, and the damage these oxygen-devils inflict. Much of this damage is complicit (directly or indirectly) in secondary conditions brought on by diabetes. It is, no doubt, because free radicals play such a large destructive role in diabetics that antioxidants – and lipoic acid in particular – have shown such beneficial results.

In Europe, where there has been a big head start in the use of lipoic acid, and in determining some of its most beneficial applications, a host of heartening results have been achieved. There, and more recently in America, the use of lipoic acid in the treatment of diabetes has shown it to be a superb adjunct in controlling symptoms of diabetes, and in preventing some of the secondary problems that ensue with that disease over time. Many of these secondary problems are directly associated with the high sugar levels diabetes brings about, and the resultant skyrocketing of free radical activity. One of the most painful and debilitating of these secondary conditions is diabetic neuropathy, which involves weakening and damage to peripheral nerve cells.

Diabetic neuropathy is itself preceded by damage to

arteries that supply these nerves with blood. There is a covering encasing the nerve, the myelin sheath, which might be likened to the covering around copper wires running through the walls of a house. When these myelin sheaths are in poor repair it often produces a feeling of numbness, or pins-and-needles, in the affected area. As the condition progresses, the discomfort frequently worsens, bringing an intense burning sensation and pain.

Lipoic acid has been used successfully in countries like Germany in combating peripheral neuropathy, and in reducing or eliminating the accompanying pain. Recent studies in the laboratory are now corroborating the excellent clinical results of lipoic acid in this application.

In one study, neuropathy was induced in rats, which then had their diets supplemented with lipoic acid. By measuring correlates such as reduced glutathione and the conductive velocity in distal nerves, it was found that "lipoic acid improves nerve blood flow, reduces oxidative stress, and improves distal nerve conduction in experimental diabetic neuropathy." (Diabetes Care, 1995 Aug).

In another study, the ALADIN study (alpha lipoic acid in non-insulin-diabetic patients), 328 individuals were involved in a double blind placebo-controlled trial that tested the effects of lipoic acid. The conclusion: "These findings substantiate that intravenous treatment with alpha-lipoic acid using a dose of 600 mg/day over 3 weeks is superior to placebo in reducing symptoms of diabetic peripheral neuropathy, without causing significant adverse reactions."

Because lipoic acid is able to improve glucose metabolism, and the delivery of glucose to the mitochondria, and as well to serve as a stalwart antioxidant in this part of the war zone, it is undoubtedly a first choice antioxidant for the diabetic. Ongoing research will almost certainly confirm and expand upon its efficacy in benefiting those with diabetes.

Skin and Wrinkles

Dr. Nicholas Perricone has a wonderful book out, "The Wrinkle Cure", that explains the importance of antioxidants and essential fatty acids in the diet to maintain proper skin health. Alpha lipoic acid is an essential ingredient in any preparation to reduce acne scars, reduce pore size, reverse lines, wrinkles and to relieve puffiness under the eyes. Dimethylaminoethanol (DMAE) and a vitamin C ester added to alpha lipoic acid will address almost every sign of aging to the skin. Alpha and beta hydroxy acids act as great exfoliants to clear the skin of dead cells and also work in conjunction with the other antioxidants

Aids and Immunity

People with AIDS, as part and parcel of their compromised immune function, also carry a high load of free radicals. This heavy load, besides taking its toll in all the typical ways we have looked at, will inflict an additional hit on those with AIDS: where the immune system has already been decimated by the AIDS virus, the free radicals will then kick the immune system while it is down. In anthropomorphising still further, one would be tempted to say: such is the nature of free radicals. But in this circumstance lipoic acid has shown once more that it can help. Clinical applications in which lipoic acid has been used as an adjunctive treatment have provided extremely positive results. A number of laboratory experiments, as well, have also shown marked benefits for the use of lipoic acid.

One study, in which HIV patients were given lipoic acid 3 times daily, 75% showed an increase in T-cells. And all of these patients showed elevated levels of glutathione, which is also a decided plus.

In vitro experiments have shown that lipoic acid is able

to prevent the replication of the HIV virus in cultured human cells. In vivo studies on humans have yet to be conducted, but it is hoped that similar results will be obtained.

Experiments so far are encouraging because they indicate that lipoic acid can help rearm the immune system. And by stimulating increased glutathione levels in the body, lipoic acid provides a second line of reinforcement, because as we will see, glutathione is crucial in promoting a healthy physiology.

Radiation

Radiation poisoning brings about an avalanche of free radicals which, when severe enough, ends up burying its victims. Literally. Such has been its effects from earliest investigations, going back to the research done on radiation by Marie Curie. She worked many hours on radium – which she and husband Pierre discovered – and later on worked more endless hours in purifying the radioactive isotope of uranium.

For her immense labors and contributions to science in the field of radiation, Madame Curie became the first person to receive two Nobel prizes. And a premature death. Which was almost certainly hastened by her constant exposure to the radioactivity, and – unbeknownst to her – the host of free radicals such exposure generated.

There have been a number of instances over the decades where radiation poisoning has either killed its victims quickly, or brought on sickness and eventual premature death. One of the more recent of these, coming in the aftermath of Chernobyl, left many people in jeopardy there. Those who continued to live in the region after the near meltdown were subjected to ongoing low levels of radiation. One way in which this exposure manifested itself was through high levels of peroxidation in the blood.

Experiments on mice prior to the Chernobyl disaster had shown lipoic acid to be highly effective in protecting mice from the deleterious effects of radiation poisoning. Treatments with lipoic acid prior to radiation exposure had, in fact, brought the death rate down from 65% to only 10% in these mice. With this kind of performance behind it, lipoic acid was called upon following the spread of Chernobyl's radioactive cloud.

In the region of Chernobyl itself, lipoic acid was administered to the children still living there after the accident. These children had been showing high levels of peroxidation, a sure sign of free radicals at work in the body. These same children, after four weeks of lipoic acid treatment, then showed peroxidation levels that had fallen to normal. Even more auspicious, their liver and kidney function had also returned to normal.

Measures are generally taken only when something is drastically wrong. So the increased free radical activity that most of us experience from our surroundings – UV radiation, air pollution, electromagnetic fields, etc. – will not usually bring us into the range shown by those in the area of Chernobyl after the accident. But although not as drastic, the effects are there. And if lipoic acid can bring free radical levels into the normal range after Chernobyl, it will almost certainly have a correspondingly salutarious effect on us as well.

Mind Your Memory

In the movie "Donnie Brasco", Johnny Depp plays an undercover FBI agent who has infiltrated the mafia and become a pal of a mafia member played by Al Pacino. At one point the FBI agent asks the mafia character what the mobsters mean when they use the phrase "fo-gedaboudit" (forget about it). The mafia character explains that the phrase may mean many things, but it doesn't really mean forget about it.

And the audience, of course, is fully aware that one does not want to forget about anything when dealing with the mob. Because if you are an undercover infiltrator, that could be fatal. And although memory may be more important in that situation, in day to day circumstances, memory today plays a larger role than ever.

As Alvin Toffler pointed out in his book "Future Shock", we live in an age of accelerated change. For one thing, we are an extremely mobile society in comparison to that of our forbears, and we move around a lot: new neighborhoods, new cities, new places of all kinds – all exacting a toll on the memory. New zip codes, new e-mail addresses, new phone numbers (which are often longer). The use of PIN numbers is mushrooming, imposing further tolls on the memory. And the list goes on.

To make matters worse, just when we arrive at a point in life such that our duties and responsibilities are more complex than ever- usually around middle age – our memory function begins to decline. Near the beginning, this mental decline is almost imperceptible. But the declines are there, and over the coming years they will increasingly make themselves felt. If its any consolation (and you know we will be referring to it shortly), this type of mental decline occurs in mice as well.

A lesser known fact is that brain function – thinking, remembering – requires huge quantities of energy. Indicative of this requirement is the occurrance of large numbers of mitochondria that are found in brain cells. It is the mitochondria that produce the energy needed by the cell, but in producing energy they produce many free radical as well. Such energy and free radical production occurs in skeletal muscles or heart muscle during a workout, and both are generated in the brain during a mental workout as well.

Fortunately, with lipoic acid present, and taking part in

the oxidative processes that "burn" sugar to give us energy, it is also on hand to put out the free radical fires generated by these oxidative processes. This means that where lipoic acid is present in the body in sufficient quantities, it is in the right place at the right time to prevent damage. Which is supremely important when it comes to the brain, because it is within the brain that the seat of consciousness exists, and it is within the brain that the formation and generation of our identity comes about. So, much of who we are and what we are depends upon mental function and memory.

Where sufficient lipoic acid is present to prevent free radical damage to brain cells, one might conclude that mental functions, including memory, will be preserved or enhanced. And that is exactly what research so far indicates.

One experiment conducted on older mice demonstrated this clearly. Since mice, like humans, experience faltering memory function as they age, they served as appropriate subjects. In the experiment, half the mice were given lipoic acid which was added to their drinking water, while half were not. After a two week period the mice were put through a maze to test for memory function. Those that had received lipoic acid performed much better than those that had not. In some cases their performance was on a par with mice half their age.

Other experiments, as well, have shown equally convincing results. Such evidence, combined with studies that have shown lipoic acid to increase the energy available in brain cells, would have the authors make the following suggestion: when it comes to protecting memory function, lipoic acid should immediately spring to mind. This is one case where you do not want to "fo-gedaboudit".

Restoring Glutathione

A case could be made that lipoic acid's most important role in the body has to do with its ability to restore glutathione.

Glutathione is of crucial importance to good health, and in stimulating the body to produce more of it – especially where it is in low supply – lipoic acid is also then of great importance as well.

The precise mechanism by which lipoic acid achieves this positive effect on glutathione levels has only recently come under the eye of scientists. Evidence of this recent research indicates "that lipoic acid induces a substantial increase in cellular reduced glutathione in cultured human Jurat T cells, C6 glial cells, NB41A3 neuroblastoma cells, and peripheral blood lymphocytes. The effect depends on metabolic reduction of lipoic acid to dihydrolipoic acid. Dihydrolipoic acid is released into the culture medium where it reduces cysteine. Cysteine thus formed is readily taken up by the neutral amino acid transport system and utilized for glutathione synthesis....Thereby lipoic acid enables the key enzyme of glutathione synthesis, gamma-glutamylcysteine synthetase, which is regulated by uptake-limited cysteine supply, to work at optimum conditions....Hence lipoic acid may have clinical relevance in restoration of severely glutathione deficient cells." (Biofactors, 6(3):321-38 1997)

Simple and Efficient...and Formidable

Because the levels of lipoic acid are more readily fortified in the body than are those of glutathione, taking lipoic acid supplements is a simple and efficient expedient in achieving higher levels of both. This will also help maintain higher levels of vitamin C and vitamin E, and Co Q-10 in the body, and offer all the benefits these antioxidants confer. Add to this the benefits lipoic acid brings from its own action in the body, including assisting in glucose metabolism and energy production, as well as neutralizing free radicals, and you can add the adjective "formidable" to its resume.

Because lipoic acid occurs only in small amounts in our foodstuffs (remember it took tons of beef hearts to get 30 mg of it), we strongly recommend it as a supplement, where most of the supplemental lipoic acid is derived from potatoes and then concentrated.

Glutathione

Master Key

You are in an old deserted building, making your way along a dark corridor, and it's like you are in a strange dream. You are not sure how you got there but you know you are trying to find someone, to rescue someone from...something – but you cannot say from what. You only know you are searching feverishly.

The corridor runs off into the darkness and there are endless doors. You try one handle but it is locked. You dash to the next door and try it. It too is locked. You spy something ahead in a dusty corner. It is a ring of old keys. Immediately you try one in the nearest locked door. It does not work in the lock. You try another key, then another. Finally one of the keys unlocks the door. Inside there is nothing.

Knowing time is crucial, you dash to the next door, but the key does not unlock this one. Again you begin trying more keys, until finally the door opens. In this room too there is nothing, only the dank air.

You hurry to the next door. The key works there also, but once more you find nothing in the room. And now you begin racing down the corridor, trying this key and that. Only now and then does a key open a door, sometimes even two or three. Where still you find nothing. And finding the right key for each door is taking forever.

Finally, as you reach the top floor you try a key and it

opens the door. And the next. And the next after that. It opens every door you try. You have found the master key.

At the last door at the end of the corridor you turn the key and the door unlocks. You push it open and in the musty gloom you see a hunched and withered figure with its back to you. It is standing before a window that is covered in cobwebs. It is an old and spindly human being, bent forward and rocking rhythmically. The back of the person's head is a patchwork of age spots and bits of thin wispy white hair.

You know somehow that this is the person you wanted to rescue and there is an anguished sorrow in your heart, for you also know that you have got there too late.

And then the figure turns, slowly, revealing a face lined with fissures and creases. The eyes are opaque and the wrinkled skin is stiff like ancient parchment, frozen in a skeleton grin. Missing teeth leave dark holes in the grin. You peer more closely and you feel the hairs go up on the back of your neck, you feel goosebumps break out on your arms – because now you can vaguely make out the aged and craggy features on the sunken face. And you see that this withered creature is you.

Master Antioxidant

Just as a master key allows you to quickly and easily open many doors in a building, so too glutathione allows you to quickly and easily open many doors to health. Glutathione is produced by the body and is found in virtually every cell in the body. In healthy people it is normally found in relatively high concentrations. Serving as an antioxidant, glutathione plays a large role in our first line of defence against free radical activity. Glutathione is multifunctional, and does everything from preventing free radical formation to assisting in the repair of damaged genes. Low levels of this powerful antioxidant tend to accompany numerous diseases, and are widely regarded as the consequence of glutathione's battling on the body's behalf to protect it against these diseases. Because it plays such a wide and varied role in the body, glutathione has often been referred to as the master antioxidant.

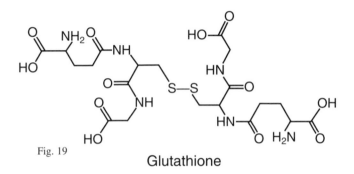

Fig. 19

Glutathione

Glutathione Pedigree

Glutathione was discovered in 1888, but like many of the antioxidants its full role was examined only sporadically over the decades, with much of the early research focusing on its benefits to the eye. In the 1980s, as research on antioxidants began its upsurge, glutathione, too, came to be more fully investigated.

Glutathione, like lipoic acid, is a thiol antioxidant, meaning it too has a sulfur component to its makeup. Another resemblance between the two is that glutathione also has an oxidized and reduced form, with the oxidized form coming about mainly from neutralizing, or reducing, free radicals. Both antioxidants occur at high levels in the mitochondria, so it is not surprising that glutathione – like lipoic acid – also plays a large part in the health of the liver and the brain. Given their resemblances, lipoic acid and glutathione might well be regarded as sister antioxidants, where lipoic acid works in conjunction with glutathione, and is able to bolster its production levels.

Glutathione, in contrast to lipoic acid, is soluble only in water, but in this medium it is the body's primary defence against free radicals. One major reason for this is that it is generally found in very high concentrations in comparison to other antioxidants. For example, there are typically a few million times more molecules of glutathione than there are of vitamin E molecules within our cells.

Glutathione might also be regarded as a primary defender in that it is in the front line of defence. As part of the Front Four, glutathione neutralizes free radicals even before they can begin their destruction. Which means that when glutathione is at optimal levels, the other antioxidants will not be as heavily burdened in their labors. And this in turn means that our bodies will sustain less by way of free radical attacks, and we will then be less susceptible to disease. In addition, we will age at a slower rate and very likely live longer.

Glutathione is made up of three constituent amino acids: cysteine, glutamic acid, and glycine. These three constituents are all found in a variety of foodstuffs (fruits, vegetables, meats), and it is important that our diet include them. The reason for this is that, although glutathione is also found in foods, much of it is generally broken down by our digestive enzymes during the process of normal digestion. Glutathione is only partially absorbed through the distal bowel (ileum). Intravenous glutathione is used to supply large quantities of this antioxidant to cell membranes but there is still a problem for cell transport into the cell.

It is for this reason that in the past, glutathione has not worked well as a supplement. However, progress has been made on this front and, as we shall see, there are supplements that will be available in the near future that are able to get around these impediments.

An Intrinsic Role

The vitamin antioxidants (A,C,E) play an integral role in the body's chemistry when serving as vitamins. As antioxidants, however, their role – vital as it is – takes on a somewhat different cast. They come into the body from the outside via our foodstuffs and supplements, and then go to work in combating free radicals. Invaluable as this is to our health, they are not, when serving as antioxidants, a truly intrinsic or inherent part of our physiology. Like hired guns, they come in, sometimes hitch rides on our proteins or travel through tissue matrices, and then disarm our enemies. But they are not produced by us, they are not born of us.

Glutathione, on the other hand, is an intrinsic part of our physiology. It is produced in the body, is found throughout the body, and is intimately and innately bound up with the biochemistry of the body. And its single most important task is in countering hydrogen peroxide, which although not truly a free radical, we have tended to regard as one. It does, after all, readily give rise to the hydroxyl radical, and it is the initiator of lipid peroxidation, and its autocatalytic chain reactions.

Working with the enzyme glutathione peroxidase (GPx), glutathione (GSH) converts hydrogen peroxide (H_2O_2) to water (H_2O).

$$2\,GSH \;+\; H_2O_2 \;\;\xrightarrow{\text{GPx}}\;\; GSSG \;+\; 2\,H_2O$$

From this we see that the reaction also converts the reduced form of glutathione (GSH) to its oxidized form, GSSG. At this point another enzyme, glutathione reductase, comes into play. It reduces the "spent" or oxidized glutathione (GSSG) back to its potent antioxidant form, GSH. Which then completes the cycle, with GSH once more armed and ready to go back into battle and convert more harmful hydrogen peroxide into harmless water.

Glutathione Cycle

Where levels are sufficiently high, glutathione is also capable of neutralizing the hydroxyl radical directly. This again oxidizes glutathione to its spent form, which must be acted upon once more by glutathione reductase to rearm it.

The work of glutathione, along with that of superoxide dismutase and catalase, is well nigh incalculable. By keeping hydrogen peroxide from beginning chain reactions of lipid peroxidation from starting, it prevents a cascade of damage. The action of glutathione is so elemental that without it we would be subject to billions of oxygen based free radical "hits" in the millions of cells of our bodies. Without this intervention we would be almost as badly off as if we had no oxygen at all.

In one experiment, the production of glutathione was artificially blocked in mice. All of them died. Glutathione is that essential to our well being.

Health, Disease, Aging

Even where glutathione is present, but only at low levels, our health invariably suffers. For when our glutathione levels are low we will not have sufficient amounts of this crucial antioxidant to fully intervene on our behalf. Over and over again we see that low levels of glutathione accompany disease and are implicated in the occurrance of disease.

From the glutathione cycle we see that it is in its reduced form (GSH) that glutathione serves as an antioxidant. When we are healthy it is in this form – ready to do battle on our behalf – that glutathione tends to predominate. When we are in good health this reduced form may be eight or ten times higher than that of the "used up" or oxidized form.

However, when we are struck down with disease, the

levels of GSH drop. In the battle, glutathione gets used up in fighting the disease. We might think of glutathione in terms of the contents of a fire extinguisher. When a kitchen fire breaks out, a fire extinguisher may be used in putting out the fire. In this operation the contents in the extinguisher are used up, their levels in the extinguisher diminish. So, too, when the body is fighting a disease. With the progression of many diseases, the levels of glutathione diminish during the battle.

Aging, too, is accompanied by decreasing levels of glutathione, as the body slips away into decline and decay. Which then leaves us more weakened still, and more vulnerable. Dr. James Balch, in "The Super Antioxidants", has written: "In relation to aging, the decline in glutathione levels appears to be more consistent in explaining age-related disorders than any other antioxidant fluctuations."

Decreasing levels with age is also the case for most hormones in the body, and great successes have been achieved in this area with hormone replacement therapy. (For those seeking detailed information on hormone replacement therapy we refer them to our previous book, "Doctors' Secrets: The Road To Longevity".) Early indications are that replacing glutathione to optimal levels will also help stave off the aging process. Certainly, results so far definitely indicate that glutathione confers strong benefits in countering various diseases, many of them age-related.

Waste Management

The levels of glutathione are highest in the liver, lungs and the lens of the eye which is lucky since these cells face the onslaught of toxins, drugs, pollutants and alcohol.

The liver is the toxic waste site in the body. It deals with cleansing the body of poisons of all kinds, including heavy metals. When it is not functioning adequately – when it has become impaired or overwhelmed – the liver becomes more of a toxic waste storage site than a disposal site. More poisons accumulate than can be dealt with and disposed of.

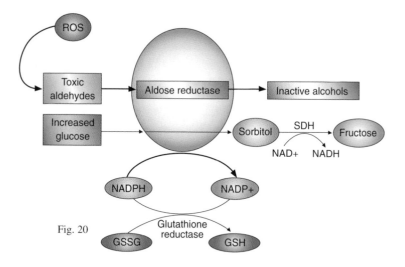

Fig. 20

Toxins and sugar managed by liver cells

Indicative of glutathione's central role in this process – in helping the liver cleanse us of poisons – are the high levels in which it is normally found in the liver. In the liver glutathione benefits us in two different ways. First, as an antioxidant, it counters the increased free radical activity that is generated by most toxins. Because glutathione has a high negative redox potential it has a powerful capacity for donating electrons. This capacity allows it to readily neutralize or reduce free radicals in the body, which means that it excels at keeping oxidative stress under control. It is this same property – at work along other physiological pathways – that allows glutathione to restore vitamin C, vitamin E, and possibly even some carotenoids.

In addition, it appears that the liver has two different reservoirs of glutathione. The first, occurring in the cell's cytoplasm, has a higher turnover rate, suggesting that it is more readily and more speedily available. The second, in the mitochondria, has a much slower turnover rate, suggesting that it is conserved there to a higher degree, probably because the mitochondria are under greater oxidative stress and cannot afford to run out of this valuable antioxidant. This double reservoir adds versatility to glutathione's deployment, and almost certainly adds to its effectiveness as an antioxidant.

The second major way that glutathione assists the liver is through its effectiveness at waste removal. Glutathione helps rid the body of the poisons accumulating there. It is instrumental in the formation of proteins called metallothionenes. These proteins are able to bind with heavy metals and other potential sulfhydryl poisons in a process known as S conjugation. In this bound state many of the poisons are then more water soluble, which allows them to be more readily carried off to the kidneys, where they are excreted in the urine.

In the normally functioning liver, the heaviest toll on glutathione results from the activity and production of the GSH transferase enzymes (GSTs). These conjugating enzymes are able to remove endotoxins (produced inside the body), and exotoxins or xenobiotics (those that come from the outside the body). These GSTs are inducible, which means that the body is able to increase production of them in order to meet stepped up quantities of poisons coming to the liver. Which again suggests that one reason the aged and the unhealthy have low levels of glutathione is that much of their glutathione is being expended in the battle against aging and disease. Because as we age, the body is less able to rid itself of toxins. And during the course of a disease, almost always the liver becomes overtaxed.

Research done on rats bears this out dramatically. In one experiment, the livers of the rats were depleted of glutathione by exposure to acetaminophen, which induced liver damage. It was found that such damage could be ameliorated by increasing the reserves of glutathione. Such damage could also be exacerbated by prior depletion, as, for example, by withholding food prior to the experiment. Further, it was found that glutathione depletion by one xenobiotic was able to predispose the liver to damage by the oxidative stress brought about by exposure to a subsequent and unrelated oxidant. A prime example of this occurs where medication – such as acetaminophen – is used in conjunction with alcohol. Here the alcohol alone might do little damage, but when acetaminophen is taken prior to the alcohol, it increases the probability of harm occurring to the liver.

Liver impairment, and liver diseases such as cirrhosis, are almost always accompanied by lowered glutathione levels. Obviously, increasing the levels of glutathione back to the normal range will surely gird the liver in its struggle. Supportive of this view are suggestions by Dr. Lester Packer: "Since lipoic acid boosts glutathione levels, it could very well be that its positive effects on liver function is actually caused by its ability to increase glutathione."

Lungs

A fact that many people are not really aware of is that the lungs, too, are an organ of excretion. Besides water vapor, their principal excretion is carbon dioxide. Carbon dioxide, at sufficient levels, is poisonous, and can bring about death.

Those who have seen the movie "Apollo 13" will recall how carbon dioxide levels were rising dangerously in the crippled space capsule. The astronauts were facing death until a ground crew, which was handed a box containing duct tape, filter parts, and other odds and ends, was able to jury-rig a makeshift filter. These were items that were aboard the space capsule and which were then assembled in a similar fashion there, where the apparatus was able to remove the carbon dioxide from the air, and keep the astronauts alive.

In addition to getting rid of poisons, the lungs also take in poisons, countless poisons – poisons that occur in the atmosphere, in unventilated buildings, and even in our own homes. Here again, indicative of its role in battling these poisons (and their related oxidative progeny), are the high levels of glutathione which are normally found in the lungs, particularly in the epithelial lining fluid (ELF) of the lower respiratory tract. Higher levels of glutathione are normal in the young and healthy. In people with chronic respiratory ailments, glutathione (in its effective form of GSH) is usually found in low levels, while the spent form of glutathione (GSSG) tends to predominate, indicative of heavy oxidative stress.

Such were the circumstances for patients in one study that were suffering from acute pulmonary respiratory distress, or ARDS. Their levels of glutathione were typically low. As an experiment, they were given a glutathione booster (N-acetyl-cysteine) intravenously. This then raised glutathione levels in their epithelial lining fluid. The effect was to speed recovery time such that they regained independent lung function and were able to leave the intensive care unit much sooner than normal.

There are some exceptions to the rule that low glutathione levels accompany a disease. Conditions such as asthma tend to generate higher levels of free radical activity. In response to this activity, these patients tend to maintain higher than normal levels of glutathione as well, by way of adaptive protection. In most conditions, however, this is not the case. In some conditions, such as idiopathic pulmonary fibrosis, the levels of glutathione in the lining of the lower respiratory tract are a scant 25% of normal, and it is thought that this may be a factor in the pathophysiology of the disease.

Although some of the evidence concerning glutathione and lung disease is indirect, the evidence is nevertheless consistent and strong. And underscored time and again is the fact that low levels of glutathione – with rare exception – accompany disease and aging. And high levels of glutathione accompany youth and health.

Immune Function

Glutathione is also intimately bound up with a healthy immune system. Where immune function is strong, high levels of glutathione are usually present as well.. Conversely, where immune function has been compromised, lower levels of glutathione are part of the picture.

Very often viral infections trigger a depletion of glutathione in immune cells. For example, patients chronically infected with the hepatitis C virus were found to have low glutathione levels in their circulating monocytes. This was also found to be the case in patients with HIV infection. Where glutathione levels can be restored to the normal range, this may well provide an ameliorating effect.

Scientific research has shown that glutathione depletion inhibits immune cell function, at times markedly. Experiments in this area show that the intracellular glutathione levels of lymphocytes were able to determine the magnitude of their immunological capacity. Other research as well has demonstrated the causal link between glutathione levels and immune function.

A significant factor in immune function attaches to T-cell number and performance. Research has shown that glutathione is required for T-cell proliferation, especially in response to mitogenic stimulation. This suggests that when some foreign invaders in the body stimulate the immune system to bring on more T-cells into the battle, it will be able to do so with greater efficacy if glutathione levels are adequate.

Glutathione is also required for other specific T-cell

functions, including DNA synthesis for cell replication, and the metabolism of interleukin-2.

In one experiment the link between glutathione levels and immune capacity was demonstrated in terms of interleukin-1 and interleukin-2. In the experiment immune cells were extracted from the blood of both younger men (35-45 years) and older men (65-84 years). The cells were then exposed to high levels of glutathione. The cells from the younger men did not exhibit much change. Those from the older men, however, showed an elevated production of interleukin-1 and interleukin-2.

Interleukin-1 serves to combat infection, while interleukin-2 is a factor in the production of new immune cells. By stimulating increased levels of both, glutathione demonstrated that it can fortify us against infection, and can also bring about increased production rates for lymphocytes.

For people with a compromised immune function – where glutathione levels have become depressed – raising the glutathione levels will also augment immune function by serving as a scavenger antioxidant. This is a task at which glutathione excels because of its high negative redox potential, which allows it to readily reduce or neutralize free radicals.

For those with a well functioning immune system, maintaining optional glutathione levels will help keep it that way. By helping maintain our immune cells at high numbers and in good working order, glutathione assists in keeping foreign invaders under control. And by keeping free radicals from forming, and neutralizing them when they do come onto the scene, glutathione provides an environment inimical to foreign invaders. Functioning in this fashion and doing double duty, glutathione is thereby able to boost the immune system in two important ways.

The Brain

Brain cells have higher numbers of mitochondria than are found in most other parts of the body. And glutathione levels tend to occur at higher levels in the mitochondria than in other parts of the cell. In the mitochondria, glutathione is in continual battle against the free radicals generated during the production of energy, which is needed in large quantities by the brain. Where there are diseases present that originate in the brain, the levels of glutathione tend to drop – again bringing to mind how the contents in the fire extinguisher are used up in fighting a fire.

Although research has not yet established an absolute causal relationship between lowered glutathione levels and some of these diseases, few scientists currently working in the field have any doubt that a causal link is present. This is especially so in cases of degenerative tissue, including degenerative brain conditions.

High levels of free radical activity are associated with a number of these conditions, including Down's Syndrome, Alzheimer's Disease, Parkinson's Disease, and others. Early research in these areas often employed antioxidants such as vitamins C and E, and more recently, lipoic acid. Glutathione, the latest to be brought forward in research here, is expected to show its effectiveness in its turn, since it has the capacity of outnumbering many of the other antioxidants. Also, glutathione is able to restore other effective antioxidants such as vitamins C and E, and glutathione serves as an exceptional antioxidant on its own.

"Too soon we get old, too late we get smart." So goes the old saying. By maintaining our youthful glutathione levels we may just be able to put the lie to this old chestnut. Intravenous glutathione has shown improvements as an adjunct treatment for Parkinson's Disease in many centers.

Cancer

About a million people per year in the U.S. are diagnosed with cancer. Sadly, a great many of these cases could have been prevented. It is estimated that up to 70% may have been induced by lifestyle.

Most people take in a number of poisons every day – even those who strive to be careful in this regard. For many, the numbers of poisons to which they are exposed is huge – poisons from exhaust fumes, from smog, from the food we eat or the water we drink, and so on. For the average person, taking in poisons is unavoidable. And a large number of these poisons, besides increasing free radical activity inside us, also act as carcinogens.

Glutathione has shown itself eminently capable of battling on both of these fronts. It excels at neutralizing free radicals in the liver and elsewhere, thereby safeguarding the nuclei of cells and their precious DNA cargo from damage. It also helps the liver with the removal of poisons, many of which are carcinogenic, getting them out of the body to where they can do no harm. In so doing glutathione removes or reduces two conditions so important in the development of cancer.

Besides working to prevent conditions that are conducive to cancer, glutathione has also been shown to have an ameliorating effect on some cancers. This has been reported in cases of ovarian cancer, where glutathione has been able to increase the efficiency of chemotherapy drugs, particularly cisplatin, and has been able to reduce the severity of side effects.

Since about half of all cancers lend themselves to treatment with radiation, one might expect positive effects from glutathione in this area as well. From the outset, the cancer will almost certainly have some aspect of free radical involvement in its inception or its progression. And once the cancer is established it will exacerbate the situation further, promoting even greater free radical activity. Finally, the radiation treatments will increase free radical activity still further yet.

Glutathione, on the other side of the ledger, is extremely efficient at negating much of this free radical activity. For this reason, and others, glutathione has shown positive results in providing relief from side effects in the treatment of cancer..

Experiments on rats have shown that glutathione may even limit the scope of some types of cancer, possibly even cure it. In one study, cancerous liver tumors were first induced in the rats. Then one group of rats was treated with glutathione while the other group received no treatment at all. For the treated rats, there was an 80% survival rate, with many of the tumors in the survivors either shrinking or disappearing altogether. For those receiving no glutathione treatment, all died. Cancer cells appear not to be able to utilize glutathione and that is why glutathione may keep normal cells healthy during cancer treatments that destroy cancer cells.

It is unlikely that such results will soon be obtained for humans. Cancer is a many headed beast and it is unlikely that any single agent or procedure will ever cure it in its many forms. But evidence suggesting that glutathione serves well as an adjunct in the treatment of certain cancers is strong. And the evidence that glutathione prevents and controls conditions conducive to cancer is well nigh incontrovertible. And that is of utmost importance.

Thus far in our practice the authors have yet to find a patient who would not rather prevent cancer than have to cure it.

Aging

Poor health usually accompanies aging, and lowered glutathione levels usually accompanies both.

Although studies on glutathione as it affects the aging process are not numerous, the evidence that has accumulated so far indicates strongly that glutathione levels do play a significant part in the process.

An experiment conducted on mosquitoes supported this point clearly. Mosquitoes were chosen for the research since, having a normal lifespan of only thirty days, they would provide results quickly. Also, prior experiments had shown that a substance called N-acetyl-cysteine, or NAC for short, would boost glutathione levels in mosquitoes anywhere from 50 to 100 percent. In the experiment, the mosquitoes with the NAC-boosted glutathione levels lived, on average, 40% longer than those without. In another experiment NAC treated fruit flies lived 26% longer than controls.

For humans who might expect to live to the age of 80, if similar results were to be obtained their life expectancy would then be increased to about 112 years of age. Of course, humans are considerably more complicated than a mosquito or fruit fly. Also we smoke, drink, and carry on with a number of unhealthy activities, so results of this magnitude might be difficult to obtain. But experiments of this sort do nevertheless suggest that keeping our glutathione levels at healthy, youthful levels will help stave off the aging process. Other research as well has tended to corroborate this conclusion, showing that glutathione levels correlate well with extending the lifespan.

Almost without exception, in human studies youth and health tend to go hand in hand with higher levels of glutathione.

Boosting Glutathione Levels

Because glutathione is a fairly large molecule, in the past it has not readily lent itself well to being used as a supplement. For one thing, it is a tripeptide, and when it gets into the digestive tract it tends to be digested. That is, it is easily broken down (as is meat or other protein) into its three constituent amino acids – cysteine, glutamic acid, and glycine.

Also, because it is not a small molecule, glutathione is not as readily absorbed into the gut as are some smaller molecules. However, where an individual does not have any impairment of the digestive tract (or other impediment to digestion), it has been shown that glutathione can be absorbed through out the small intestine. Further, in a process employing compression – where glutathione is compressed into the heart of a pill – glutathione is kept safe from the digestive processes of the stomach and upper intestine. Arriving molecularly intact, glutathione is then available for absorption through a healthy small intestine.

Antioxidant supplements of this sort are about to enter the marketplace, where they will serve as another adjunct in battling free radical activity. In addition, there are other supplements that are also able to boost the levels of glutathione.

N-Acetyl-L-Cysteine (NAC) (Mucomyst)

Another way of maintaining high levels of glutathione is by taking supplements in the form of glutathione's three principal constituents, cysteine, glutamic acid, or glycine. Of the three, the most limiting factor by far is cysteine. If there is a shortage in the assembly line, it is most often cysteine that is lacking. One reason for this is that it occurs only in small amounts in foods.

Taking cysteine as L-cysteine has been shown to produce some toxicity. The way around this is by taking cysteine into the body by way of a related substance called N-acetyl-L-cysteine, or NAC. NAC is well absorbed by the body, is very safe, and in numerous studies has shown good results in raising the levels of glutathione.

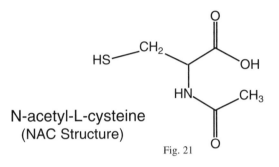

**N-acetyl-L-cysteine
(NAC Structure)**

Fig. 21

Another reason cysteine is important is that cysteine is the component that brings with it the all important sulfur atom, and it is this atom that plays such a crucial part in the oxidation-reduction reactions by which free radicals are neutralized. NAC has been used for many years as an intravenous medicine to boost glutathione levels in the liver to prevent damage from acetaminophen overdoses. It also is an excellent inhalant for the lungs to prevent lung damage from toxins and has been used for many years as a mucolytic (breaks up mucus) agent for diseases like cystic fibrosis for many years. Recently we have seen NAC intravenously drop a damaged liver enzyme count by 50% in 24 hours even 72 hours after an acetaminophen overdose in a teenager patient. An antioxidant this powerful should be a consideration for all of us fearing free radical damage. N-acetyl-L-cysteine has vasodilator properties and appears to protect the kidneys if given before angiography by reducing oxidative damage on renal tubular cells as reported by Dr. J.H. Burgess, Senior Cardiologist, Montreal General Hospital.

Other Glutathione Boosters

Other supplements may include forms of methionine, which the body is able to convert to cysteine; glutamine, which the body can convert to glutamic acid; and glycine. And once the three building blocks are in the body and on the production line, they may then be assembled into the glutathione molecule. Also undenatured whey (dairy product) proteins have cystine present which is two cysteines joined together and seem very well absorbed orally. The cystine manages to get to the cells and provides cysteine for increased intracellular glutathione production.

Lipoic acid, as well, has shown an impressive effectiveness at increasing levels of glutathione. And given that the two of them work well together, lipoic acid is well worth keeping in mind when attempting to maintain glutathione levels.

However, the simplest route to maintaining glutathione levels would be to follow a diet which supplies either glutathione or the three peptides that comprise it. In the case of glutathione itself, much of it in food will be broken down by digestion into the three peptides, absorbed, and then used as building blocks by the body in reconstructing the glutathione molecule

As we approach middle age, diet alone will not likely be sufficient to maintain optimal levels of glutathione. To a good diet we might want to add a supplement of NAC, but simpler still will be to add a state of the art antioxidant preparation that contains both lipoic acid and glutathione, one with the glutathione compressed in the center so as to allow safe passage through the initial digestive processes. And that should take care of it. For most people, this will assure high glutathione levels (as well as lipoic acid levels), and in turn, will serve the body well in preventing disease, achieving optimal health, and slowing the aging process.

A Fundamental Thing

Glutathione is almost as fundamental in the workings of the body as is oxygen. It is necessary for life. Without it, like the mice in the experiment that had the production of glutathione blocked, we would not last long. If, like those mice, our production of glutathione was blocked by some drug, we might limp along for a time – if some meager amounts of it were supplied in our diet. But even with that, our prospects would be poor. And if no glutathione was supplied by the diet our prospects would fade to nothing. Glutathione is that fundamental a thing in the body.

Although oxygen, too, is fundamental to our existence, it is a double edged sword: it both gives life and then works to erode it through the free radicals it generates. Glutathione, on the other hand, works in only one direction – to promote life. It does this through its many functions in the body, but especially in countering free radical activity. Where we maintain optimal levels of glutathione in the body, we will be well guarded against disease, and the aging process.

SUPEROXIDE DISMUTASE AND CATALASE

Superoxide Dismutase is an antioxidant enzyme that works at the cellular level. It is a large molecule that can now be produced by recombinant DNA technology and can be given by intravenous infusion experimentally and even may be absorbed through the jejunum and ileum parts of the small bowel. Intestinal absorption has yet to be proven but would constitute a medical breakthrough. Many companies are testing methods of increasing SOD production or administration of the oral enzyme for the antioxidant effect. Many studies have shown benefits for osteoarthritis patients by preventing cartilage damage thus stopping many of the degenerative changes from the joint free radicals. Intra articular injections of SOD has even been successful as a treatment for TMJ (temporal mandibular joint) arthritis.

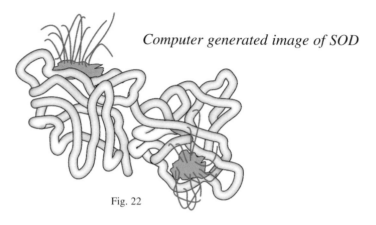

Computer generated image of SOD

Fig. 22

Following brain injury, there is a brain edema or swelling that is resulting from leaking blood vessels associated with superoxide free radicals. SOD has shown promise in preventing this swelling. SOD has reduced the cystitis associated with bladder cancer radiation therapy. Single intratracheal doses of recombinant SOD has a protective effect against lung injury in premature babies with respiratory distress syndrome. Topical SOD has been used with promise to prevent burn induced skin lesions in adults.

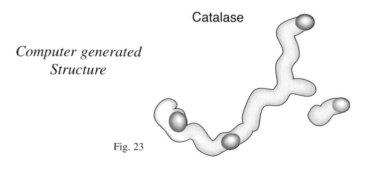

Catalase

Computer generated Structure

Fig. 23

As far as rats go, there are countless experiments extolling the benefits of SOD. Stomach injury in rats with stress has been prevented by SOD and has also increased the lifespan of rats exposed to hemorrhagic shock. SOD has been shown to minimize the damage of ischemic/reperfusion liver damage and kidney damage in rats. Even rabbits have had spinal cord improvements up to a week following oxygen deprivation if treated with SOD. Mice had increased survival rates from influenza by more than 30% if treated even later with SOD. Many lung damage trials in animals have shown SOD protection. In humans, 3000 mg/day intravenous recombinant SOD has helped multiple trauma patients improve cardiovascular and pulmonary function.

An Enzyme Extends Life

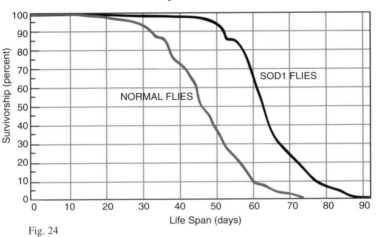

Fig. 24

Superoxide treated fleas live longer

Again an article in Science magazine last year announced that wild-type worms (Caenorhabditis elegans) treated with superoxide dismutase/catalase increased mean lifespan by 44%. The conclusion was that in this organism (more simple than humans but with 88% of the same DNA!) treatment of reactive oxygen species (ROS) with antioxidants prolongs life. Remember that catalase turns the dangerous hydrogen peroxide (produced by superoxide dismutase from superoxide) into oxygen and water. A very necessary second step reaction.

Selenium: The Honorary Antioxidant

Although not a bona fide antioxidant, selenium plays a more important role in the antioxidant scheme of things than many actual antioxidants. One reason for this is that in the case of some antioxidants – the proanthocyanidins, for example – if a particular one happens to be missing, there might be a dozen others present similar to it, which could fill in for it in its role as an antioxidant. But for selenium, nothing else can do what it does. Fulfilling one of its most important functions, selenium serves as a unique and necessary constituent of glutathione peroxidase. Selenium is also a unique and necessary constituent of other enzymes involved in the production of glutathione.

Without selenium, the entire glutathione cycle comes to a halt. Which allows hydrogen peroxide – and the free radicals it generates – a free hand to inflict damage upon us. Since it plays such a necessary part in the battle against free radicals, we are well justified in regarding selenium as an honorary antioxidant.

The Main Mineral

Chief amongst the minerals involved with the antioxidant team is selenium. Not only is selenium necessary in the formation of glutathione peroxidase, but it is also a necessary constituent of other enzymes that play a role in the manufacture of glutathione itself. Which is why we include the chapter on selenium here, following the chapter on glutathione.

Although discovered in 1817, the importance of selenium to human health has only come to be appreciated in the last few decades. And it was only in 1990 that it was formally recognized as an essential trace element by the Food and Drug Administration (FDA). It was recognised by vets to be essential for animal health and has been included in salt blocks for cattle and horses for many years.

The prime importance of selenium derives from its role in the glutathione cycle. Just as sodium is a necessary constituent of sodium chloride (table salt), so too selenium is a necessary constituent of a number of enzymes in the body. Chief amongst these are certain enzymes that promote the production of glutathione, and as well, the enzyme glutathione peroxidase (GPx). Without the selenium present, these enzymes cannot be produced. It is like the rope in a tug-of-war contest. There may be the many participants on hand for a tug-of-war, but without the rope, they are just people standing in line. Only with the addition of the rope can the event become a tug-of-war. And so it is with selenium – without it these necessary enzymes cannot be produced. They remain pre-enzymic components just standing in line.

Without sufficient selenium available, glutathione production is cut back. The low levels of glutathione, in turn, leave us weakened, vulnerable to numerous health risks, and to an accelerated aging process but selenium toxicity has also been described so don't take too much.

Without sufficient selenium on hand, the levels of glutathione peroxidase are also adversely affected, which cripples the body in its attempt to limit the harm inflicted by hydrogen peroxide. Where hydrogen peroxide is given free reign, the end result is that there is no end result. A chain reaction ensues, where free radicals produce more free radicals in an exponential explosion.

Another important feature concerning selenium is that it works in synergism with vitamin E, where each tends to enhance the effectiveness of the other.

Given the important role selenium plays in the glutathione cycle, and its enhancement of vitamin E, selenium is a natural in promoting heart health.

Heart Health

An experiment conducted by Dr. Avram of the Rambam Medical Center in Haifa, Israel, used selenium supplements to increase glutathione levels. These supplements, in fact, brought about a 33% increase in glutathione activity. This in turn brought about a 46% decrease in LDL oxidation. Without the oxidized LDLs, the reduced incidence of plaque is a natural consequence. And a reduced risk of high blood pressure, and heart attack.

Results of this sort are highly in keeping with statistical studies conducted in the U.S. and elsewhere. Repeated investigations have shown that people living in parts of America where the soil was rich in selenium, have less heart disease than people living in areas where the soil was selenium poor.

One study conducted in Finland demonstrated similar results, except that this study was concerned with water supplies. Here, people living in areas with higher concentrations of selenium in the drinking water had appreciably lower death rates than those living where selenium in the water was low.

Again, when one considers the crucial role selenium plays as a constituent of glutathione peroxidase, and thence in preventing lipid peroxidation (and the ensuing chain reactions), such results are almost what one would expect.

Selenium is also necessary for certain antioxidant enzymes involved in detoxifying rancid fats in lipid membranes.

Although selenium's role in human platelet cells is only now being investigated, it is thought to play a role here too. The platelet cells are responsible for the clotting of blood, and they tend to have a high selenium content. A preliminary conclusion is that selenium may help prevent unwanted blood clots in the body.

Immune System

Selenium also plays a large role in the immune system. This role has been investigated most intensively as it relates to the HIV virus.

Selenium is necessary for optimal immune function. As a unique component of enzymes related to glutathione production, selenium like glutathione – affects the performance of T-cells. And it is the T-cells that bear much of the brunt when the immune system is under attack in AIDS patients. Selenium has also been shown to affect the activity of interleukin 2, which also helps arm the immune system against foreign invaders.

As the disease progresses in AIDS patients, their T-cells take a beating and their numbers diminish. Correspondingly, selenium levels drop as well. In fact, selenium levels may be regarded as an indicator of the disease's progress in the body. Thus, as the disease overcomes more and more of the body's defences, the selenium levels correspondingly diminish. The one exception to this correlation occurs in the early stages of the disease, where selenium levels tend to be low as well.

Since selenium compounds have shown they can inhibit the proliferation of the HIV virus in vitro, the above anomaly is not what one would expect. There is also much evidence to suggest that oxidative stress tends to promote HIV replication in humans, and that a number of antioxidants are able to inhibit the process. This again causes one to wonder why, then, low levels of selenium tend to occur both in the early stages of HIV development, and in the later stages. Dr. Ethan Will Taylor, a pathologist at the University of Georgia, has offered an explanation concerning this anomaly.

Dr. Taylor postulates that the declining levels of selenium, rather than being the result of the disease's progression, were part of the cause. Dr. Taylor believes the data suggests that the virus, via an involved series of genetic and physio-logical events, may require selenium for a particular genetic need. If it gets the selenium, a particular gene for replication does not become expressed, and the virus does not reproduce itself. But once the selenium supply becomes diminished, some of the virus cells that do not get selenium will become active, and will begin replicating. This would explain why there are lower selenium levels during the early period of the disease – it is being used up by the virus while at the same time it is keeping the virus somewhat in check.

There are signs on some peoples' desks that say: "Give me coffee and you won't get hurt!" If the HIV virus had a similar sign perhaps it would read: "Give me selenium and you won't get hurt!"

Cancer Connection

There is a growing body of evidence which supports the role of selenium as a cancer fighter. As in the case of glu-tathione, the initial clue to selenium's benefits here derive from the correlation between low levels of selenium and high rates of cancer.

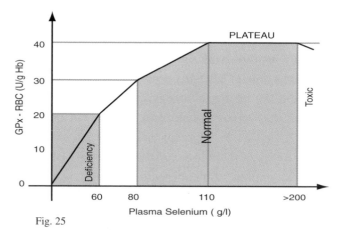

Fig. 25

Ideal Selenium Levels

One well known study linking low selenium levels to cancer was conducted by Dr. Walter C. Willet of Harvard. The study was carried out at numerous research centers throughout the U.S. in 1973. In the study, blood samples were collected from 4,480 men in fourteen different areas across the U.S. At the time the blood samples were taken, none of the men showed any signs of cancer.

In the five years that followed, 111 men developed cancer. From the men who had not developed the disease, 210 were selected for comparison, being matched for age and lifestyle to those with the disease.

A comparison of the selenium levels in the blood samples was telling. Those who had the lowest selenium levels were twice as likely to have developed the disease!

In another study, done at Cornell University, low selenium levels were also strongly linked to the risk of skin cancer. It was found that those with low selenium levels were over five times more likely to have skin cancer than those in the group with the highest levels.

Magnificent Failure

There have been experiments conducted over the centuries that have failed in what they were intended to prove – and yet they were nevertheless, magnificent failures. One such endeavor was the Michelson-Morley experiment, which demonstrated that the speed of light was constant, regardless of the motion of its source. This was, of course, a bizarre and unexpected result. But it was this magnificent failure that ultimately led Albert Einstein to his famous theory of relativity.

Another magnificent failure, admittedly on not so grand a scale, occurred in a study conducted on the effects of selenium levels on the recurrence of skin cancer. Sponsored by the National Cancer Institute and involving 1312 patients, the study did not show the expected correlation between low selenium levels and a recurrence of skin cancer. However, the data from the experiment indicated something even more surprising for those in the study who were taking selenium supplements: lower rates for lung cancer by 46%, for prostate cancer by 72%, for esophageal cancer by 67%, and for colon cancer by 62%. Overall there was a 50% reduction in the number of deaths from cancer. A magnificent failure!

The term Pyhrric victory applies to victories where the cost was so high as to almost negate the positive aspects of the victory itself. If there was a term to describe the circumstance where the positive aspects far outweighed a defeat, the above experiment would certainly exemplify it. And as well, it would certainly underscore the need for selenium in the diet.

A Need For Selenium

We need selenium to stay healthy, and to stay alive. Even governments have finally come to recognize this.

We need selenium to produce enzymes that assist in the production of glutathione. Which is, at least in part, how selenium is able to raise levels of glutathione in the body.

We need selenium to produce glutathione peroxidase, and without it we lose one of the most effective ways in which the body can prevent hydrogen peroxide from rampaging out of control.

We need selenium to enhance the work of vitamin E.

Without selenium we fall into stagnating health, and then failing health.

It is as simple as that – we need selenium.

Coenzyme Q-10: The Heartfelt Antioxidant

A catalyst is a substance that promotes or facilitates a chemical reaction, often by speeding it up or allowing it to proceed under less stringent conditions. An enzyme is, in contradistinction, a biochemical catalyst. It promotes or facilitates a particular biochemical reaction in a living organism. And a coenzyme assists an enzyme in promoting a reaction. It works with an enzyme and helps it do its job.

Coenzyme Q-10 is, as its name suggests, a coenzyme. But it is more often referred to by the shortened form of its name, CoQ-10.

Although CoQ-10 was discovered in 1957, the means of producing large quantities of it did not come about until the 1980s. It was originally available from beef hearts but is now available synthetically. With more abundant supplies becoming available, research into CoQ-10 accelerated, spearheaded by the efforts of Dr. Karl Folkers. Its chemical name is 2,3-dimethoxy-5-methyl-6-decaprenyl-1,4-benzoquinone. Studies have shown most vegetarians and also patients taking statin cholesterol lowering medicines to be low in CoQ-10.

Much of the initial research has shown that CoQ-10 is of great benefit to the cardiovascular system, such that many of its positive effects are felt in the heart. For this reason we feel that CoQ-10 might be thought of as the heartfelt antioxidant.

Dual Function

CoQ-10 has a dual function in the body. It serves as a remarkable antioxidant, and it also assists in reactions dealing with energy production. In this regard it is somewhat reminiscent of lipoic acid.

Like lipoic acid, as well, CoQ-10 is produced by the body and is found in virtually every cell in the body. Since it is a quinone, and since it is ubiquitous (everywhere) in the body, CoQ-10 is also known as ubiquinone and was even once known as vitamin Q.

CoQ-10 also shares a strong characteristic found in vitamin E – it is fat soluble. Because of that it is readily found in the lipid matrix of cell membranes, which in part will account for the benefits it confers on the cardiovascular system.

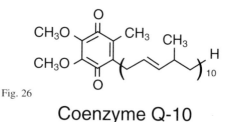

Fig. 26

Coenzyme Q-10

Like so many of the hormones and antioxidants produced by the body, the levels of CoQ-10 decline as we age. Further, diminished levels of CoQ-10 tend to accompany certain diseases, with the two foremost in this regard being heart disease and cancer.

Energy Production

CoQ-10 assists in the production of energy, specifically in the Krebs Cycle. This is a process in which a substance called ATP is produced, the ATP then serving as fuel for the cells of the body.

Although the roles for CoQ-10 and lipoic acid are particular unto themselves, there are two important parallels between them: both are involved in energy production, and both are ideally poised in the mitochondria to mop up the free radicals generated there as the unwanted by-products of the energy production.

Consequent to that, CoQ-10 confers its most pronounced benefits in parts of the body where energy production is highest. These include the heart, the brain, and the skeletal muscles. Of these, due no doubt to its own physiological idiosyncrasies, CoQ-10 has shown superlative benefits in combating heart disease.

The Indefatigable Heart

If the brain is the most intriguing organ in the body, the heart is the most indefatigable. It beats about 60 or 70 times per minute, or 100,000 times a day, and 2 or 3 billion times throughout a normal human lifespan. The heart may be stopped briefly during heart operations, or it may stop briefly under other rare and unusual circumstances. But other than these few instances, while we are alive, the heart never stops beating. Because when it stops, we stop.

Over and over again the correlation between low levels of CoQ-10 and heart disease come to the fore. In fact a correspondence between the two has been found in between half and three quarters of all heart patients. Where there is heart disease, most of the time there are also low levels of CoQ-10 to be found.

Given the fact that low levels of CoQ-10 accompany such a large proportion of heart disease, early researchers suspected a causal relationship between the two. On that assumption, it was reasonable to assume further that replenishing the levels of CoQ-10 would ease the disease. The evidence has since borne out this assumption with resounding success.

Ease The Disease

The first experiment using CoQ-10 to treat heart disease was carried out in 1965 by a Japanese physician. It was an inspired success and today over six million people in Japan use CoQ-10 in treating or preventing heart disease.

Some years later in the 1980s, once CoQ-10 became available in quantity, the research of Dr. Karl Folkers forged ahead. From the 1970s until his death in 1997 he was at the forefront of research in the use of CoQ-10 to treat heart disease, and during his latter years, in other areas as well. Much of the research carried out under his auspices was done at the Institute for Biomedical Research, at the University of Texas. Other important studies were conducted by Dr. Peter Langsjoen at the Langsjoen Clinic in Tyler, Texas.

In one study, conducted jointly by Dr. Folkers and Dr. Langsjoen, the results were both impressive and promising. The study involved patients with cardiomyopathy, a condition where some of the heart muscle has become dysfunctional and damaged. It is a serious condition which can lead to heart failure. These patients were treated either with their regular medication, with their medication along with CoQ-10, or with CoQ-10 alone. The striking result was that those patients treated with CoQ-10, either alone or with their standard medication, lived – on average – three years longer than those not taking CoQ-10.

Another large study was conducted at the Langsjoen Clinic, where 424 patients served as subjects. All suffered from a range of cardiovascular problems, including cardiomyopathy, valve problems, and high blood pressure. All patients were treated with CoQ-10 in addition to their regular medications.

Using a standard developed by the New York Heart Association, and widely recognized as the premier standard for assessing heart conditions, the results were evaluated at the end of the study. These results showed that over 50% of the patients had shown considerable improvement, over 25% had shown strong improvement, and a smaller group had shown a most striking improvement. More impressive still, about half of the patients had been able to stop taking anywhere from one to three of their regular medications during the study.

The latter result reflects an important secondary benefit in addition to improving cardiovascular performance. Where many medications often bring serious side effects with them, CoQ-10 has shown none of these. In all studies so far it has come out clean. But since it has shown that it can replace some medications while achieving better results, it also eliminates the possibility of serious side effects. This is an added plus.

Similar positive results have been mirrored in other studies conducted throughout the world. In Japan, where initial investigations into CoQ-10 were first begun, one study showed that CoQ-10 could speed recovery in heart patients. The study, conducted at the Hamamatsu School of Medicine, tested CoQ-10 against a placebo. At the completion of the study it was found that over half of those treated with CoQ-10 experienced a reduced frequency of angina attacks, used less nitroglycerine in combating pain, and showed greater endurance on the treadmill. Dr. Stephen Sinatra, cardiologist, has promoted through his informative newsletter, the benefits of CoQ-10.

Dr. Jeejeebhoy, cardiologist at William Osler Health Centre says "If the cell is depleted of carnitine and CoQ-10, which are essential for energy production, you can imagine the cell is not as capable of producing as much energy". But increasing the level of these proteins in the myocardium could improve myocardial function. Canadian researchers showed that taking oral CoQ-10 led to increased concentrations in heart muscle as proved by biopsy. This was presented in scientific sessions at the latest meeting of the American College of Cardiology.

Data of this sort continues to pile up, all of it strongly supporting the contention that CoQ-10 is indeed the heartfelt antioxidant.

The Brain

Initial research and success with CoQ-10 occurred mainly in the area of cardiovascular disease. However, more recent investigations have begun to focus on its effects in other parts of the body as well. Since CoQ-10 has shown positive results in one area of high energy production – namely the heart – researchers have begun to look at the benefits of CoQ-10 in another area of high energy production, the brain. Indicative of the brain's high energy needs are the large numbers of mitochondria found there. Early results are showing that, indeed, CoQ-10 works its benefits in this part of the body as well.

Data from research in Poland has shown that CoQ-10 is instrumental in preventing oxidative damage in the brain. This is important because the oxidation of LDLs, and attendant attacks on arterial membranes in the brain, may ultimately bring about memory loss, stroke, and even cancer.

Research conducted at the Massachusetts General Hospital under the auspices of Dr. Flint Beal shows that CoQ-10 can also protect brain cells and their mitochondria against damage. In this research, mice were used that had been bred to develop amyotrophic lateral sclerosis, which is also known as ALS or Lou Gehrig's disease and more recently Stephen Hawking's disease.

Accompanying ALS, as is the case for many brain diseases, are low levels of antioxidants and high levels of free radical activity. When the mice in the experiment were given injections of a substance called malonate, they typically developed lesions in the brain. These lesions generally become quite large, destroying brain tissue as they grow, and in the end bring about a rapid death.

However, when the mice were administered CoQ-10 along with the malonate, the brain damage was much less pronounced, and the mice lived a substantial eight days longer.

Research has also indicated that CoQ-10 has a connection with Parkinson's disease, and an application here. It has been shown that levels of CoQ-10 were low in untreated Parkinson's patients, as were enzymes that CoQ-10 helps regulate. Also, there are diminished levels of dopamine that occur in these patients. Since dopamine is necessary in the proper transmission of nerve signals, where it is in low supply it may interfere with normal brain function. CoQ-10 has shown that it is instrumental in ameliorating all of these conditions by reducing oxidative damage.

Gum Disease

CoQ-10, like some of the other antioxidants we have examined (vitamins A and C, for example), has shown a particular effectiveness in combating gum disease.

Although dental health has taken huge leaps forward in past decades, gum disease is one area where progress has lagged. It is estimated that over a half of all patients seen by dentists in the U.S. show some signs of gum disease. Not surprisingly then, gum disease is the leading cause of tooth loss in the U.S. Many dentists and doctors correlate periodontal disease inversely to longevity.

Many of the more serious cases of gum disease tend to occur in those who are getting on in years. One reason for this is that with age, the body is less able to effect proper tissue maintenance and repair. Compounding the problem are the lower levels of antioxidants that almost always accompany aging. In the case of gum disease, low levels of CoQ-10 were frequently found to be a part of the picture. One study showed that those with gum disease even showed markedly low levels of CoQ-10 in their saliva.

Research into the effects of CoQ-10 has shown that it can reduce and prevent problems in the gums. One study employed CoQ-10, either taken orally or applied onto the surface of the gums. CoQ-10 was omitted in a second group. Patients receiving CoQ-10 showed a recovery rate that was three times faster than for those not receiving it.

Given the efficacy shown by CoQ-10 in promoting healthy gums, we recommend it highly in this application. In addition, other antioxidants such as vitamins A and C, in combination with CoQ-10, would be more effective still. When it comes to antioxidants, teamwork almost always provides the best work.

Cancer

The benefits of CoQ-10 with respect to cancer maybe both preventive and ameliorative. As to a cure for cancer, it is unlikely that any one substance or any one drug will ever serve as a cure for cancer. And that goes for the antioxidants as well. However, antioxidants do reduce the risk of cancer. And, importantly, antioxidants are invaluable by way of adjunctive treatment. They reduce the severity of the symptoms of some cancers, and the suffering and discomfort associated with the radiation and drugs used in treating cancer. None of this will substitute for your doctor's prescribed treatment of standard cancer therapy. Please follow the advice of your doctor if you have cancer.

In the case of CoQ-10, studies have shown that it can enhance the performance of the body's immune system, particularly in the T-cells. Since the immune system plays an active role in destroying rogue cancer cells early in their proliferation, where CoQ-10 boosts the immune system and helps maintain it against depletion, it also helps guard us against cancer by improving T lymphocyte cell ratios of T4/T8.

CoQ-10 should not be used with the anti-cancer drug

called adriamycin. CoQ-10 may increase tissue levels of a potentially toxic metabolite of adriamycin. But CoQ-10 may alleviate the toxic effects on the heart from epirubicin, a chemotherapy for breast cancer. With high dose treatment with CoQ-10 there have been reports of headaches, heartburn, involuntary movements, fatigue and some urine changes but all these mild effects disappear after reducing the dose.

Other studies conducted under the auspices of Dr. Karl Folkers have shown early results indicating direct benefits in fighting cancer itself. Some of these studies were small, and used CoQ-10 as an adjunct with conventional treatment. That being said, the results were, nevertheless, very favorable.

In one of these studies, which involved 32 women with breast cancer, the cases were all extremely serious. It was expected that at least a few deaths would occur during the study. The good news is that none of them did. And of the 32 women, none showed any signs of the cancer spreading, while six showed signs of partial remission.

To emphasize once more, besides CoQ-10, other antioxidants and minerals were used in addition to conventional treatment in the above study. However, this again underscores two elementary thoughts that the authors cannot emphasize enough: because antioxidants work at an elementary level in aiding the body, they have an almost universal application; and when it comes to the efficacy of antioxidants, the best work is teamwork.

Antioxidant Summary

Oxygen based free radicals take a number of forms, and derive from a number of sources. They damage us by damaging tissues, cells, and parts of cells.

Fortunately, there are substances called antioxidants,

which are able to neutralize the free radicals, and they come in an even greater variety of forms. They too derive from a number of sources, and are generally most effective when working in conjunction with one another, as a team.

At the forefront of this antioxidant team are various enzymes that are able to counter the destructive free radicals, often before they can even begin to harm us. The most important of these are the enzymes that react with hydrogen peroxide, converting it to harmless water. They do their work inside the cell and in our new classification we call them "The intra cellular endogenous antioxidants". These enzymes include superoxide dismutase (SOD), catalase (Cat), and glutathione peroxidase (GPx). The latter, glutathione peroxidase, works with another antioxidant, glutathione, in rendering hydrogen peroxide harmless.

Because these four antioxidants are something of a pre-emptive strike force, and are on the front line in halting and preventing free radical activity, we have also named them the Front Four.

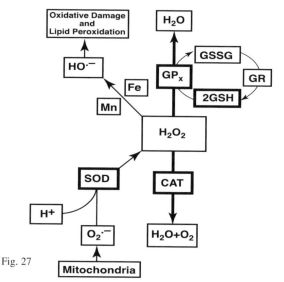

Fig. 27

The preemptive Front Four Antioxidants

These four, the three enzymes along with glutathione, are all produced by the body. Therefore, two of the best ways of keeping them at optimal levels are by availing ourselves of a varied and nutritional diet, and by taking these enzymes in appropriate supplements. If we include a wide variety of foodstuffs in our diet, we will provide the body with the many building blocks it needs in producing not only these enzymes, but many other necessary substances as well.

As we age, our production of these antioxidants – and others – will almost always go into decline. As we come up to middle age, we can offset this decline with supplements that improve SOD, Cat, and glutathione levels in our cells.

Two other antioxidants produced by the body are lipoic acid and CoQ-10. These two, along with glutathione, all present some difficulty as to optimizing their levels in the body through diet alone. Lipoic acid and CoQ-10 are generally found in small amounts in food, and compounding that, they too tend to be produced in ever declining amounts as we age.

The glutathione that is found in food tends to be broken down into its constituent peptides in the upper digestive tract. Also, the most important of these, cysteine, tends to occur at fairly low levels in foods.

Here again, as we go through middle age and beyond, adding supplements of lipoic acid, CoQ-10 and NAC (which supplies cysteine) offers a simple and effective solution. In addition we may wish to use a multioxidant which has glutathione compressed at its core. All the while, continuing with a nutritional diet, of course.

In choosing our supplements, one important factor will have to do with fortifying ourselves against and preventing the diseases or conditions for which we are most at risk.

Besides the antioxidants produced by the body, there are those which we acquire only from without, from what we ingest. These include the vitamins A, C, and E (the ACEs), as well as the carotenoids and the flavonoids. All are superb scavenger antioxidants. That is, they travel through the body like scavengers, and where they encounter a free radical, they neutralize it, rendering it harmless. We call these "The extra cellular antioxidants" for the sake of simplicity as they range freely throughout the body fluids and do their work everywhere and not just in the cell.

With the exception of vitamin A, we can rarely get too much of these scavenger antioxidants. And in modern times with modern lifestyles, we can almost always use more – especially for the average North American. Fast foods, processed foods, depleted foods, contaminated foods, eating on the run – all contribute to the fact that there are few people today in North America who follow a varied and well rounded diet. And this at a time when the sources of free radicals and free radical activity are at an all time high.

So here again, supplements serve as an ideal adjunct to diet. A top quality multi-vitamin, along with supplements that provide for a range of carotenoids and flavonoids, and we will certainly be well fortified with scavenger antioxidants. Which will leave us well armed and well guarded against free radical destructiveness.

Many of the antioxidants work together in synergism. And some antioxidants are able to restore or recycle other antioxidants. Such is the case for vitamin E, which is able to restore vitamin C; and lipoic acid, which is able to restore both of them and glutathione too. Glutathione, for its part, can restore vitamin C.

This synergism amongst antioxidants points up most strongly the importance in not only maintaining high levels of antioxidant, but a wide variety of them as well.

So it comes down to this: a nutritional, well balanced diet; well chosen supplements to maintain optimal levels of antioxidants; a top quality multi-vitamin. By maintaining a regime that incorporates these few elements we provide ourselves – simply and inexpensively – with the best health care plan there is: prevention. Through such a plan we will add wellness to our years, and years to our lives.

Since antioxidants have demonstrated an ability to guard us against a range of diseases, and since free radical activity and disease both tend to exacerbate and accelerate the aging process, the best way to slow down the free radicals and to slow down the aging process is to put the free radicals into neutral. And the best way to do this is to maintain optimal levels of antioxidants. Antioxidants are the best way to shift the free radicals into neutral, and thereby keep them from fast tracking us to the grave.

Classification of Antioxidants

PRIMARY — Prevents the formation of new free radicals (Superoxide Dismutase, Catalase, Glutathione Peroxidase (GPx), Transferrin, Ferritin) "The intracellulars"

SECONDARY — Removes free radicals to prevent chain reactions (Beta-carotene, Vitamin C, Vitamin E, Uric acid, Albumin, Bilirubin, Lipoic acid) "The extracellulars"

TERTIARY — Repairs cell damage from free radicals (i.e. DNA repair by Methionine sulfoxide reductase and Vitamin C)

"The key appears to be striking the right balance (of antioxidants and minerals)"

–Dr. Ranjit Chandra, Professor Memorial University

Notes

SECTION V

Disease

"We know that most degenerative diseases are linked to free radical damage. That means diseases like arthritis, cataracts, diabetes or any disease where some part of your body is slowly falling apart. They [free radicals] can also attack your brain and central nervous system, causing disorders like multiple sclerosis and Alzheimer's disease. ROS [free radicals] have been strongly linked to heart disease and all types of cancer. They also weaken our immune system in various ways."

–Dr. James F. Balch

"And so from hour to hour we ripe and ripe, And then, from hour to hour, we rot and rot."

–Shakespeare (As You Like It)

Disease

DISEASE, AGING, DEATH

Nietchze wrote: "What does not kill me makes me stronger."

Now, you may think Nietchze is pietchze, but his thought here is only half true. Certainly, when a soft hand is put to work, it grows stronger and more calloused. And when a child contracts measles, the child develops an immunity and is no longer vulnerable to the disease.

However, there are a great many things that do not kill us, and neither do they make us stronger. They make us weaker.

A Thousand Cuts

"The world – each day it cuts you, on the last day it kills you." These words reflect the flip side of the Nietchze quote. Many afflictions and many diseases do not necessarily kill us, but very often they do harm us and make us weaker. And in the end many of them do shorten our lives – they do kill us.

For those of us who are not taken down quickly, at a young age, the latter part of life is like the death of a thousand cuts. The march to the grave is wrought by aging that weakens us, cuts us. It makes us more vulnerable to disease. In turn, disease too weakens us, cuts us, and in the latter part of our lives hastens the aging process. The two play off each other, each augmenting the effects of the other. Each of them producing a pattern of alternating footprints, marking our way to the grave.

A Bursting Bubble

Much infectious disease has been conquered – or was thought to be. But new, more virulent bugs are beginning to raise their heads. Many of these like Bordetella pertussis (whooping cough) and tuberculosis (TB) and others resistant to antibiotics are rehaunting us. And this at a time when a large demographic bubble of baby boomers are growing older, and more susceptible to disease. And the bubble is about to burst.

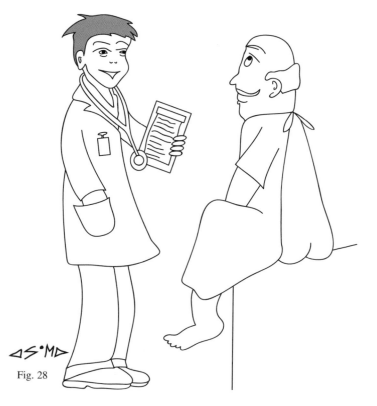

Fig. 28

I've got good news and bad news — the good news is you're not a hypochondriac!

For we do not die of old age – not really. Certainly the process of aging weakens us, and sets us up for the coupe de grace. But aging only prepares the way, along with other forms of the thousand cuts: the diseases we catch, some of which weaken us; the accidents we have, some of which weaken us; the poisons we take in over the years, most of which weaken us; and the free radicals we generate over the years, all of which weaken us. And all the time the clock is ticking.

Ticking Clock

We are made something like a clock, a wind-up clock, and once the spring unwinds, the clock stops ticking. Our days are numbered.

In the section on aging we saw how free radicals play a major role in our decline. They do this through their destructiveness both directly, and by undermining other mechanisms that play a part in the aging process, intensifying their effects at impelling us along the path to our demise.

In this section on disease we will see how free radicals promote disease, either from its inception or through its progression in the body, or both. We will see how, by promoting disease in the body, the free radicals weaken the springs in our inner clock until finally our clock, too, stops ticking.

Cancer

Cancer may not be the number one cause of death in America, but it is, arguably, the ugliest. It is rarely quick, it is often protracted, and it almost always brings with it pain and mental suffering. Some of the pain and suffering comes as an intrinsic part of the disease, some comes with the treatment for the disease, and a great deal of it comes from the mental anguish the disease inflicts – the baleful foreboding, the uncertainty.

And although it is not yet the number one killer, with the gains that cancer has been making, many in the medical field are certain that it will achieve that dubious distinction early in this century.

The worst of it is that much of this horrible disease could be prevented.

It is estimated that smoking alone accounts for about a third of all cancers, and diet for perhaps another third. To be sure, genetics lays the foundation for the entire potential of how we develop and what we may be predisposed to. But in the case of cancer, lifestyle is by far the most significant factor for most people.

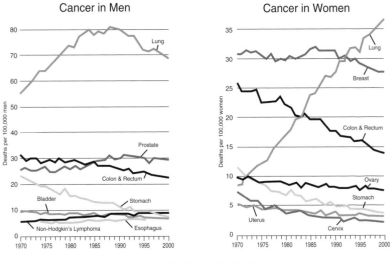

Fig. 29   Source: National Cancer Institute of Canada

The Development of Cancer

The development of neoplasia, or tumor growth, proceeds through the following three stages: initiation, promotion, and progression.

The first stage, initiation, is characterized by an irreversible, specific alteration in the DNA (blueprint) of a particular cell. This alteration may result from any number of causes, or from a combination of causes. Viral factors, carcinogens, or radiation, for instance, may serve as agents that induce these DNA alterations. The alterations themselves may take the form of gene deletions, gene insertions, gene splices, and so on. Once the DNA has undergone this permanent alteration, it leads to the next stage: progression.

Progression is characterized by the tendency toward expansion of the initiated cell, and to the expression of the gene alteration in the cell and those of its progeny. So, although the altered DNA in one of these cells cannot be reversed, with the DNA being returned to its original state, the effects of this genetic alteration can be countered in this second stage. That is, such a cell may be checked or curtailed in the expression of its altered material, and in its replication.

It is in this second phase, in the promotion phase, that free radical activity shows its strongest effects. Although some free radicals may act as weak carcinogens, and show some capacity by way of inducing initiation, by far the strongest effects of free radicals are felt in the promotion stage.

For example, a substance called phorbol mistrate promotes tumor formation by bringing about breaks in chromosomal strands. It has been found that this damage to chromosomes is mediated by free radical activity. Which means that free radicals play an active role in bringing about such damage to the chromosomes.

As noted earlier, the research of Dr. Ames suggests that rat cells sustain about 100,000 free radical "hits" each day, while for humans the number of hits to each cell is about 10,000 per day. Each of these hits represents a free radical inflicting damage to some part of the cell, including the cell's genetic material.

Concomitant with this damage are DNA alterations, or DNA oxidative lesions. And although repair enzymes remove most of these lesions, they do not remove all of them. Over time this damage tends to accumulate, such that in an old rat of about two years of age there are about 2 million DNA lesions per cell, while in a young adult rat there are only 1 million lesions per cell.

Further, free radical attacks on DNA can produce dozens of different abnormal chemical entities, which are in addition to those produced by free radical attacks on proteins and fats. Some of this DNA damage manifests itself in cross linkages in the chromosomal strands, both within the same chromosome and between different chromosomes.

At this point in time most people will have seen pictorial representations of the DNA double helix: the two intertwined helical strands coiling around each other like the railings of a circular staircase, with what appear to be horizontal stairs between the two coiling strands that join them together.

The "stairs" that hold the two strands together consist of four chemical compounds: guanine, cytosine, adenine, and thymine. Normally the guanine on one strand joins up with or pairs with cystine on the other strand, while adenine pairs up with thymine.

Aberrations to this pattern may sometimes occur. Research conducted by Floyd et al indicates that a tumor promoter generated by free radical activity can produce DNA alterations in these pairings. Specifically, through the oxidative action of free radicals, guanine may be converted to a substance called 8-hydroxyguanine, which instead of pairing with cytosine, may pair with adenine. And this may, in turn, induce further substitutions.

Since changes of this sort represent a scrambling of the genetic information, they are very likely responsible for at least part of the carcinogenesis that results from free radical damage to DNA.

Other research as well strongly supports the thesis that free radical damage does indeed contribute to the development of cancer.

Antioxidants, on the other hand, have been shown to work against tumor formation by acting as anticarcinogens.

Antioxidants and Cancer

Because humans have a lengthy lifespan, direct experiments evaluating the effects of antioxidants on cancer prevention in humans will, of necessity, require a long time as well. Most cancers develop over many years, and tend to occur in the latter part of our lives. Also, since we are not captive animals in cages, it is difficult to set up experiments with humans that control for all factors. Further, it would be immoral to withhold from a control group the substance that was expected to be the favored alternative in preventing a disease such as cancer. That being said, there is nevertheless strong evidence supporting the role of antioxidants in cancer prevention.

We have already examined the evidence provided by a natural laboratory situation concerning genistein in soy products. With the use of these products over many years in Japan, and their near absence in the American diet, the "experiment" had already been conducted. It was just a matter of collecting the data. And the data has shown that genistein played a substantial role in preventing both breast cancer and prostate cancer.

In a review of over 200 studies, Block et al have reported consistent correlations between low antioxidant intake and higher risks for cancer. By way of example, research has shown that the one fourth of the population with the lowest dietary intake of fruits and vegetables had approximately twice the incidence of cancer as did the one fourth who had the highest intake of fruits and vegetables.

This survey has also found that most studies support the role of vitamin C in preventing non-hormone dependant cancers. The protective effect was such that those with the lowest intake of vitamin C had twice the chance of developing cancer.

In a separate review of the literature, Gershoff has found similar results demonstrating the link between vitamin C and cancer prevention.

In a study conducted by Blot et al, 30,000 Chinese people were given antioxidant supplements of vitamin E, beta-carotene, and selenium. They showed a 13% reduced risk of cancer when compared to those who had received no supplements.

Gridley et al has also reported results showing that vitamin E is able to reduce the risk of oral and pharyngeal cancers.

Selenium, too, has demonstrated its role in cancer prevention. In over 55 studies conducted on lab animals, selenium supplements have produced a reduced incidence of cancer.

Statistical studies on selenium in humans also provide solid results. Where selenium levels are low, the incidence of cancer is high. And vice-versa.

Almost certainly this has to do with the role of selenium as a necessary constituent of glutathione peroxidase, and in turn, the crucial role of glutathione peroxidase in the glutathione cycle.

It is, at this time, virtually certain that free radicals play a significant role in the development in cancer, and that antioxidants, by countering free radicals and free radical activity, play a significant role in the prevention of cancer.

Research over the next decade and beyond will undoubtedly corroborate the positive results already obtained through past research, and supply the details of the mechanisms and biochemistry involved.

Causative Factors

Cancer is the end result of accumulated mutations in the DNA of our cells, which at some point are then able to achieve expression through the biochemical or replicative process of the cell. Most of these mutations occur in the somatic cells of the body, which means that they will be found only in the cells which comprise part of the cancer. Less than 1% of all human cancers have a direct hereditary cause.

Heredity, however, does play a significant role in cancer susceptibility. This is particularly the case in subsets of breast cancer or colorectal cancer.

Attempts to effect cures or prevention through genetic means are at present largely experimental. However, progress is being made on this front, which bodes well for major breakthroughs in the near and intermediate future.

Reflective of the genetic influence is the role particular hormones play in the incidence of cancer. This is certainly the case for endometrial, breast, prostate, and ovarian cancers. In this area, hormone replacement therapy and hormonal regulation will play a role in reducing the susceptibility to cancers of these kinds.

Inflammation, with its attendant high levels of free radicals, has also been linked to cancer. Phagocytes at the site of the inflammation produce large quantities of cytokines and also free radicals and as we have seen, represent a significant causal aspect in carcinogenesis.

In this regard, Weitzman and Gordon have set forth evidence for this conclusion in the following:

a) In cells exposed to activated neutrophils or hydrogen peroxide, DNA strand breaks developed at a rapid rate.

b) Bacteria and mammalian cells experienced mutations when exposed to human neutrophils and macrophages.

c) The cells of mice in tissue culture became malignant when exposed to human neutrophils, or to cellular substance that would generate free radicals.

Research conducted by Dr. Zhuang has demonstrated that the nitric oxide radical produced by macrophages was able to bring about genetic mutation in a gene called the hprt gene. This team has also shown that other infectious agents as well – such as Helicobacter pylori – bring about inflammatory disorders that increase the likelihood of stomach cancer development. Here again, the elevated levels of free radical activity is implicated.

Environment and Lifestyle

The environment brings a number of causative factors to bear in the development of cancer.

Pollution of all kinds, with an emphasis on auto exhaust, is one obvious factor. Some of the environmental factors are often beyond our control in an everyday, practical sense. We cannot all move to the top of Mt. Everest. However, there are some very important factors over which we can affect a large measure of control. And these involve aspects of our lifestyle.

Diet

One of the most significant factors over which we may exercise control involves our diet.

The typical diet followed by our cave ancestors was one to which their bodies had become attuned over many thousands of years, and through this evolutionary process, was a diet to which they were well suited.

Present day humans have virtually the same kind of body as our cave ancestors, but the modern diet – particularly in North America – is radically different in just two generations. For one thing, our present day diet is thought to be much higher in fats, especially as a proportion of our total daily calories. And the proportion of saturated to unsaturated fats is higher as well. Another significant difference is that we take in perhaps a third of the fiber and a quarter of the vitamin C consumed by our ancestors. The PALEO or STONE AGE DIET is worth a discussion here.

There are cancers in which diet plays a highly significant role. These include colorectal cancer, breast cancer, prostate cancer, stomach cancer and lung cancer.

As to the effect of diet on free radical generation, and thence to cancer promotion, the dietary sins also include sins of omission as well as sins of commission. Extremely important is what we do not eat, as well as the unhealthy things we do eat. Invariably we will generate free radicals in the body. But if we are not eating foods that supply the antioxidants to counter free radical activity, we are leaving the door open to cancer.

As we will see in a brief overview of the more prevalent and the more deadly of cancers, by reducing free radical activity in the body, and by following a diet that provides for a healthy supply of antioxidants, we will reduce the risks of some of these cancers.

Smoking

Another huge factor – perhaps the greatest – affecting the risk of cancer lies in the use of tobacco products – especially smoking. It is estimated that smoking is a major factor in about a third of all cancers, and in about a quarter of all coronary heart disease.

Smoking contributes to cancer of the lungs, breast, mouth, larynx, kidney, urinary tract, esophagus, stomach, and pancreas. That doesn't leave much out. And for the die-hards and old timers who are still using products such as chewing tobacco and snuff, the risk for oral cancer is greatly increased.

Notwithstanding that the health risks of smoking are widely known, in 1985 there were nearly 20 million people in the U.S. who smoked heavily. In some high schools today 20% of the teenagers are trying the habit.

Although the detailed biochemistry has not been worked out, there is no doubt that smoking kills. Even the tobacco companies can no longer deny this fact.

Included in the deadly contents of cigarette smoke are carcinogens, free radicals, chemicals that increase free radical activity, and other poisons. C. Borek (Antioxidants and Cancer) estimates that a single puff of cigarette smoke results in more than a billion oxyradicals.

As in the case of an unhealthy diet, smoking too increases the risks for some of the major cancers we will look at and this is of deep concern in developing countries and even some European countries.

Colorectal Cancer

Colorectal cancer is the second most common of the visceral cancers. Heredity is a factor in this form of cancer. An individual is at higher risk if a parent or sibling has had colorectal cancer.

But the most important factor, and one which we can do something about, involves diet. A high fat diet, which is often coupled with obesity, increases the risk for colorectal cancer considerably. This is borne out by statistics which show that men who weigh 40% above average, have a 35% greater likelihood of developing cancer, especially colorectal cancer.

There are also increased risks for colorectal cancer in obese women, but the risk is not as pronounced as for men. However, obesity in women, especially when combined with a high fat diet, also predisposes them to hormone related cancers.

It has been surmised that the presence of salicylic acid (ASA) in fruits and vegetables may explain why vegetarians have less heart disease and less bowel cancer than meat eaters as seen in a Scottish study in the Journal of Clinical Pathology.

Alcohol and smoking also affect the chances of developing colorectal cancer. The risks increase with increased alcohol intake, while smoking is not as significant a factor in this cancer.

Low fiber in the diet, too, adds to the risk of colorectal cancer. High fiber, on the other hand, reduces the risk. It reduces the time fecal matter takes to move through us. This not only shortens the time that potential carcinogens have in which to act on the mucosal lining of the colon, but it also dilutes the stool and reduces the fecal pH, both of which have an inhibitory effect on carcinogenesis.

Antioxidants have shown a definite benefit in preventing a number of prominent cancers, including colorectal cancer. One of the more interesting studies in this regard was conducted by Alabaster et al.

This research examined the effects of beta-carotene in rats on high fat and variable fiber diets. After being on these diets for some time, half the rats were given bi-weekly injections of a carcinogen, azoxymethane, while the other half were given injections of a saline solution.

The results showed that the beta-carotene and the high fiber diets – both together and alone – protected the rats on the high fat diet from cancer. Specifically, the beta-carotene and wheat bran protected them against abnormal crypt foci, and against benign and malignant tumors.

Another study, equally interesting, was conducted by Chinery et al, and it too had striking results. Here vitamin E, along with an antioxidant called pyrrolidinedithiocarbamate, was able to induce apoptosis in colorectal cancer cells by bringing into production in these cells a substance that arrests the cell cycle activity, causing the cell to die off.

There are a number of studies that have shown the benefits of antioxidants in preventing colorectal cancer. Current studies coming forth at present are beginning to show in more detail how these antioxidants work their beneficial effects.

Breast Cancer

Breast cancer, after skin cancer, is the most common cancer in women. And only lung cancer in women causes more deaths.

Heredity is definitely a factor in some breast cancers. Certain genes (such as BRCA 1 or BRCA 2) have been identified as two that bring with them an increased risk for breast cancer. This risk, over a lifetime, is about 85 percent. The presence of these genes in individuals also brings a greater risk for colon and prostate cancer, when compared with the general population.

Obesity and a high fat diet also increase the chances for breast cancer. Exercise, on the other hand, reduces the risk.

We have seen that hormones also play a significant role in the development of breast cancer, especially for women who have never given birth, and for those who have had their first pregnancy after the age of thirty.

It has been shown (Heber et al) that estradiol levels are significantly affected by diet. In this study, 75% of the women that were put on a low fat diet showed a decrease in estradiol levels. The lower estradiol levels would in turn carry a lowered risk for breast cancer.

Other studies indicate that vegetarians, too, in addition to having less body fat, also have lower serum estradiol levels.

Data amassed by Huang et al indicates that where women avoid gaining weight in adulthood, they will be at lower risk for breast cancer after menopause.

Obviously, then, where women avoid a high fat diet and avoid becoming overweight, they will take a giant step in avoiding breast cancer as well.

Current theory holds that metabolites of estradiol may take the form of free radicals. Oxidative stress is also implicated in the metastasis or spreading of cancers as well. It is thought that, under free radical attack, cells undergo a loss of adhesion, which means that they will be more susceptible to being detached, and then able to move to other sites. And this means a spreading of cancer to other parts of the body.

The antioxidants at the top of the list that have shown a protective role in preventing breast cancer are vitamins A, C, and E – the ACEs. Early research indicates that Co Q-10 will have a preventive effect in this area as well.

Prostate Cancer

Prostate cancer, one of the most common cancers, occurs at almost twice the rate of either lung cancer or breast cancer.

Numerous factors are involved in the initiation and progression of prostate cancer from its initial stem cell source. As a result, the incidence and mortality associated with prostate cancer vary considerably throughout the world. We saw this most notably in our examination of genistein, where in Japan, the rate of latent prostate cancer was very similar to that in the U.S., while the rate for the fully developed disease was much lower. In keeping with these figures, the Japanese mortality rate was only one fifth of that for American men.

Although the etiology of prostate cancer has only recently been investigated in detail, already free radical activity is showing up as a factor here too, resulting from the redox recycling of hormones. This is in agreement with data indicating that the hydroxyl radical can bring about DNA alterations (e.g. 8-hydroxyadenine and 8-hydroxyguanine) that have been associated with other malignancies. Research conducted by Malins et al indicates that DNA alterations are a causative factor in transforming normal prostate tissue into a benign prostatic hyperplasia. And looking one step further down the causal chain, this same research group regards the hydroxyl radical as the chief culprit in producing these DNA alterations. We are both members of the Andropause Society and recently traveled to Berlin in 2002 to discuss the latest prostate cancer research.

Risk Factors

Heredity, age, and race all play a part in the incidence of prostate cancer. Carriers of the BRCA 1 and BRCA 2 gene mutations are at higher risk, as are older men and men of

African American descent. Men in Japan and China are much less at risk. Obviously, these are risk factors over which the individual has no control.

Other risk factors over which the individual may exercise considerable control include diet, obesity, sexual activity, infectious agents, and toxic metals.

As for dietary factors, Giovanucci et al reported a risk factor for animal fats and red meat in the diet, while those from dairy products and fish were not particularly significant here. Risks for advanced prostate cancer are also associated with saturated and monosaturated fats.

Antioxidant Assist

Although vitamin A may be of use in the prevention of prostate cancer, this effect has not been conclusively established. Since much of the research here has focused on vitamin A obtained from the diet, and since vitamin A may be obtained from both vegetable and animal sources, clear cut results for vitamin A's preventive effects have not been obtained. That is, the preventive effects of vitamin A obtained from animal sources may have been offset by the promotion of the disease by these animal products.

Lycopene, on the other hand, has shown a definite preventive effect for prostate cancer. Although a carotenoid, lycopene is one of the few that may not be converted to vitamin A. One might be led to speculate that its own idiosyncratic chemical properties in this regard are also the ones that confer its preventive properties with respect to prostate cancer.

Long term studies have shown that vitamin E, particularly in the form of alpha tocopherol, has accompanied a decreased risk for prostate cancer – and a lower mortality rate as well.

Beta-carotene, too, has shown some positive effects in this area, but not as definitively as in the case of lycopene or vitamin E.

Low levels of the enzyme antioxidants have also been implicated in the development of prostate cancer. In studies conducted by Baker et al, it was found that tumors were often accompanied by decreased levels of superoxide dismutase (SOD) and catalase (CAT). Once more referring to our fire extinguisher analogy, where the fire retardant is used up fighting the fire, we might also regard the diminished enzyme levels accompanying prostate cancer as a depletion that occurs in fighting the disease. Further details on the physiological mechanisms involved will undoubtedly be forthcoming with research done in the near future.

In the meantime, maintaining optimal levels of lycopene, vitamin E, selenium and beta-carotene, by means of diet or supplements, is certainly one major way in which males can reduce the risk factor for prostate cancer. Increasing superoxide dismutase and catalase will almost certainly help in this regard as well.

Lung Cancer

Lung cancer is the most common visceral cancer in men. In women, lung cancer is second only to breast cancer as a cause of death. And as more women take up smoking, more of them are now succumbing to the disease. This factor alone offers compelling evidence of smoking as a major cause of lung cancer.

Other risk factors for lung cancer include heredity, where some individuals have a greater predisposition to the disease; diet, where a diet deficient in fruits and vegetables (and the antioxidants they contain) plays a role; and occupation, where exposure to radiation, heavy metals, asbestos, as well as other pollutants have an effect. All have demonstrated a definite causative link to cancer.

But the greatest risk for lung cancer comes from smoking. And just as genistein and tofu provided scientists with a ready made "experiment", so too for smoking. There are huge groups of people who smoke, and others who are similar in virtually all other ways who do not. It was merely a matter of collecting the evidence. And the evidence is overwhelming, uncontestable even, so that now even the cigarette companies no longer deny it: smoking plays a huge causative role in lung cancer.

In the case of women, for example, when few of them smoked, fewer of them developed lung cancer. As more women began to smoke, their rates for lung cancer began to rise.

Other studies show that the rates for lung cancer also rise with the number of cigarettes smoked daily.

Laboratory evidence also weighs in with telling results that implicate smoking – and the countless toxins it brings – in the development of cancer. Many of the constituent substances of cigarette smoke have been shown directly to produce tumors and other cancers in animals

Free Radicals and Lung Cancer

There are countless free radicals generated by one puff on a cigarette. Borek puts the number at "more than a billion oxyradicals in each puff."

Research has shown that smoking has been linked with activated phagocytes, which in turn serve as an additional source of oxidative stress. Some of this research has also demonstrated an increased role played by oxidative stress in smokers.

Dr. Frei has shown that plasma exposed to cigarette smoke in the gas phase induces the formation of lipid hydroperoxides. This has been demonstrated in a number of ways, including the measurement and comparison of serum levels for malondialdehyde in smokers and non-smokers, where higher levels are indicative of lipid peroxidation. Pentene excretion in the alveolar breath of the two groups also corroborates the role of smoking as a factor in the formation of free radicals.

Research has been conducted that also links cigarette smoke to oxidative DNA damage, as indicated by the increased production of the aberrant 8-hydroxydioxy-guanine, along with increased basal DNA damage to circulating lymphocytes.

In addition, other oxidants are produced by the autooxidation of phenolic agents found in cigarette smoke, and these have been shown to bring about an increase in tumor cell invasion and metastasis.

The central message from this mountain of research is clear: smoking – with its host of carcinogens and free radicals – is an incontrovertible cause of lung cancer, and lung cancer is responsible for about a third of all deaths today. To put it another way: smoking is a loaded gun that kills, and one of its deadly bullets takes the form of free radicals.

Antioxidants and Lung Cancer

As surely as free radicals kill through their promotion of lung cancer, antioxidants protect against this deadly disease. This has been shown in study after study.

Fruits and vegetables, with their many and varied antioxidants, have shown in a host of studies that they offer strong protective effects in preventing lung cancer.

The preventive effect conferred by antioxidants has been

especially well documented for vitamin C but only for naturally acquired vitamin C to date. Higher levels of vitamin C supplementation will react with cadmium in cigarette smoke and this combination can be lethal to DNA. Smoking invariably produces reduced levels of vitamin C in smokers. Attendant with these lower levels are higher rates for lung cancer. Where vitamin C levels are increased through higher intake of fruits and vegetables rich in vitamin C, significant protective effects have been reported.

In a study conducted by Halst et al, it was found that those who consumed less than 90 mg of vitamin C daily were about one and a half times more likely to develop lung cancer when compared to those taking 140 mg per day. Particularly striking, those who had a daily vitamin C intake of less than 50 mg per day were more than four times as likely to develop lung cancer as those who took over 50 mg per day.

Other studies have shown that fruits and vegetables rich in vitamins C and E provide protection against lung cancer, as do dietary sources of carotenoids and flavonoids although some studies have shown contradictory results showing little benefit.

Smoking, from the host of free radicals it introduces into the body, provides some of the best evidence we have in illuminating their destructive effects on the body. Here, too, the protective effects conferred by antioxidants have been supported by research.

Certainly, the best thing a smoker can do to avoid cancer is to quit smoking. The second best thing would be to increase the intake of fruits and vegetables, especially those rich in vitamin C, vitamin E and consider other antioxidant supplements.

Since smoking also introduces other carcinogens into the body that can overwork the liver, a smoker would not be remiss in safeguarding this organ by the use of additional supplements that include lipoic acid and glutathione.

The latter two suggestions, of course, comprise a strong prescription for non smokers as well.

In Short

We have looked at some of the major forms of cancer, and certainly at some of the major killers. Although there are many cancers we did not look at, the following summary will almost certainly apply to them as well.

The research shows that free radical activity plays a significant role in the development of cancer. This was underscored in the case of lung cancer, where cigarette smoke, which is laden with free radicals, played a large role in the occurrance of lung cancer.

Antioxidants, conversely, offer a protective effect against cancer, with particular antioxidants showing a more pronounced effect in protecting against particular cancers. This protective effect has been shown for selenium as well. This very likely derives from the fact that selenium is a necessary component of glutathione peroxidase, which is instrumental in combating hydrogen peroxide and the free radicals it may engender.

A wide range of fruits and vegetables, which themselves contain a range of antioxidants, have shown this protective effect. Again, certain fruits and vegetable were found to be more effective against certain cancers.

Animal fats in the diet, and obesity, are other cancer promoters. Reducing these in the diet and increasing fruits and vegetables, then, will offer a number of benefits in reducing the risk for cancer along a number of pathways.

Smoking, too, greatly increases the risk for several

major cancers. Obviously, quitting smoking is the best thing a smoker can do in reducing the attendant risk.

Cancer is like the great white shark of diseases. It strikes fear into the hearts of almost everyone. Like the great white shark it can attack almost any part of the body, with highly destructive, and often deadly, results. Cutting down on fats, avoiding obesity, quitting smoking – all will serve as a shark net to keep the sharks away. But perhaps the most beneficial single thing we can do is to maintain high levels of antioxidants, both through increasing our intake of fruits and vegetables, and our intake of appropriate antioxidant supplements.

Cardiovascular Disease

If cancer is the great white shark of diseases, cardiovascular disease is the octopus. It can occur most dramatically in the heart, or like the tentacles of an octopus, it can spread itself along the veins and arteries, reaching throughout the body.

Heart Attack and Stroke Death Rates

(Death rates, age-adjusted to the European standard population)

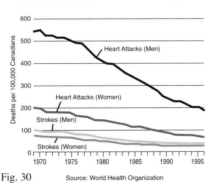

Fig. 30   Source: World Health Organization

And although cancer is the ugliest killer, cardiovascular disease is the most prevalent. It accounts for 40% of all mortality in the western world, and is the leading cause of death in the United States.

The underlying condition that gives rise to much of cardiovascular disease is atherosclerosis. It is atherosclerosis that so often precedes coronary heart disease, stroke, gangrene of the extremities, and it also plays a role in hypertension or high blood pressure.

Atherosclerosis

Atherosclerosis, sometimes referred to as "hardening of the arteries", is characterized by the accumulation of plaque on the inner endothelial layer of artery walls.

Some risk factors for atherosclerosis and subsequent cardiovascular disease include age, sex, and a family history for heart disease. These are factors over which we have no control.

Other factors over which we may exercise some control include smoking, obesity, cholesterol and triglyceride levels, glucose levels and the levels of homocysteine.

There are factors such as blood serum levels of fibrinogen, total leukocyte count, C-reactive protein that matter.

What we will examine are the factors over which we may exercise considerable control, and concerning which, free radical activity is thought to play a large and significant role. Besides free radical activity, and in conjunction with this activity, are factors such as high levels of the bad cholesterol (LDL) and triglycerides, and low levels of the good cholesterol (HDL). These factors are important because it is the oxidizing effect of free radicals on the LDLs that play a determining role in the development of atherosclerosis.

Our discussion of these factors as they effect the development of atherosclerosis will represent an oversimplification of the total picture, but it will give a general idea of how this condition comes about.

Atherosclerotic Lesions: Plaque

The role of free radicals in the development of athero-sclerosis is now generally accepted and there are few scientists in the field today who do not consider it to be an accurate representation of how atherosclerosis gets a foothold and then progresses.

Atherosclerosis involves the buildup of plaque on the inner endothelial lining of artery walls, which occurs as follows.

The blood coursing through our arteries carries a great many things, including varying kinds of cholesterols, which themselves occur at varying levels. Two of the main kinds of cholesterol are the low density lipoproteins (LDLs), and the high density lipoproteins (HDLs). To remember that the LDL is the bad cholesterol, we might think of the L as standing for Lethal. For HDL, the good cholesterol, we might think of the H as standing for Healthy.

Also found in the blood are white blood cells called monocytes, as well as the more differentiated white blood cells called macrophages. The macrophages are large cells that resemble amoebas, and a large part of their job in protecting us consists of ingesting foreign material. The macrophages are also able to ingest unoxidized LDLs, but sensors on their surface limit the amount. These sensors are thrown off by oxidized LDLs, and the macrophages are able to ingest in large quantities becoming foam cells.

And finally, there are varying levels of free radicals being carried along in the blood.

Where lifestyle – such as a high fat diet – and genetic predisposition bring about elevated levels of LDL in the blood, and where lifestyle and environment also bring about high levels of free radicals in the blood, we have the beginnings of a toxic soup – and atherosclerosis.

RISKS FOR 'HARDENING OF THE ARTERIES' (ATHEROSCLEROSIS)

A   Constitutional Factors
   Age
   Sex
   Familial predisposition

B   Acquired and Metabolic Factors
   Increased serum cholesterol
   Increased serum LDL
   Decreased serum HDL
   Increased cholesterol/HDL ratio
   Increased plasma fibrinogen
   Increased plasma Factor VII
   Increased serum homocysteine
   Inflammation (e.g. herpes virus, chlamydia, CMV)
   Increased blood neutrophil count
   Increased serum triglycerides
   Increased hematocrit/viscosity
   Increased C-reactive protein
   Increased tissue plasminogen activator
   Increased iron stores

C   Miscellaneous Factors
   Smoking
   Obesity
   Hypertension
   Diabetes

"The discovery that homocysteine may be a risk factor for atherosclerosis and that levels are affected by both diet and inexpensive vitamins offers potential hope in the area of ischemic heart disease prevention."

Dr. J. Genest, Director of Cardiology, McGill

Oxidative Chain of Events

The superoxide radical is one of the initiators of the oxidative process that ultimately produces atherosclerosis. Many of these radicals result from energy production in the mitochondria, where an errant electron reacts with oxygen. The superoxide radical can itself serve as an oxidative agent, and – as importantly – it can serve as a reactant in the production of hydrogen peroxide. Via the Fenton reaction, hydrogen peroxide can then give rise to the hydroxyl radical, which in turn may initiate lipid peroxidation. The end product of this free radical activity is oxidized LDL.

More recently implicated in the oxidation of lipids is the nitric oxide radical. Combining with the superoxide radical it can produce peroxynitrite. Although not a true free radical, peroxynitrite, it is a highly destructive oxidative agent. Recent research conducted by Buttery et al has shown that an enzyme present in macrophages and other white blood cells, and which is linked to peroxynitrite activity, is present in atherosclerotic lesions.

Once the oxidized LDL is on the scene, the development of atherosclerosis moves forward. Some of the initial research in this area was conducted by Goldstein et al, and it indicates that in the development of atherosclerosis the following chain of events takes place.

Where the oxidation of LDL is minimal it is able to act on the endothelial cells lining the artery. This stimulates these cells to secrete two different substances. One of them promotes the adhesion of monocytes to their cell surface, from which they will afterwards migrate to the subendothelial space. It also promotes the adhesion of T-cells, further adding to the atherosclerotic matrix. The second substance secreted by the endothelial cell promotes the differentiation of monocytes into macrophages. The macrophages further oxidize the LDLs, which then allows the macrophages to increase greatly the quantity of oxidized LDL they are able to ingest. In addition, since the oxidized LDL are somewhat toxic to macrophages, it tends to limit their motility. Eventually the macrophages become bloated and enlarged – they have become transformed into foam cells.

The endothelial cells, too, are susceptible to the oxidative effects of free radicals. Li et al have shown that these oxidative effects are able to bring about apoptosis in endothelial cells. In the case of appoptosis (or cell death) caused by the superoxide radical, the addition of catalase or superoxide dismutase did not have an ameliorating effect. However, where the apoptosis of the endothelial cells was caused by hydrogen peroxide, the apoptosis was reduced. Which is what one might expect since it is on hydrogen peroxide that these two antioxidant enzymes are designed to operate. Apoptosis (cell death) itself accelerates and exacerbates the inflammatory process through the release of toxic cytokines causing even more cell death, rupture, more cytokines, more inflammation and often a clotting cascade leading to disaster.

Another piece of evidence linking free radical activity and endothelial cell death is indicated by the fact that not only do hydroxyl radicals bring about cell death, but the more hydroxyl radicals are involved, the more cell death ensues.

As the foam cells aggregate they attract other entities as well – besides the dead endothelial cells – and they form "colonies". As these colonies grow and spread they give rise to lesions. And with a sufficient buildup of this sort, the arterial wall becomes lined with plaque, characterizing the condition known as atherosclerosis. Ready to undergo the cascade noted above.

It was the evidence showing that oxidized LDL were responsible for the development of foam cells that finally led to the free radical hypothesis that was put forth by Steinberg et al.

Further evidence corroborating the free radical theory, as it pertains to the development of atherosclerosis, derives from a great many studies and experiments, conducted in a number of fields.

In laboratory studies, for instance, oxidized LDL extracted from atherosclerotic lesions is in every way identical with that produced in vitro.

Other research has shown that where there are specific serum levels of antioxidants present, their levels will drop in proportion to the quantities of free radicals they trap.

Work conducted in the field has repeatedly demonstrated that where people have a high dietary intake of antioxidants, they have a lower incidence of heart disease. This inverse relationship has also been shown for plasma levels of antioxidants.

Autoantibodies present that have been generated in response to oxidized LDL are found in atherosclerotic lesions and in the serum of laboratory animals and in humans.

Additional research on lab animals has produced equally corroborative results: in rabbits and primates there was a diminished incidence of atherosclerosis accompanying the increased uptake of antioxidants.

The evidence for the free radical theory of atherosclerosis is now incontrovertible. The evidence for this theory is solid and extensive. But it is still a theory, for scientists are ever cautious, and rightly so. As a further example of this caution, after all these years of corroborative evidence, the theory of relativity is still a theory. An initial study out of Seattle, Washington suggested that specific antioxidants reduced the effectiveness of Statin (anticholesterol) medications. Dr. McLeod and Dr. White have shown in their studies that a proper balanced antioxidant combination actually helps lower LDL cholesterol levels when combined with a Statin drug. In a study in the New England Journal of Medicine (Nov 2001) a simple antioxidant did not confer any benefit for lipid lowering for patients taking a Statin and niacin. In fact there seemed to be best regression of cholesterol plaques in the group taking the Statin and niacin without the simple antioxidant. And the controversy rages on from those that think all antioxidants are not unique in their duties. We, the authors, have noted that conducting trials with just single antioxidants prevent these substances from realizing their potential as antioxidants.

Cholesterol Lowering Drugs and Antioxidants

A Boston, Brigham and Women's Hospital study of effects of vitamin C and vitamin E on progression of transplant-associated arteriosclerosis (Lancet Mar 2002, JC Fang et al) showed that in 40 pravastatin (cholesterol lowering drug) treated patients receiving vitamin C 500 mg and vitamin E 400 IU, each twice daily, that these antioxidants retard the progression of coronary athersclerosis when compared to controls.

An example of data from a study done by Dr. D. McLeod and Dr. P. White showed the effects on lipid profile in October 2001 for patients on lipid lowering agents combined with a more complete antioxidant product after only one week, normalized for no diet and lifestyle change.

Study: Dr. D. McLeod and Dr. P. White

THE CONTINUING STUDY BY DR. MCLEOD AND DR. WHITE SHOWS: ON AVERAGE THE DROP IN TOTAL CHOLESTEROL WITH VITAMIN SUPPLEMENTS WAS 0.20 mmol/L WHICH WAS A 3.4% DECLINE WHICH IS A CONTRADICTION TO RESULTS FROM SEATTLE WHICH USED A LIMITED ANTIOXIDANT PROTOCOL.

ON AVERAGE THE DROP IN LDL CHOLESTEROL WITH ANTIOXIDANT SUPPLEMENTS WAS 0.47 mmol/L AFTER ONE WEEK OF USE. THIS IS A DECLINE OF 12% SHOWING BENEFICIAL EFFECTS OF ANTIOXIDANTS COMBINED WITH STATINS, FOR MORE THAN TWENTY PATIENTS.

Ischemia

Ischemia refers to the interruption or restriction of blood flow to some part of an organ or tissue. A major cause of ischemia is the buildup of plaque in an artery. Where this occurs in the coronary arteries and they become clogged with plaque, a sudden interruption of blood flow may occur, resulting in a heart attack.

Such a buildup of plaque may also occur in the carotid arteries, which supply the brain with blood. When this produces a sudden and severe interruption of blood flow to the brain, the result is stroke. Stroke may also occur when arteries in the brain undergo a similar process.

Ischemic – Reperfusion Injury

The tissue damage that occurs as the result of ischemia is largely due to a shortage of oxygen being delivered to the tissue involved. This alone, where ischemia is protracted and severe, is sufficient to bring about the death of cells but even then takes time. However, a great deal more injury often occurs with the restoration of flood flow to the tissue, and this is called reperfusion injury.

Where ischemic-reperfusion injury occurs, a number of physiological events ensue. As oxygenated blood floods back into the tissue, the cells lose their ability to maintain a proper ionic balance in the membrane. This ultimately results in the cell not being able to produce ATP, which is the fuel source for the cell. A further result, following a lengthy and complex chain of biochemical reactions, is the production of free radicals, particularly the superoxide radical. Accompanying these physiological events is cell damage, cell death, and tissue damage. When this damage occurs in the heart, the muscle tissue often loses much of its contractile function. Where this condition is prolonged and extensive, the result is death.

SUPEROXIDE AND URIC ACID FORMATION WITH OXYGEN

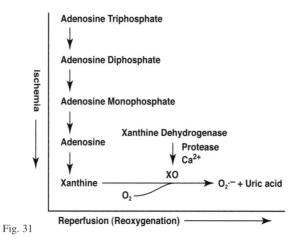

Fig. 31

There are numerous studies which offer strong evidence of free radical involvement in reperfusion injury. Boli et al demonstrated that the production of free radicals continued for up to three hours after reperfusion was initiated. In another experiment, Boli and McCay showed that the administration of superoxide dismutase and catalase not only attenuated the production of free radicals, but was also conducive to an improved cardiac recovery.

Clearly, in experiments of the latter sort, the fact that antioxidants were able to reduce the extent of free radical production and damage in reperfusion injury attests to both the presence and the involvement of free radicals in this injury. And in the case of heart attack and stroke, antioxidants also demonstrate conclusively their effectiveness in limiting free radical damage.

Antioxidants and Cardiovascular Disease

From our discussion of the individual antioxidants, we have already seen the effectiveness of many of them in combating cardiovascular disease, and in ameliorating cardiovascular damage and disease.

Experiments conducted by Esterbauer et al have shown that where vitamin E was used to counter in vitro LDL oxidation, the resistance to oxidation increased with increases of vitamin E. Clearly, this experiment – and numerous others – show how vitamin E is able to reduce LDL in a test tube.

As for in vivo (in the body) experiments, where antioxidants are tested for their effectiveness in living organisms, these too abound. Prasad and Kaltra, in their investigations on the effect of vitamin E in rabbits that were on a high cholesterol diet, demonstrated positive results in vivo. The rabbits receiving vitamin E were much less affected by symptoms and signs of atherogenesis than were the rabbits that had received no vitamin E. Specifically, they had lower blood and tissue levels of malondialdehyde, which is a clear indicator of lipid peroxidation. In addition, microscopically and macroscopically, the rabbits receiving vitamin E showed fewer signs of atherosclerosis in the aorta.

Similar positive results have been obtained for a number of the antioxidants we have examined earlier. Vitamin E, of course, is front and center, being fat soluble and able to permeate lipid membranes lining the arteries. This allows it to get in and counter free radical activity there. Lipoic acid, too, is fat soluble, and plays a strong role in combating cardiovascular disease.

Vitamin C also showed an effectiveness in this area. Although not fat soluble, vitamin C is able to restore vitamin E after it has neutralized a free radical in the lipid medium of the arterial membrane, allowing vitamin E to go back in and do more of the same. This ability to restore vitamin E is also a feature of lipoic acid, making it a double threat to free radicals.

The flavonoids, as well, are very high profile in the battle against heart disease. This was illustrated impressively by means of the French paradox, where people in France were able to offset the effects of widespread cigarette smoking and high fat diets. Research on this front showed that the flavonoids in wine – a beverage widely consumed in France – conferred strong preventive effects for cardiovascular disease. Research from others have shown similar results for varying flavonoids from other sources. Of particular merit are the proanthocyanidins in pycnogenol and grapeseed extract, and quercetin obtained from onion and garlic. Genistein, found in soy products, especially tofu, besides protecting against breast and prostate cancer, also offers protection against cardiovascular disease.

CoQ-10 has been equally impressive in promoting heart health.

The carotenoids, too, have made a contribution, with diets high in a mixture of carotenoids offering protection against cardiovascular disease.

The literature is replete with studies and experiments demonstrating the preventive effects of antioxidants in helping us guard against cardiovascular disease. Rather than catalogue these studies here, we refer the reader to the bibliography-reference section in the book for further material.

Chelation and Cardiovascular Disease

Everyone has now heard about the benefits of chelation. But does everyone believe in the ability of chelation to reverse atherosclerosis? Unlikely is the answer if you interview most of the medical doctors in North America. EDTA (ethylenediamine tetraacetic acid) is the cornerstone of chelation therapy in our country and this compound has been available to us for decades as a method of binding metals in our body like lead, mercury, arsenic and cadmium to allow them to be eliminated safely. As we now know many transition metals like copper and iron can be harmful in excess quantities and pesticides like dioxin can act as terrible free radicals stealing electrons from important molecules in our body. Chelation therapy was the brainchild of Dr. Carlos Lamar in the 1960's and has literally hundreds of thousands of anecdotal successes to its credit. But what about the studies to back it up say the physicians? Intravenous EDTA should not be confined to just the use of treating atherosclerosis say many of its proponents but should be used when ever antioxidants may be necessary to help alleviate disease. Oral chelation or suppository chelation may be the future answer for most as oral EDTA is absorbed (18%) as shown in the literature with even better absorption rectally. Many improved oral chelators will be available in the future and hopefully studies will be double blind to prove the effectiveness of the whole idea of "chelation". EDTA can be toxic if used inappropriately since it can cause kidney problems, sodium loads, low calcium and even low blood sugar. Guldager et al did not find benefit in treadmill testing of patients with narrowed leg arteries when comparing placebo to EDTA treated patients. A study of cardiologist's patients from Calgary, Alberta (JAMA 2002, Knudtson et al) showed that 84 ischemic heart disease patients did not improve with exercise capacity or quality of life after only 27 weeks of chelation treatment when compared to controls of placebo treatment. The study was flawed, the numbers were small and more treatments were needed say the chelators. This recent Canadian study of coronary patients treated with EDTA was presented to the American College of Cardiology. Many say that these results are biased since cardiologists have a vested interest in mechanical methods of cleaning arteries. It is surely accepted that free radicals, metals and toxins play a part in disease and super antioxidants will be necessary to battle many of these damaging particles. The logic is that chelation whether it be oral, by suppository or by intravenous will be important in the future as it is refined and guidelines for its use are explored with proper studies. But chelation is certainly not the panacea for illness but is just another brushstroke that makes up the total picture of the health puzzle.

A Summing Up

Cardiovascular disease is the number one killer in America today. In no other area of illness and disease has the record shown more clearly the link between free radicals and cardiovascular disease.

In this area a great deal of the biochemistry has already been worked out, with more data coming forward daily.

Almost as conclusively, the protective effects of numerous antioxidants against cardiovascular disease has also been demonstrated. Thus far there may be less detail worked out for the physiological mechanisms involved, but the big picture leaves no doubt: many of the antioxidants have the power to prevent and ameliorate cardiovascular disease. And the detailed biochemistry, as it comes forward from current research, invariably tends to corroborate this conclusion, putting more and more of the detail in place. It is just a matter of time until the all the detail is worked out and we have the full picture before us. Unfortunately some studies have come up with controversial conclusions regarding antioxidant protection. The "Hope Study" did not show protection from cardiovascular events like heart attack and stroke with vitamin E but it showed there was a lower incidence of cancer in the vitamin E group. Vitamin E alone does not appear to confer a benefit on the heart as an antioxidant (and we would not expect it to alone) and thus the result of the study. Vitamins are essential to life and can never be contraindicated in patients in proper dosages.

Diabetes

We will examine diabetes at this point in the book following the chapters on cancer and cardiovascular disease for two reasons: diabetes – like cancer and heart disease – is especially affected by lifestyle, where obesity is a major indictable offender; and secondly, diabetes in North America is presently occurring in epidemic proportions. This is especially so for one form of the disease.

There are two types of diabetes mellitus. Type 1 diabetes, which is also called insulin dependent diabetes mellitus, or juvenile onset diabetes; and Type 2 diabetes mellitus, which is also called non-insulin dependent diabetes mellitus, or adult onset diabetes. Both are characterized by an inability to properly metabolize carbohydrate, fat, and protein, with poor sugar metabolism predominating. In diabetics, not enough of the glucose in the blood can get into the body's cells for use in energy production. Diabetes with its extra free radical production speeds up the aging process and is of particular interest to Dr. White and Dr. McLeod.

Type 1 and Type 2

In Type 1 diabetes, the islets of Langerhans in the pancreas, which normally supply the body with insulin, secrete almost none. Since a principal function of insulin is to facilitate the entry of blood glucose into the cell, where there is little insulin being produced by the body, there is little of it to assist sugar molecules into the cell. Which means that much of the sugar stays in the blood, bringing on further complications. Associated with this form of diabetes are muscle and fat loss, and very high levels of glucose in the blood. Type 1 diabetes, as its alternate name suggests, manifests itself early in life.

Type 2 diabetes, on the other hand, tends to occur later

in life. It is often preceded by or accompanied by obesity, which is a strong causative factor in the disease, and which itself is epidemic in America today. In some Type 2 diabetics, initially the body can produce enough insulin, but there is a resistance to it so it is no longer efficient at escorting sugar across the cellular membrane and into the cell. As a result, sugar metabolism is compromised.

Besides obesity, another major factor affecting the development of diabetes – and the secondary conditions that the disease brings on – is the role of free radicals, and their destructive effects.

Free Radicals and Diabetes

There is a considerable body of evidence indicating that free radical activity plays a significant role in the etiology of the disease. There is even more evidence showing free radical complicity in the secondary conditions that result from the disease.

In the past it was a debatable point as to whether free radicals were the result of the disease, or were part of its cause. Recent evidence is now leaning in support of the latter conclusion: free radicals do appear to play a causative role – at least partially – in the occurrence of diabetes.

Much of the initial research implicating free radicals in the development of diabetes was based on the effects of two drugs known as alloxam and streptozotocin, or STZ. These two drugs can produce Type 1 diabetes in animals by destroying the islets of Langerhans in the pancreas of these animals. In addition, alloxan goes through a number of reactions which ultimately give rise to hydrogen peroxide, and as well, the superoxide and hydroxyl radicals.

Research has also shown that the oxidative damage from alloxan is abetted by its ability to first join with sulfur based antioxidants and vitamin C, thereby depleting their supply and their ability to exercise damage control. It has also been shown that low levels of glutathione peroxidase also allows alloxan to more readily inflict damage. Further, in vitro and in vivo studies show that oxidative damage caused by alloxan can be inhibited by hydroxyl radical scavengers, metal chelating compounds, and fat soluble antioxidants.

Slonim and others were able to attenuate the development of diabetes in mice with the use of vitamin E. Cowden et al were able to prevent the development of alloxan-induced diabetes by administering the synthetic free radical scavenger called butylated hydroxyanisole. As further evidence still, it has been shown that adding exogenous superoxide dismutase and catalase brings a further reduction in damage done by alloxan.

The detailed biochemistry in the foregoing studies tends, cumulatively, to suggest that the alloxan-induced diabetes does proceed from oxidative action.

There is also evidence indicating that oxidative processes are involved in STZ-induced diabetes. Here, nitric oxide, reacting with the superoxide radical to produce peroxynitrite, also appears to be part of the oxidative process.

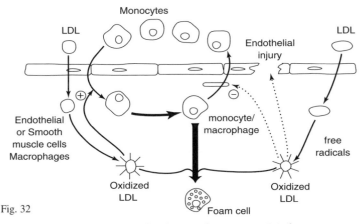

Fig. 32

Development of Atherosclerosis in Diabetes

In STZ-induced diabetes in rats, research has shown that the rate of induced disease was decreased by the use of vitamin E, and this result was dose dependent. Which means that the higher amounts of vitamin E administered, the higher were the reduction rates.

As for secondary conditions brought about by diabetes, there is an even greater indictment of free radicals in their development. And in combating some of these conditions there is heartening evidence that the administration of antioxidants can be of great benefit.

Secondary Conditions

Concomitant with elevated levels of free radical activity are the advanced glycation end products, or AGEs. Simply put, AGEs come into being when certain proteins are conjoined with certain sugars. And the process is mediated by oxidative stress.

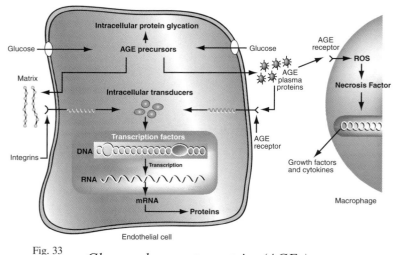

Fig. 33

Glucose damage to proteins (AGEs)

Where the formation of AGEs proceeds along a particular biochemical pathway, they bring about a complex cross-linked protein structure. This cross-linkage is responsible for a number of problems, including a loss of elasticity in connective tissue, which can affect the skin as well as various internal organs. The effect of AGEs may even manifest themselves at the cellular level by decreasing the elasticity of the extracellular compartment, impeding the inflow and outflow of nutrients and waste products respectively.

Some of the chemistry involved in the production AGEs has also shown links to atherogenesis in diabetics. Here the AGEs in arteries can trap LDL and accelerate the development of atherosclerosis. From recent research in this area, AGEs are now thought to be a major factor in the pathogenesis of various complications in diabetics.

Oxidative stress also plays a role in peripheral neuropathy in diabetics. In the peripheral nerves, diabetics exhibit lower levels of antioxidant enzyme activity than do non-diabetics.

Diabetic retinopathy and diabetic nephropathy are two other secondary conditions where oxidative stress plays a role as well.

In preventing diabetes, and in slowing the development of secondary conditions associated with diabetes, and in ameliorating the symptoms of these conditions, antioxidant treatment is of great value.

Antioxidant Relief

Depressed levels of vitamin C are invariably found in diabetics, even where there is a normal quantity of vitamin C in the diet. Therefore, vitamin C supplements are definitely in order. Vitamin C resembles in structure, the glucose molecule, and even is transported into the cell via insulin. There is some competition between sugar (glucose) and vitamin C for this transport. You can see that if the glucose levels are high, then the transport system is overwhelmed by sugar and the vitamin C doesn't get into the cells. Our antioxidant team approach will suffer.

Also, in sugar metabolism a by-product called sorbitol is formed. It, too, is thought to play a role in diabetic complications by raising levels of aldose reductase. In the non-diabetic sorbitol is broken down, so that the levels of sorbitol do not rise out of control. The sorbitol levels in the diabetic, however, tend to be elevated. Here too vitamin C is of value, since it helps in keeping sorbitol levels under control.

Vitamin E has also demonstrated strong benefit to the diabetic. Where atherosclerosis and other cardiovascular problems often result from diabetes, vitamin E helps by preventing or at least diminishing the severity of these diseases.

Lipoic acid, too, confers a definite benefit in controlling the symptoms and complications of diabetes, particularly in the case of peripheral neuropathy. In this painful and distressing condition in the peripheral nerves, research has shown that lipoic acid is able to reduce nerve damage, and – very importantly – to provide a merciful reduction in the excruciating pain that can accompany this condition.

In general, since diabetes is invariably accompanied by high levels of free radical activity, maintaining a wide variety of antioxidant intake via fruits and vegetables, as well as supplements that provide for a range of antioxidants, is highly recommended for an optimal health. The remarkable thiazolidinediones such as Avandia and Actos make us more sensitive to insulin allowing better glucose control in diabetics.

Lung Disease

We have seen that oxygen, besides being necessary for life, can also be injurious to life. And inhaled at sufficient concentrations, it can be deadly. And since we take in oxygen via the lungs, they are the organs directly in the line of fire of the oxygen bullets.

The injurious effects of oxygen on the lungs have been demonstrated over the decades. Evidence of this damaging effect began with Lorrain Smith, a Belfast physician who demonstrated that rodents exposed to high concentrations of oxygen developed pulmonary congestion, and symptoms resembling pneumonia.

Experiments of this sort continued over the years, and in 1967 the research of Nash et al demonstrated conclusively the toxic effects of oxygen on humans. This research showed that the higher the concentration of oxygen inhaled preceding death – and the more of it – the greater the pulmonary damage that was done. The pulmonary changes were detectable both macroscopically and microscopically.

Throughout these decades of research, the implication of free radical activity as destructive agents that bring about disease has become more and more obvious. And since the lungs are the organs by which we take in oxygen from the atmosphere – and any pollutants it contains – they are particularly vulnerable.

Lung Cancer, Oxygen, and Free Radicals

In examining lung cancer we saw the pronounced effects of free radicals on the lungs, especially as derived from cigarette smoke. Other major sources of free radicals impacting on the lungs were those from air pollution and pollutants at the workplace.

Numerous studies have shown that free radicals play an important part in oxygen toxicity. For example, research indicates that increased oxygen tension brings about higher concentrations of both the superoxide radical and hydrogen peroxide. Also, where oxygen was supplied at 85% concentration, malonaldehyde (a distinctive marker for lipid peroxidation) reached levels that were 2.5 times that of normal. (Freeman et al).

Other research has demonstrated that where rats are subjected to higher oxygen levels, they can develop a certain tolerance to it. In these rats, there has also been reported an increase in the activity for levels of the antioxidant enzymes such as superoxide dismutase (SOD), glutathione peroxidase (GPx), glutathione reductase (GRed), and in glutathione as well. The obvious conclusion here is that in making the adjustment to the higher oxygen levels, the cells in the rats increased the production of these antioxidant enzymes by way of defending against the increased oxygen and its damaging effects.

Lung Diseases

Just as free radical activity played a significant role in the development of lung cancer, free radicals are also a factor in a number of other forms of lung disease.

- Adult respiratory distress syndrome (ARDS)
- Asbestosis, silicosis
- Asthma
- Preterm respiratory distress syndrome/bronchopulmonary dysplasia
- Cancer
- Chronic obstructive pulmonary disease
- Emphysema
- Pneumonia
- Pulmonary edema (shock, sepsis, pneumonia)
- Others (idiopathic interstitial fibrosis, immune complexes, etc.)

In premature babies that are often maintained on a higher than normal (hyperoxic) concentration of oxygen, free radical damage to lung tissue has been reported. Complicit in this damage are underdeveloped antioxidant defences.

In adult respiratory distress syndrome (ARDS), free radicals have also been strongly implicated. Some of the free radical activity has been attributed to activated neutrophils. In these neutrophils, which are immune cells, free radicals are often used as a matter of course in defending against foreign substances and foreign invaders. Several studies, including those done by Kelly et al have shown that through stimulation by specific antibodies, neutrophils then greatly increase their production rate of free radicals, and in so doing, they too contribute to the oxidative stress and the destructive inflammation.

Other studies indicate that activated neutrophils, through their ability to bring about increased hypochlorous acid levels, were able to alter pulmonary circulation.

Studies conducted by Leff et al demonstrated that intratracheal administration of interleukin-1 alpha produced the following: an influx of neutrophils into the lungs; an increase in the level of spent glutathione (GSSG); an increase in hydrogen peroxide; and defects in the cellular structure of the lungs accompanied this influx.

Emphysema

For emphysema as well, there is almost overwhelming evidence implicating free radicals as a causative factor. In this disease the evidence also suggests that proteases are involved. Proteases are enzymes that dissolve protein, and are kept in check by protease inhibitors.

The research indicates that free radicals, from cigarette smoke and air pollution, besides the damage they do along other physiological pathways, also increase the action of proteolitic enzymes. This is particularly so in the case of neutrophil proteases. (We have seen that these neutrophils tend to gather in higher numbers in the lungs in response to oxidative stress.) Here the oxidation of the protease inhibitor alters its structure to that of a much less active and much less effective form. This gives the proteases the upper hand, allowing them to proceed in the destruction of protein. The end result of this prolonged activity is emphysema.

Chronic Obstructive Pulmonary Disease

Free radicals have also been found to play a part in chronic obstructive pulmonary disease (COPD). As in the case of emphysema, the role of cigarette smoke – with its huge numbers of free radicals – has figured largely in the research into COPD.

The heavy load of free radicals in cigarette smoke correlates closely with the higher numbers of macrophages and neutrophils in the alveoli in the lungs of smokers. In turn, the macrophages and neutrophils add further to the quantity of free radicals present.

In the research, one measurement indicative of antioxidant function is the plasma Trolox equivalent antioxidant capacity, or TEAC. Findings reported by Rahman et al indicate that in healthy chronic smokers, the plasma TEAC was significantly reduced. At the same time, markers for increased lipid peroxidation were evident. The lowered plasma TEAC numbers were also accompanied by greater quantities of the superoxide radicals released by activated neutrophils.

Other recent research has used the levels of exhaled hydrogen peroxide as a measure of free radical activity. In one study, these levels were compared for three groups: unstable COPD patients; stable COPD patients; and a control group. Here the hydrogen peroxide levels were lowest for the control group, higher for the stable COPD patients, and highest for the unstable COPD patients. At present, Dr. Bill

Arkinstall, respirologist, Canada is investigating the benefits of Human Growth Hormone on a group of COPD patients.

Asthma

Asthma, now recognized as an inflammatory disorder of the airways, has been occurring in ever increasing numbers over recent years. From 1980 to 1987, the cases of asthma reported by physicians in those under twenty years of age increased by 43 percent. As in the case for inflammatory disease in general, free radical activity in asthma is regarded as a strong causative factor.

A number of studies, including those by Owen et al, have found various indicators for higher levels of lipid peroxidation in asthma patients when compared with non-asthmatics. As well, asthma patients have shown lower plasma TEAC figures.

Research has also implicated nitric oxide as a factor in the pathogenesis of asthma.

For asthmatics, higher counts for macrophages and neutrophils have also been found. Which will account – at least in part – for higher levels of free radical activity in asthmatics.

As for other pulmonary disorders, cigarette smoke and other forms of air pollution is complicit in the development of asthma.

Antioxidants and Lung Disease

Dr. Stephen van Eeden, respirologist, writes in the Journal of the American College of Cardiology, that typical city air pollution from cars is a risk factor for stroke and heart attack. Rabbits were exposed to typical pollutants and compared to controls. Inflammation and constriction of blood vessels occurred in rabbits and human subjects as published in Circulation journal this year. Smoke and particulate matter causes vascular changes.

Smoking goes hand in hand with so much of lung disease. Depressed levels of certain antioxidants tend to go hand in hand with both. The research indicates that antioxidants can be of benefit in the treatment of many lung diseases.

In hyperoxia experiments, where lab animals were exposed to high oxygen concentrations, toxicity and tissue damage from free radical activity occurs. However, treatment with antioxidants in numerous experiments have been shown to produce a sizeable reduction in the toxicity and damage. Some of the antioxidants that have produced such results are: vitamins C and E, N-acetyl-cysteine (NAC), selenium, zinc, allopurinol, and dimethyl sulfoxide.

Research on ARDS has shown that treatment with antioxidants may be particularly helpful here. Leff et al found that the use of NAC in ARDS patients diminished cell damage, decreased the "spent" glutathione (GSSG) levels, and decreased the levels of hydrogen peroxide in the exhaled breath – all of which is indicative of a reduction in free radical activity and injury.

Other free radical scavengers have also shown beneficial effects in ARDS. These include a synthetic compound that exhibits SOD-like properties.

In emphysema, antioxidants have demonstrated a beneficial role as well.

Two measures of lung capacity and lung health are: the forced expiratory volume (FEV), and the forced vital expiratory capacity (FVC). Britton et al have shown a strong correlation to exist between the dietary intake of antioxidants and lung capacity. Those who had a greater intake of vitamins C and E had much better scores for both the FEV and the FVC tests.

In asthma, too, there is ample evidence that antioxidants can offer an improvement. Studies have shown that a diet low in vitamin C increases the risk for asthma. And those with asthma who have a lower dietary intake of vitamin C, also have more severe symptoms of the disease, especially the wheezing. In a survey done on asthma studies, it was found that most studies showed that supplementation with vitamin C will bring about significant improvement in those with this disease.

Liver Disease

There is an impressive and growing body of work implicating free radicals as an important causative factor in liver disease. Some of the research has involved the use of particular chemicals, chemicals which were known to bring about oxidative stress. A considerable part of the research has focused on a variety of liver disorders, where again the known effect of which is increased free radical activity.

The Research

Some of the early research investigated the effects of a chemical called carbon tetrachloride on the livers in rats. Through a particular biochemical pathway this substance produced the trichlormethyl peroxyl radical, which in turn initiated lipid peroxidation.

From this early work, and other research since, the effects of this free radical activity in the liver include the following: a depletion of sulfur based antioxidants such as glutathione; protein oxidation; and a disruption of the intracellular calcium balance.

We have seen that one of the indicators for genetic damage was DNA fragmentation. Also, where the normal pairings of the "steps" between the two strands of the DNA double helix was altered, one of the "mutated steps" that brought about this altering was 8-hydroxy-2-deoxyguanosine. Both of these indicators have been found in livers where free radical activity has been heightened, providing strong evidence of DNA damage.

Along with signs of DNA damage are signs of lipid peroxidation. Malonaldehyde has been found, as well as other substances such as 4 hydroxy-2-nonenal, whose presence is a definite marker for lipid peroxidation.

Hartley et al conducted experiments which demonstrated that induced oxidative stress diminished liver viability, and at the same time reduced glutathione levels. In addition, there were increases in the protein carbonyl levels, which is an indicator of protein oxidation – and aging.

In experiments conducted by Kanecko et al, further evidence has been adduced supporting the conclusion that oxidative stress brings about DNA damage. Here again, where oxidative stress was induced, the indicator found was 8-hydroxy-2-deoxyguanosine. Other research by this group, employed both dietary restrictions and vitamin E depletion. These conditions produced decreased glutathione levels in the mitochondria of the liver, and increased levels of lipid peroxidation.

Alcohol

It has long been known that an overuse of alcohol harms the liver. It has only more recently become known that much of this damage comes as the result of the increased oxidative stress that excessive alcohol consumption induces. Here again, there is an impressive and growing body of evidence supporting this conclusion. The following is a dicussion of the mechanism of this followed by paradoxical research about alcohol.

The oxidative stress, taking the form of lipid peroxidation, comes about in one of two ways – by enhancing the production of free radicals, or by depleting the liver of its endogenous antioxidants. Here too, indicators of increased lipid peroxidation in high alcohol users have been found. Some of these include: malonaldehyde; pentane in the exhaled breath; conjugated dienes; and 4-hydroxynonenal. All are indicators of lipid peroxidation, and these indicators have been found repeatedly at elevated levels in alcoholics.

There are a number of biochemical pathways by which alcohol (ethanol) may produce oxidative stress. Two of the resultant oxidants are the superoxide radical and hydrogen peroxide. Other by-products of these pathways include acetaldehyde, which works to deplete the availability of glutathione in the liver, reducing the liver's defence against oxidative damage.

Cahil et al report that some of the effects of alcohol-induced oxidative stress include changes in the mitochondrial DNA. In their research, rats were put on a diet that included high alcohol consumption. These rats showed a 21% increase in the levels of 8-hydroxy-2-deoxyguanosine indicating DNA damage..

Other studies show that the oxidative stress induced by excessive alcohol consumption can bring on a number of damaging conditions, including an impaired permeability of the mitochondrial membrane in liver cells, as well as depleted glutathione levels, and even an increased rate of apoptosis.

Research into a variety of liver disorders also indicates that where the liver is affected by infection, heavy metals, etc., it is also afflicted by increased oxidative stress.

In one interesting experiment, a group of rats were exposed to cigarette smoke over a period of 90 days. At the end of this time the rats were found to exhibit the various markers for increased lipid peroxidation: malonaldehyde, conjugated dienes, hydroperoxides, and free fatty acids. Concomitant with the increased free radical activity were depressed levels for various antioxidants such as vitamins C and E, as well as superoxide dismutase and catalase.

Rats in which fatty livers had been induced also manifested higher levels of lipid peroxidation, particularly when subjected to acute alcohol intoxication.

Accompanying many liver disorders is a condition called fibrogenesis. This condition is characterized by increased amounts of connective tissue that is undergoing a fibrotic degeneration. Here, too, numerous researchers – beginning with Chojkier et al in 1989 – have provided evidence indicating a strong link between fibrogenesis and lipid peroxidation.

Interestingly, a city of Bapin, China, harbors some of our healthiest longevity residents. The secret here is reputed to be daily drinking of rice wine, snake wine and a soup made from cannabis seeds. The Old Age Science Research Centre in Beijing says that the 4,500 foot elevation and clean river water helps keep this 300,000 population, older and healthier than all other comparison communities. Maybe they just don't worry, they stay happy.

Alcohol: The Supreme Paradox

As the human race continues its headlong dash into the twenty-first century, along with the clarion cry of evidence-based action, perhaps it is time to reflect on what many of our ancestors knew (particularly the Scots, of course) with regards to alcohol. Alcohol, far from being the bete noir, painted by so many in the last century, it is now being viewed in a new light as results are published from highly respected scientific institutions.

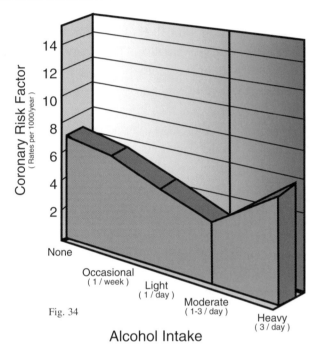

Fig. 34

We call this "The Supreme Paradox" as in a significant number of patients or individuals who chronically consume alcohol in significant amounts there is associated liver damage that includes fatty liver, alcoholic hepatitis and ultimately hepatic cirrhosis. However, paradoxically there is an equally large group of individuals in whom moderate chronic alcohol ingestion fails to produce cirrhosis or any other hepatic disorder. Not only that, but it bestows upon them health benefits. The reasons for this are associated with variations in the cellular chemistry of the individual which is essentially genetically determined whereby the relative toxicity of alcohol varies from one individual to another. Certainly abundant evidence has accumulated over the past thirty years that heavy chronic alcohol intake can result in increased oxidative stress in the liver, and not just in the liver but in many target tissues. DiLucio in 1966 in a very elegant scientific paper showed that alcohol-induced fatty liver problems could be at least in part prevented by certain anti-oxidants. What he said was that liver damage was caused by alcohol-mediated lipid peroxidation. The chemistry is quite complex and we will not go into it here but others have shown that liver and serum lipid peroxide levels in alcoholics with biopsy proven fatty livers are higher than those in non-alcoholics even though the latter may be drinking moderately. Doctors now warn their patients about alcohol when liver enzymes are elevated in blood tests but perhaps the future will give us the test that will predict the optimal amount of alcohol that will be best for each of us.

Alcohol seems to induce increased activities of catalase, glutathione reductase, glutathione S-transferase and glutathione and again somewhat paradoxically, reduce the activities of glutathione peroxidase and glucose-6-phosphate dehydrogenase. In studies, it has been suggested that the enhancement of the liver anti-oxidant system in chronically alcohol-fed but otherwise well-nourished rats and humans, might be a protective mechanism against alcohol-induced oxidative stress. Interesting! Can we therefore surmise, then, those in which the anti-oxidant levels do not increase are the ones that are going to run into trouble and those where there is a good increase in the anti-oxidants will maintain a healthy liver?

It is not just the liver that is subject to alcohol-induced oxidative damage. It is other organs that suffer as well, particularly the gastrointestinal tract and brain. And again, protective mechanisms with anti-oxidants have been demonstrated in many studies.

As already shown, excessive alcohol consumption has been associated with increased cancer rates particularly at the level of six or more drinks per day. This is felt to be again due to the oxidative stress that alcohol puts on the cell and particularly the cellular DNA where DNA is a natural target for free radical attack. Significant increases in the levels of abnormal DNA bases causing fragmentation of both mitochondrial and nuclear DNA have been demonstrated in the cells of heavy alcohol users.

So... where does all this lead us? It is certainly interesting that more than moderate alcohol consumption can lead to significant and serious problems but the paradox is that light to moderate alcohol consumption has been shown to be significantly protective when it comes to the risk of coronary artery disease, myocardial infarction and strokes. In many of us, moderate alcohol consumption does not appear to cause an imbalance of the liver enzymes or the intracellular oxidative reactions and may be beneficial and helps to explain the French paradox which we mentioned earlier in the book, not just the paradox of alcohol itself.

The paradox of alcohol itself is how can something in moderate amounts be so beneficial when it can be so damaging in greater amounts to some of us. The line can be fairly fine.

The key word for alcohol use is moderation. It must also be made clear that there are contra-indications for alcohol consumption and among these are pregnancy, women at high risk of breast cancer, a history of alcoholism, uncontrolled hypertension and certain concomitant medications. You should always check with your health care professional when taking any medication or nutriceutical with alcohol. Having said all that, in a recent report, "Beer, Wine and Spirits: Advising Patients about Moderate Drinking", a leading panel of cardiologists agreed that "again, the best evidence suggests any alcoholic beverage – beer, wine or spirits – used in moderation reduces the risks of heart disease and ischemic stroke, and physicians can counsel patients accordingly, recognizing that alcohol is contra-indicated for some individuals".

So again.... The good news is that observational studies of large cohorts show mild to moderate alcohol consumption is associated with a relative coronary artery disease risk reduction of 30 – 50 %, a similar risk reduction for acute myocardial infarction (heart attack) and angina (chest pain from narrowing of the coronary arteries), as well as a 24% risk reduction for all strokes, mostly due to ischemic events.

There is still more good news. Reported data explains how alcohol in beer and other drinks raises levels of HDL cholesterol and decreases the activity of cholesterol ester-transfer protein (CETP) preventing the transfer of HDL molecules to LDL (low density lipoprotein) or VLDL (very low density lipoprotein) cholesterol. There is also a reduction in the activation of those little sticky mini blood corpuscles called platelets, and therefore clotting factor activity is less so the blood will not clot as easily inside the arteries. Fibrinogen (another factor in blood clotting) levels are also lowered. A study from the Lancet Jan 26, 2002 showed that 1-3 drinks of alcohol per day may lower the risk for Alzheimer's and vascular dementia in older people.

So, what is moderate alcohol consumption? We consider this to be no more than one to two drinks per day for the average woman, and no more than two to three drinks per day for the average male. People who are significantly smaller than average should drink less, those who are larger should not drink more.

What is a standard drink, you might ask. A standard drink has now been defined as equal to one twelve ounce (375 ml) 5% alcohol beer, or a five ounce (156 ml) glass of wine 10 – 13% alcohol, or 1.5 ounces (47 ml) of 40% alcohol spirits. So now you know. Again we caution those who should not be drinking alcohol in any form. Otherwise, bon vivre as we raise our glasses to a long and healthy life and most of us feel no guilt with our glass of wine, pint of beer or dram of Scotch on daily occasions.

Antioxidant Assist

Since many disorders of the liver are at least in part the result of free radical activity, for many of these disorders antioxidants are of considerable benefit, either by way of prevention or amelioration.

Vitamin E supplementation, for example, has been shown to prevent fibrogenesis in patients with hepatitis C.

In the rats with fatty livers, a synthetic free radical scavenger produced a significant reduction in lipid peroxidation, as measured in this case by thiobarbituric acid-reactive substances (TBARS), and triglycerides. This suggests that quite likely other antioxidants such as vitamin E and alpha lipoic acid will show this kind of effect here, too.

The activation of certain specialized cells in the liver known as Kupffer cells has also been implicated in the pathogenesis of a number of liver disorders. Research by Bellazzo et al has shown that N-acetylcysteine (NAC) – a primary contributor to glutathione – and vitamin E were both able to inhibit this activation of Kupffer cells. The researchers suggest that not only was this indicative of the antioxidant being effective in reducing free radical activity, but that the antioxidants may also be fortifying the liver itself in its fight against oxidative stress and endotoxins.

Certainly in this regard, Dr. Berkson has shown that alpha lipoic acid is of immense benefit where the liver is under attack from toxins and free radicals resulting from mushroom poisoning.

In a comprehensive study, Chen and Tappel investigated the effects of multiple antioxidants in preventing lipid peroxidation. Using a range of diets that were either deficient in, or were supplemented with, a variety of antioxidant combinations, they obtained the following conclusive results. Particular antioxidants were shown to protect against lipid peroxidation, and in certain combinations their protective effects were much greater. Thus, in diets where two or three of the antioxidants were demonstrably effective, the most effective of all was the diet that was supplemented with vitamins C and E, selenium, Trolox, NAC, CoQ-10, various catechins, beta-carotene, and zeaxanthin, taken altogether. This experiment demonstrates most emphatically a point we cannot emphasize too often: When it comes to antioxidants, variety is the spice of life.

In Summary

The liver is a sort of clearing house for all manner of toxins and wastes. It is probably the most complex organ – physiologically – that we possess. Because it deals with so much of the garbage that comes into the body, it is susceptible to numerous diseases.

Many of the toxins in the liver have the effect of increasing free radical activity, which plays a considerable part in the development of many liver diseases. Conversely, many of the antioxidants offer protection against this free radical activity, and in providing an ameliorating effect where some of these diseases are already in progress.

Some of the most effective antioxidants where the liver is concerned are lipoic acid, glutathione, glutathione constituents such as NAC, and vitamin E.

Besides working as a superb antioxidant in the liver, glutathione also has the ability to join with toxic heavy metals and carry them off to be excreted in the urine. In this regard glutathione is something like a "bouncer" or chelator, ridding the liver of undesirables.

When it comes to liver protection, the above antioxidants are a must. We recommend alpha lipoic acid supplement before challenging your liver with alcohol. Milk thistle or silymarin is also added for extra liver antioxidant protection.

Kidney Disease

There is solid evidence that free radicals play an important role in the pathogenesis of many kidney diseases. In general, this comes about where free radical activity is able to overcome the antioxidant defences in the kidney and bring on cellular damage.

We see evidence of this as part of the aging effect on the kidneys. In research conducted by de la Asuncion, Millan, Pla, et al, for instance, the ratio of "spent" or reduced glutathione (GSSG) to potent glutathione (GSH) in aging rats compared to young rats was telling – an amazing 540 percent! Which means that there was a great deal less of the glutathione in its effective form, and a great deal more of it in its "used up" form in the kidney. (For the liver and brain the ratios were 600% and 320% respectively.) Obviously the old rats were no longer able to maintain an efficient antioxidant defense system – particularly as we see here in the case of glutathione. And this growing inefficiency shows up in the numbers for humans, where more of the older people become afflicted with serious kidney disease than do young people.

Another indicator of the link between kidney disease and free radical activity is found in a study done by Rajbala. Here, children with a kidney condition called nephrotic syndrome had lower levels of superoxide dismutase (SOD) activity, and lower levels of vitamins C and E. Concomitant with that were higher levels of malonaldehyde, an indicator of oxidative stress.

Free Radicals and the Glomerulus

The kidneys, like the liver, cleanse waste from the body. They do this by filtering out metabolic and other wastes through microscopic tubules called nephrons, of which there are about 1 million per kidney.

One part of each nephron consists of capillaries coiled about a part of a nephron, and this entwined mass is called the glomerulus. This is the action spot, where much of the waste is transferred across from blood to kidney urine. Because it is an action spot, problems tend to arise in the glomerulus. And these problems – in part – arise from free radical activity.

One problem that may occur in the glomerulus stems from the infiltration of phagocytes such as monocytes and neutrophils. These are immune cells that are capable of using free radicals as part of their weaponry in combating foreign substances and foreign invaders.

That the action of the monocytes and neutrophils, and their quivers of free radical arrows, are a source of damage in the kidney is supported by an experiment conducted by Rehan. Here the monocytes and neutrophils were reduced in number by selective depletion. With their reduction in number was a concomitant reduction in glomerular damage.

The damage by these macrophages in the glomerulus was originally thought to be caused by the release of certain enzymes. But recent evidence now indicates that much of the glomerular damage derives from the release of free radicals by these immune cells. These releases tend to occur as respiratory bursts, which are likely brought on by various immunological stimuli.

In a disease called glomerulonephritis, Falk et al have reported that one of the chief radicals released is the superoxide radical. These radicals are released as a response of the immune cells to autoantibodies.

A separate study conducted by this same group also looked at the other side of the ledger. In this study, glomerlular injury was induced in rats by the injection of sheep antibodies. In the group of rats that were also given injections of catalase there was a 75% reduction in glomerular injury.

Nitric oxide has also been linked to kidney disease. It too can be produced by macrophages for use in defending the body against foreign invaders. Where it is produced to excess, nitric oxide can do more harm than good. This is especially so when, in reaction with the superoxide radical, it forms peroxynitrite, which is a particularly destructive entity. Where peroxynitrite brings about tyrosine nitration and hydroxyl radical formation, these can also function as contributory factors in the development of numerous kidney diseases. Included among them are immune-mediated glomerulonephritis, postischemic renal injury, and obstructive nephropathy.

In all, there are several renal conditions that have detailed evidence which implicates free radicals in their development.

Antioxidant Assist

Free radicals play a significant role in many kidney disorders. On the plus side, antioxidants also play a significant and beneficial role in this area.

We have seen that catalase in one experiment was able to reduce glomerular injury by 75 percent.

Other studies also show a protective effect for a number of antioxidants.

In a study conducted on rats, a condition called protein-uria was induced similar to the problem that develops in diabetic patients. One consequence of this condition is glomerular injury, which can be detected by attendant observable changes in its structure. In the group of rats where catalase was also administered, proteinuria was prevented.

In a recent experiment, renal epithelial cells were grown in culture. The cells were then subjected to conditions in which oxygen availability was greatly reduced. Afterwards oxygen was reintroduced, producing increased oxidative stress in the cells. However, where dimethyl sulfoxide – a free radical scavenger – was supplied, the oxidative stress was greatly inhibited.

In a separate part of this experiment, the antioxidants in green tea were supplied, and a similar reduction in oxidative stress was observed.

Another recent in vivo study examined the effects of antioxidants in patients with chronic renal failure. In this study, patients exhibited elevated levels of malonaldehyde, which is a standard indicator of lipid peroxidation. They also showed depressed levels of polyunsaturated fatty acids, and they had low levels of vitamin E in their red blood cells.

One group was placed on a low protein diet, supplemented with amino and keto acids, along with the vitamins A, C, and E. This group afterwards showed a reversal of the undesired indicators: reduced malonaldehyde levels, and increased levels of polyunsaturated fatty acids. Also, the vitamin E levels in their red blood cells were raised.

Summary

The research has shown that there are several kidney diseases in which free radical activity plays a sizeable role. Many other kidney diseases have yet to be examined, or are only now being researched. It is expected that many of the conditions currently being researched will also show free radical involvement.

For their part, antioxidants have been shown to play both a preventive and ameliorating role in conditions of the kidney. Thus far, the antioxidant enzymes such as superoxide dismutase and especially catalase, appear to show strong effects in this area, along with the vitamins A, C, and E.

Future research will almost certainly supply further detail and refinement concerning the applicability of antioxidants in kidney disease.

Neurodegenerative Disease

The word "dotage" refers to the feeble mindedness that sometimes comes with advancing age. There are a number of neurodegenerative diseases that may bring about the memory loss and diminished cognitive performance that is part of this impairment. Some of these include Alzheimer's disease, Parkinson's disease, Amyotrophic lateral syndrome (ALS) or Lou Gehrig's disease, and multiple sclerosis.

Although the causes of these diseases are still poorly understood, more is being discovered about them every year. And one central thread weaving its way through these conditions and tying them together is the heightened presence of free radicals where these diseases occur, and the contributory effects of free radicals as causative factors in the incidence of neurodegenerative disease.

Conditions Conducive to Damage

There are a number of underlying circumstances that are conducive to free radical activity in the central nervous system. To begin with, the central nervous system requires large quantities of energy for its operations. This means that the neurons have higher numbers of mitochondria than are found in cells making up other parts of the body. The mitochondria are the power plants of a cell, and produce the energy needed by the cell for its normal functioning. During energy production, errant electrons sometimes escape from the normal biochemical pathways involved in energy production. These errant electrons and are often taken up by oxygen that is also present in these reactions – producing free radicals. In addition, there are a number of other biochemical pathways which may generate free radicals. Since the brain has higher energy needs, it also produces more free radicals per unit weight than any other organ in the body.

Conversely, there are lower levels of antioxidants (such as glutathione, for example) found in the brain. Also in brain cells, there are lower levels of activity for the antioxidant enzymes such as superoxide dismutase (SOD), catalase (Cat), and glutathione peroxidase (GPx).

Contributing to the increased chance of free radical damage taking place in these neurons is the fact that much of the brain tissue is susceptible to the oxidative action of free radicals. These include vulnerable constituents such as the catecholamines and the polyunsaturated fatty acids making up parts of cell membranes.

Once damaged, since neurons don't normally reproduce, damaged nerve cells may be with us for life, and accumulate over the years.

Exacerbating matters still further is the complexity of the central nervous system. This maze of interconnecting nerve fibres has been compared to the large switching center of a telephone company. Where irreparable damage accumulates in the nerve fibres, the intended transmissions or nerve impulses may be blocked, or incorrectly sent.

The end result of such damage shows up in the latter part of our lives as a deteriorating memory and a diminished capacity to think clearly. Ultimately, a pervasive disorientation is the case, and a near total loss of identity.

FREE RADICAL DISEASES AFFECTING THE NERVOUS SYSTEM

- Amyotrophic lateral sclerosis
- Alzheimer's disease
- Down's syndrome
- Ischemia/reperfusion injury
- Mitochondrial DNA disorders
- Multiple sclerosis
- Parkinson's disease

Certainly, in any of the neurodegenerative diseases there are causative factors that have been posited besides those attributed to the action of free radicals on the central nervous system. But for the purposes of this book we will limit ourselves mainly to the oxidative factors as they have manifested themselves in these diseases.

Indicators of Free Radical Activity

There is a great deal of research pointing to oxidative stress as a factor in diseases of the central nervous system.

As an indirect pointer, only moderate levels of superoxide dismutase and glutathione peroxidase have been found in the brain, and very low levels of catalase. This suggests that the brain does not have a strong corps of antioxidant enzymes with which to take on excessive free radicals. Also, the reduced or potent form of glutathione is found at much lower levels in aging rats compared to those of young rats. This is important because glutathione and glutathione peroxidase work as a team in neutralizing hydrogen peroxide. More important still, are findings which indicate that young mice under oxidative stress were better able to increase the availability of glutathione in the brain than were older mice, where the evidence indicates that the older mice were struggling to make more. This, too, suggests most strongly that the aging brain is more susceptible to oxidative damage than is the young brain.

One indicator of lipid peroxidation is thiobarbituric acid-reactive substances, or TBARS. These have been found at consistently higher levels in older rats compared to those found in young rats.

Carbonyl compounds, also found at higher levels in aging brain cells, are also indicative of lipid peroxidation, and the research has demonstrated the damage that they are capable of inflicting on cerebral endothelial cells.

Research has also shown that overly high iron levels are a factor in various neurodegenerative diseases. And although iron is necessary in a number of physiological functions, in excess it can be instrumental in bringing about extensive lipid peroxidation.

The age pigments, particularly lipofuscin, are found at increasingly higher concentrations as we age. They are a product of lipid peroxidation and are found at highest concentrations in brain, liver, and heart tissue. In human glial cells, which are a specialized kind of brain cell, oxidative stress has been reported as a major factor in the production of lipofuscin which can be measured.

Free radical activity has been measured by Electron Spin Resonance (ESR) measuring the unpaired electron's magnetic field. Luminol can be added to free radical substances to cause measurable light emission. Also proteins reactions with cysteine, proline, tyrosine and tryptophan produce products that can be measured.

Nitric oxide, which performs a number of beneficial functions in the body (including that of neurotransmitter in the brain) can also be injurious. Under certain conditions nitric oxide can cause damage by reacting with the superoxide radical to form the extremely harmful oxidizer, peroxynitrite. Peroxynitrite is capable of acting upon protein to form undesirable chemicals called nitrotyrosines.

Taken altogether, the evidence amassed to date leaves little doubt in the minds of scientists that free radicals play a significant and damaging role in neurodegenerative diseases.

Alzheimer's Disease
(Ronald Reagan's Disease)

Alzheimer's disease is one of the most debilitating of diseases because in the end it steals away our identity, our way of life, our very selves. It erodes memory function and cognitive function until we do not recognize family members we have loved throughout a lifetime, and in the final stages we do not even recognize ourselves. In America it is currently the single greatest cause of older people being admitted into nursing homes. It is estimated that 50% of 80 year old Americans are showing signs of Alzheimer's disease.

The symptoms of Alzheimer's disease – progressive memory loss and dementia – tend to manifest themselves around middle age and beyond. Although a genetic factor appears to be involved, it is not a sizeable factor. Interestingly, similar pathologic changes in the brains of Alzheimer's patients also tend to occur in those with Down's syndrome that live beyond the age of thirty-five.

In the past, aluminum toxicity was thought to be a major factor in Alzheimer's, but the evidence for this was inconsistent. Currently, the evidence suggests a combination of contributory factors. These include the accumulation of a protein precursor in the brain called beta-amyloid, as well as oxidative damage, impaired calcium balance, and impaired energy metabolism.

The "Nun Study" started in 1986, follows 678 U.S. School Sisters of Notre Dame, funded by the National Institute of Aging was analysed by Dr. David Snowdon for keys to the Alzheimer's puzzle. The website www.nunstudy.org summarizes the findings. The eldest, brightest Nuns appeared to possess deep spirituality with positive outlook and community networking involving regular contact with friends and family. High linguistic ability in early life, preventing depression and stroke and continuing to exercise your brain with mental pursuits seems to protect against Alzheimer's disease. Studies of the Nuns suggested that folic acid levels correlated with elderly brain health and that lycopene levels correlated with elderly physical function. There was no relationship of amalgam teeth fillings or aluminum to brain deterioration. The Oxford University Project to Investigate Memory and Aging (OPTIMA study) agreed that low levels of folic acid may be linked to a higher risk of Alzheimer's and brain atrophy.

Free Radicals as a Contributory Factor

The complicity of free radicals as a causative factor in Alzheimer's disease was put forth by Volicer and Crino in 1990. They hypothesized that Alzheimer's disease is an acceleration of the aging process in parts of the brain that have become progressively damaged by free radicals that were generated by metabolic functions. This was based on a number of studies, some of which involved interesting experiments using gerbils.

It had been found that normal, older gerbils had twice the oxidized protein in the brain compared to young gerbils. They also exhibited lower activity levels for glutamine synthetase (GS) and neural protease (NP). These substances are required for the synthesis of glutamine and the degradation of oxidized proteins respectively. Further, in a maze test which measures spatial and short-term memory, the older gerbils made twice as many errors.

That these errors were linked to oxidative damage was shown in another experiment in which the protein oxidation was reversed in the older gerbils by use of a substance (PBN) that was able to neutralize the free radicals to form a stable compound. This resulted in a reduction of oxidized protein and an elevation in glutamine synthetase and neural protease activity – and a reduction in the number of errors made by the gerbils in the maze. When PBN supplementation was halted the error rate increased, and the improved results reverted to those that were originally found in the older gerbils.

Futher Evidence

Another study that indicts free radical activity as a factor in Alzheimer's disease involves a protein called beta-amyloid. It has been shown that beta-amyloid will fragment in aqueous solution, and in so doing generates free radical peptides. It has also been shown that these fragments are toxic to cultured neurons, and as well, that they inactivate glutamine synthetase and creatine kinase, both of which are necessary to normal functioning of the brain, and for reducing the levels of harmful oxidized protein.

Another curious aspect of beta-amyloid is also under investigation. In cases of Alzheimer's disease where there is a genetic factor involved (as indicated in part by family history), it is due to a genetic defect on chromosome 21. Interestingly, the gene coding for beta-amyloid is also on gene 21, although not at the same location. This tends to suggest another avenue for future research by exploring some of the pathology found in Alzheimer's disease that is also found in Down's syndrome, where in the latter, chromosome 21 is also involved.

In addition, beta-amyloid has also been shown to stimulate nitric oxide production in astrocytes, which are star shaped neuroglial cells in the brain. Nitric oxide, as we know, may lead to the subsequent formation of the highly destructive peroxynitrite. Other research has indicated a correlation between higher nitrotyrosine levels in Alzheimer's patients compared to those of a similar age that do not have the disease.

Further evidence indicative of free radical activity as a causative factor in Alzheimer's disease include:

- decreased levels of superoxide dismutase (SOD) found in various parts of the brain;
- decreased glutamine synthetase activity in the frontal cortex;
- increased iron levels in the brain which can lead to hydroxyl radical generation;
- higher than normal levels of lipofuscin, the aging pigment that stiffens tissues.

With respect to the last point, in vitro studies have also shown that lipofuscin production is increased by iron and decreased by various antioxidants.

Finally, it has been demonstrated that vitamin E inhibits the cytotoxic effects of the beta-amyloid protein and its fragments.

Antioxidants and Alzheimer's Disease

There are many studies that offer strong evidence that antioxidants play a significant role in preventing Alzheimer's disease. This is not surprising since free radical activity is also a major factor in its occurrence.

The most obvious point to be made is that antioxidants are found at much lower levels in Alzheimer's disease. Dr. Jeandel has shown that this is certainly the case for serum levels of vitamins A, C, and E, as well as for zinc and transferrin.

NEUROLOGICAL DISEASES AND ALZHEIMERS'S DISEASE

- Presence of Cu/Zn-SOD gene on chromosome 21
- Beta-amyloid fragments generate free radicals
- Increased protein and lipid oxidation products in frontal cortex
- Decreased antioxidant levels in Alzheimer's patients
- Decreased superoxide dismutase in frontal cortex, hippocampus and cerebellum
- Decreased glutamine synthetase activity in frontal cortex
- Increased iron levels in frontal cortex
- Increased lipofuscin in AD brain tissue
- In vitro lipofuscin production increased by iron and decreased by antioxidants
- Presence of catalase and superoxide dismutase antibodies in neuritic plaques
- Vitamin E inhibits cytotoxic effects of beta-amyloid

We have also seen that the beta-amyloid protein fragments are toxic to brain cells, and can cause cell damage or cell death. Research by Behl et al has shown that vitamin E is able to inhibit cell damage and cell death induced by these protein fragments.

Crucial to learning and memory are certain receptor cells in the brain called muscarinic cholinergic receptors. A number of researchers have shown that Alzheimer's patients exhibit a significant loss of these receptor neurons. The loss of these receptors reduces the volume of neural transmission, and very likely accounts for at least some of the memory loss in Alzheimer's patients. Current pharmaceutical therapies attempt to increase the amount of the neurotransmitter, acetylcholine in the brain. This only partly makes up for the loss of acetylcholine receptors seen in Alzheimer's but this treatment is only of temporary benefit.

Frey et al have shown that a certain endogenous inhibitor is able to prevent the receptor cells from carrying out their proper function, and that the levels of these inhibitors in Alzheimer's patients are three times the levels found in those without the disease. Most importantly, these researchers – and others – have found that glutathione plays a significant role in this process. In addition, they have reported that a form of vitamin E (Trolox) is able to block the action of this harmful inhibitor. This was also found to be the case for other substances acting as free radical scavengers, such as manganese and EDTA (ethylenediamine tetra-acetic acid).

All of this suggests most strongly that antioxidants such as vitamin E and glutathione, will provide beneficial thera-peutic effects in Alzheimer's patients by protecting these cru-cial receptors. Other research as well has shown the positive therapeutic benefits of CoQ-10 in the treatment of Alzheimer's disease.

Parkinson's Disease (Michael Fox's Disease)

Parkinson's disease is another of the neurodegenerative disorders that occurs most often around middle age and beyond. The symptoms of Parkinson's include a short, quick gate, a slowness in voluntary movements, rigidity, and tremor at rest. Associated with the disease is a pallor in a part of the brain known as the substantia nigra, which is where much of the malfunctioning that gives rise to this disease is located. At the microscopic level, a loss of pigmented neurons has been observed. Also associated with Parkinson's is a depletion of dopamine in another part of the brain called the corpus striatum, which results from the neuronal loss in the substantia nigra.

Why these abnormalities arise, bringing on the clinical symptoms of the disease, is not really known. A number of theories have been put forth but none fully accounts for the initiation or progression of the disease. What is known, however, is that oxidative stress is a principal factor in the pathogenesis of the Parkinson's.

Free Radical Involvement

As is the case for many of the neurodegenerative diseases, there is solid evidence that free radicals play a significant and substantial role in Parkinson's disease. The presence and the effects of free radicals have most often been found in the substantia nigra, the region of the brain where other abnormalities associated with Parkinson's also occur.

Findings by Dexter et al have shown that in Parkinson's patients, the levels of polyunsaturated fatty acids in the substantia nigra are lower than in other parts of the brain, and were also lower in comparison with those who did not have the disease.

Lipid peroxidation was also found to be higher in Parkinson's patients, as indicated by higher levels of malonaldehyde, which is a definite marker for this oxidative activity. The elevated levels of lipid peroxidation were shown to continue right up to the time of death. This free radical activity is thought to result from a variety of sources.

In abnormalities concerning dopamine production and storage, where the turnover rate is increased, dopamine may go through a particular oxidative pathway involving monoamine oxidase. This pathway also produces hydrogen peroxide. Furthermore, L-dopa in nerve tissue brought about increases in oxidized or "spent" glutathione (GSSG), which is also suggestive of increased hydrogen peroxide production.

The neurons where dopamime is active have also been shown to contain pigments of lipofuscin and other polymers. This waste pigment is thought to be derived from some of the products of dopamine oxidation. Some of these components undergo further oxidation, which again generates hydrogen peroxide.

Other substances, too, have been implicated in generating oxidative stress, and in producing symptoms not unlike those found in Parkinson's disease. The neurotoxin MPTP, for example, as it undergoes reduction via a particular chemical pathway, is transformed into a radical. In the process, the superoxide radical is also generated.

Corroboration of this is indicated by the research of Hung and Lee. They found that MPTP increased lipid peroxidation in mice, and as well, produced diminished levels of glutathione in the substantia nigra region of the brain. Other research has shown that MPTP can also bring about increased free radical activity in human neuroblastoma cells.

Symptoms resembling those of Parkinson's disease – and a corresponding increase in oxidative stress- have also been reported in cases of manganese poisoning, and in the use of street drugs such as methamphetamine (ICE), and methylenedioxy-methamphetamine (Ecstasy).

The upshot of the above studies indicates that no matter

how the symptoms of Parkinson's disease come about, there is invariably an increase in free radical activity, particularly in the form of lipid peroxidation. Regardless of whether the symptoms indicative of Parkinson's are "naturally" occurring, or have been induced by toxins or drugs, increased oxidative stress is attendant as well.

Antioxidants and Parkinson's Disease

Antioxidants also play an important role in Parkinson's disease. This role is often reflected in the decreased levels of many antioxidants in the affected parts of the brain.

In the case of the enzyme antioxidants, research has shown that Parkinson's patients exhibit low levels of catalase activity and only modest levels for glutathione peroxidase and superoxide dismutase. Recent reports also indicate that superoxide dismutase activity decreases as Parkinson's disease progresses.

In one interesting experiment, Barker et al measured the effects of glutathione depletion in the brains of rats. They reported that with glutathione depleted by 60%, the activity of glutathione reductase was correspondingly reduced by 40%.

The research of Seaton et al focused on a substance in the brain called NADH ubiquinone reductase (or complex 1), which tends to occur at reduced levels in the substantia nigra of Parkinson's patients. Some of this reduction may be due to complex 1 inhibitors. The research by this group has shown that these inhibitors can bring about apoptosis (cell death) in brain cells that are involved in dopamine activity. However, it was shown that this cell death was much reduced where the cells were pretreated with antioxidants such as NAC (N-acetylcysteine) and alpha lipoic acid.

Investigations have also shown that glutathione tends to

occur at reduced levels (40% less) in Parkinson's patients. Reports indicate that glutathione is able to deactivate a harmful product of lipid peroxidation called HNE. It does this by joining onto it through a process called S conjugation. The tentative conclusion from these studies, and others, is that glutathione occurs at reduced levels in Parkinson's patients because it is being used up in combating oxidative stress, and the toxic substances generated by this oxidative stress. A corollary conclusion is that antioxidants may be of therapeutic value in the treatment of Parkinson's.

An experiment conducted by Lancelot et al entailed inducing lesions and increased hydroxyl radicals in the brains of rats. It was then shown that the administration of a substance acting as a scavenger antioxidant was able to attenuate both the lesions and the generation rate of hydroxyl radicals. The conclusion here again is that scavenger antioxidants will be of therapeutic benefit in the treatment of this disease. Our experience has shown us tremendous benefits in treating our Parkinson's patients with intravenous glutathione.

Consistent with these results are field studies which employed antioxidants on Parkinson's patients. In some of these studies, vitamin E was used along with an oxidase inhibitor such as deprenyl, with positive results. Although these studies were uncontrolled, they do suggest that treatment with antioxidants is of significant benefit to Parkinson's patients, and may extend their lives as well.

Certainly the fat soluble antioxidants such as vitamin E and alpha lipoic acid will be of most benefit in the treatment of Parkinson's patients, while vitamin C and glutathione will assist by helping to restore them as they become oxidized in neutralizing free radicals. In addition, since the enzyme antioxidants tend to occur at reduced levels in these patients, supplementation with these antioxidants may be helpful as well.

Research taking place at the present time will likely provide more definitive conclusions in this regard over the next few years.

Multiple Sclerosis

Multiple sclerosis, or MS, is a progressive disease of the central nervous system that affects the myelin sheaths that encase nerve fibres in the body. As the disease progresses the myelin sheath deteriorates, and this is thought to impair proper conduction of nerve impulses. There is no effective treatment available for MS to date, although there are a number of hypotheses concerning the disease. As lecturing doctors, we are consistently asked for our advice about M.S. We have little to offer at this time but helping to counter the damaging effects of free radicals and look with anticipation at recent reports of the benefits of using minocin to improve outcomes of this terrible affliction. (What do you think, Dr. Merkin?)

It is thought that the immune system is involved in MS. This hypothesis is supported by evidence indicating that activated macrophages release toxins that bring about a deterioration in the myelin sheath. Thus far, however, attempts to combat the deterioration in the myelin sheath by manipulating the immune response have produced little by way of positive results.

Recent reports also indicate a possible genetic basis to Parkinson's.

Since the myelin sheaths consist of both protein and lipid components, this raises the possibility of free radical involvement, with the oxidative processes here resulting in both protein degradation and lipid peroxidation.

Reports by Bowen were amongst the first to present evidence supporting free radical involvement in the pathogenesis of MS. Since then further data has been presented. Using the accumulated data, LeVine has proposed a persuasive hypothesis implicating free radical activity as a contributory factor in MS. This theory suggests that there is a cooperative role between the immune system and free radicals generated in the myelin itself, effecting the deterioration that then occurs in the myelin sheaths.

Cooper, going one step further, suggests that free radicals actually initiate the disease. He theorizes that free radicals, in damaging the myelin, set in motion biochemical events that also initiate and promote T-cell activity.

Whatever details and corroboration future research may bring, the present data is strongly supportive of free radical activity in one way or another. Consonant with this thought is data from the research of Korpela et al, which indicates that serum lipid peroxidation levels were higher in patients with active progressive MS compared to those for whom the disease was in remission, and in comparison with the controls who did not have the disease. Similar results were obtained for TBARS, which are another indicator of lipid peroxidation.

Still other research has shown that pentane and ethane – which also serve as markers of lipid peroxidation – were at higher levels in the exhaled breath of those with MS.

In vitro studies conducted in the laboratory offer still further corroborative evidence suggestive of free radical activity in MS. One study by Konat and Wiggins has shown that loss of normal protein in myelin tended to increase with increased accumulations of lipid peroxides.

Research dealing with nitric oxide further implicates free radicals in MS. In a condition resembling MS in mice, it was found that peroxynitrite was generated very early in the development of the disease, and tended to increase as the disease progressed. Hooper et al used uric acid, which is a scavenger antioxidant, to treat the condition. This research group found that uric acid was able to reduce the outward signs and symptoms of the disease.

Based on recent reports, it appears likely that further corroborative evidence concerning the beneficial use of other antioxidants will be forthcoming with future research, and that antioxidants will be shown to produce at least an ameliorative effect in MS.

Lou Gehrig's Disease (Stephen Hawking's Disease)

Amyotrophic lateral sclerosis, also known as ALS or Lou Gehrig's disease, is another terrible disease that typically afflicts people who are middle aged and beyond. The disease is characterized by a progressive degeneration of motor neurons that over time brings on increasing paralysis. The neurons affected include certain cells found in the spinal cord, in the brainstem, and in parts of the cerebral cortex. Death usually occurs within five years of the onset of the disease.

Although the causes of ALS are still incompletely known, a few theories about the disease have been put forth. None to date has been completely supported by current data. However, in recent years evidence has been accumulating which tends to indicate strongly a free radical involvement in the disease.

Approximately 10% of ALS is inherited. In these cases many patients also have various mutations in the gene that encodes for one form of superoxide dismutase (SOD). Also, people who are heterozygous for the SOD mutations exhibit reduced levels of SOD activity in their brains and in their red blood cells, where this activity is less than 50% of normal.

In addition, research by Robberecht indicates that those with familial ALS show reduced activity for this form of

SOD as well. More importantly, this group has shown that this abnormal enzyme activity is detectable in red blood cells years before the symptoms actually manifest themselves clinically in the carriers of the disease.

It has also been reported (Przedborski et al) that in parts of the cerebral cortex affected by ALS, those with the disease had significantly lower levels of glutathione peroxidase.

Research by Ferrante et al, in a multi-faceted study, focused on indicators of oxidative damage in the cerebral cortex of ALS patients. These indicators of oxidative damage in the cerebral cortex were compared to levels found in other parts of the brain. There were also comparisons of these indicators made between those with ALS, those with other diseases of the central nervous system, and as well, with control subjects free of disease. Indicators for oxidative protein damage (protein carbonyl) and for DNA alterations (8-hydroxy-2-deoxyguanosine) were found to be elevated in the cerebral cortex of those with sporadic ALS. In the spinal cord similar results were obtained in both sporadic and familial ALS.

The superoxide radical is most likely involved in ALS as well, where it may react with nitric oxide to produce peroxynitrite. The peroxynitrite then reacts with SOD, generating products that bring about damage in the form of protein nitration. It is this latter damage that is thought to produce the gradual injury to the motor neurons that is responsible for ALS.

Other research (Kisby et al) indicates that in ALS patients, the protein repair mechanisms are faulty. This suggests that ALS patients may be deficient in repairing oxidative DNA damage. Diets high in certain amino acids have shown some promise for treatment in the past and this may be from their antioxidant effects.

The data from these studies, and others, convincingly

points to free radical damage as an initiator of the degeneration in motor neurons found in ALS patients.

Antioxidant Involvement

We have seen that antioxidant enzymes tend to occur at reduced levels in those with ALS.

Research on mice with a form of ALS was conducted by Gurney et al. This research indicates that vitamin E is also a casualty in the battle against free radical activity in ALS. It was found that the expression of the mutant SOD gene resulted in increased oxidative stress in the brain and spinal cord, accompanied by a depletion of vitamin E. However, with dietary supplementation of vitamin E, the onset of the disease was delayed and its progression slowed.

In the case of ALS, it will be left to future research to amplify the involvement of free radicals in greater detail, and to investigate where antioxidants may be of further therapeutic benefit.

Summary of Neurodegenerative Disease

Some of the more prominent neurodegenerative diseases have a number of elements in common. For one thing, many of these diseases tend to make their appearance around middle age or later. In addition, most are still poorly understood, which also means that at present there is little by way of truly effective or curative treatment.

One aspect concerning these diseases that is fairly well understood – and which today is virtually beyond any doubt – is that free radicals play a highly significant role in their development. In some cases it may soon be shown that free radicals even play a role in the initiation of the diseases. Some aspects of free radical activity in these diseases, and the biochemistry involved, have already been worked out, and more will undoubtedly be coming forth in the near future.

Attendant with free radical activity in neurodegenerative disease, are commonly found reduced levels of many antioxidants in those with the disease, most pronouncedly in the nerve tissue affected by a particular disease. The antioxidant enzymes such as superoxide dismutase, catalase, and glutathione peroxidase are those most often cited in this regard, as are glutathione and the fat soluble antioxidant, vitamin E.

Not surprisingly then, that a number of antioxidants have shown beneficial results in reducing free radical activity under laboratory conditions. Some, such as vitamin E and CoQ-10, have also proved beneficial in ameliorating conditions such as Alzheimer's and Parkinson's diseases. Research into the use of antioxidants in the treatment of neurodegenerative disease has not been all that extensive to date, but results so far indicate an expanding role in their use for the future. Certainly, since free radical activity occurs at high levels in the incidence of these diseases, it would seem reasonable that antioxidants may confer preventive benefits as well. Many neurologists continue to prescribe vitamin E as a useful adjunct to many sparse treatment options.

Inflammatory Disease (Arthritis)

Inflammatory disease is characterized by redness and swelling, and is often accompanied by heat, pain, and loss of function. It may be caused by tissue injury resulting from a number of causes, including microbial infection, physical trauma, burns, chemicals such as toxins or caustic substances. Inflammatory conditions may also occur as the result of necrotic tissue or immunologic reactions.

The inflammation may be regarded as acute or as chronic.

Acute Inflammation

In the cases of acute inflammation, the symptoms are of short duration, lasting no more than a few days. During this period the body's defences come into play, largely through the activity of the immune system. In the initial period following injury or infection, for example, the body will increase blood flow to the site, and the immune system will usher increased numbers of leukocytes (white blood cells) to the area as well. Neutrophils are the most numerous defenders brought to bear on foreign invaders during this initial period, followed afterwards by monocytes.

The body counters foreign invaders first by identifying them as foreign. Macrophages produce a protein that adheres to the foreign invaders, making it easier for the immune cells to adhere to these invaders, and in the end engulf them.

During this process, free radicals are employed as weapons by the immune cells to weaken or kill invaders such as bacteria. Following phagocytosis, where the bacteria are engulfed by cells such as macrophages, the bacteria are killed and broken down. The leukocytes, too, often decompose.

During phagocytosis an enzyme called NADH oxidase is activated, which then brings about a respiratory burst, whereby superoxide radicals are generated. These may then be converted to hydrogen peroxide. Either of these may then be used in destroying invaders such as bacteria.

However necessary this defence system may be in defending us and keeping us alive, it greatly increases the free radical load in the body. And this increased load takes its toll.

Where there are insufficient levels of antioxidants present in the body to neutralize this surfeit of free radicals on hand after the microscopic battle, we become subject to the many forms of damage that free radicals may inflict on our own cells.

To be sure, sustaining free radical damage is preferable to dying or being severely weakened by disease. But maintaining optimal levels of antioxidants in the body provides a secondary line of defence to counter the free radicals that are on hand after the bacteria have been vanquished.

Chronic Inflammation

The hunched stance, the slow and halting steps – these are certain indicators of advancing age, and of chronic inflammatory disease. And unlike sunken eyes or wrinkled skin, these symptoms are detectable even from a distance.

Chronic inflammatory disease may persist over many days, many years, or often a lifetime. In the form of arthritis – an umbrella term for over a hundred different conditions – the connective tissue becomes inflamed and swollen in the joints. Often the cartilage degenerates and wears away, leaving bone grinding on bone.

Although the cause of arthritis is not known, evidence suggests that free radicals play a central role in either its initiation or its development. Certainly, once the condition is progressing, free radicals occur at higher numbers in the affected areas, exacerbating the swelling and degeneration. And where the positioning of a swollen joint impedes blood flow, once the joint is flexed and blood flow is restored and rushes back into the area, even more free radicals are generated. Here again we see an incidence of reperfusion injury, which becomes part of a cyclical process: the free radical activity adds to the swelling, and the swelling induces more free radical activity.

Another factor that is thought to be involved in arthritis comes in the form of adhesion proteins. These are proteins used by the immune cells which allow them to attach to bacteria and the like. Evidence suggests that an over abundance of these proteins are also a contributing factor to inflammatory disease. Cytokines are substances released causing further inflammation. These substances can be suppressed by using anti-inflammatory medicines like Ibuprofen, Naproxen or the newer Cox-2 inhibitors like Vioxx or Celebrex. A diet high in omega-3 fatty acids (fish oils) will lead to less production of arachidonic acid which comes from omega-6 fatty acids in the diet (corn oil, safflower oil and soyabean oil).

Autoimmunity is also a circumstance which figures strongly in the development of rheumatoid arthritis. Autoimmunity occurs where the body's immune system loses the sensitivity to differentiate between some of the cells of the body it is supposed to protect, and foreign invaders, and begins to attack the cells of the body as well. As we look at the immune system shortly, we will see that free radicals also play a role in autoimmunity.

Maintaining an optimal antioxidant profile will certainly help in the prevention of inflammatory diseases such as arthritis. Since patients with arthritis have been found to exhibit lower levels of vitamin E, calcium, zinc, and folic acid, it would make sense to maintain healthy levels of these substances as a preventive measure. Also, vitamins A, C, and E – the ACEs – all contribute to healthy tissue formation and maintenance. Vitamin C is especially important in the production of connective tissue such as cartilage. Most importantly for those suffering the pain of arthritis, studies have shown that vitamin E, besides playing a preventive role, is also able to reduce the symptoms of arthritis.

The Immune System

The immune system is our defence system. It defends us against attack both from without and from within. The various constituents of the immune system are able to protect us against foreign invaders, such as viruses and bacteria. They are also able to protect us from ourselves by attacking our own defective cells such as potential cancer cells.

As we come into middle age, the immune system generally goes into decline. By the time we reach old age the immune system has become greatly weakened, and in some people is almost defunct.

There is a great deal of evidence suggesting that the hormonal decline accompanying middle age is also a major causative factor in the decline of immune function. Another important factor affecting immune function decline is that of free radical activity.

Crash Course

A crash course on the immune system would include a mention of some of its more prominent foot soldiers – the leukocytes or white blood cells. It is these cells that actually do battle for us on the front lines.

Some of these include neutrophils, natural killer (NK) cells, and T-cells. The neutrophils operate by engulfing foreign invaders of almost any kind in a process called phagocytosis. Natural killer (NK) cells are most effective in combating rogue cancer cells. And T-cells are the specialists in battling viruses.

In addition to these components, there are immune factors such as interleukin-2 (IL-2), which is produced by T-cells and serves to promote further T-cell proliferation and activity. Other immune factors include tumor necrosis factor, which is a type of protein that is able to kill cancer cells; and immunoglobulin G (IgG), which is an antibody produced by lymphocytes and serves in identifying and clearing foreign matter.

Production Line

Other components of the immune system consist of the bone marrow of long bones, the lymphatics, the spleen, and the thymus gland. All of these play a role as part of the production line in providing the foot soldiers, or in maintaining them.

The tissues in the marrow of long bones produce stem cells. The stem cells evolve into what are called progenitor cells, which are relatively undifferentiated. Over time the progenitor cells differentiate into the various red and white blood cells. Tissues of the lymphatic system produce lymphocytes, a white blood cell involved in acquired immunity.

The thymus gland plays a most important part in the immune system – and in aging. The thymus gland begins shrinking almost from the time we are born, and by the age of sixty, the thymus has shriveled away to almost nothing.

The thymus produces various protein hormones, some which are becoming commercially available and some show promise in treating hepatitis A, hepatitis C, AIDS, herpes and fungal infections. But perhaps the most important function of the thymus is the role it plays in the development of T-cells. Besides producing immune cells of its own, the thymus serves as an incubator for cells generated in the bone marrow. It is in the thymus gland that these cells continue their development and differentiation, until they have matured into fully capable warriors, ready to do battle on our behalf.

The decline of the immune system undoubtedly plays a causative role in aging, and death. And free radicals play a major role in the decline of the immune system.

As we age, immune function declines. We become more susceptible to disease from the outside, such as infectious disease. We also become more susceptible to disease from the inside, such as cancer. And where these diseases do not kill us outright, they most often expedite the aging process, wearing us down and weakening us.

Thus, as we move past middle age, the decline of the immune system hastens our own general physical decline. And when there is insufficient defence left, we are left to the assault of an overwhelming infection. And we die.

So it is that infectious disease is a major cause of death in the elderly.

Free Radicals and the Decline

There are a number of factors that affect immune function, and its decline in our advancing years. Certainly, hormonal influences constitute a major factor. For instance, declining levels of human growth hormone (HGH) have a pronounced effect on a declining immune function. This is also the case for DHEA (dehydroepiandrosterone).

Another important factor in the weakening of the immune system stems from free radical activity. This is not surprising, since free radicals are able to attack virtually any part of a cell and virtually any cell in the body. And that includes cells and tissues involved in immune function.

The involution (shriveling) of the thymus gland over the years is almost certainly abetted by free radical activity. And this decline of the thymus bears directly on the strength and quantity of immune cells (such as T-cells), and quantity of immune factors (such as IL-2).

There is abundant evidence indicating that various immune cells – especially T-cells – are significantly and adversely affected by free radical activity. For example, research has shown that various antioxidants are able to stimulate T-cell activity. This brings about increased production of IL-2, which in turn stimulates further T-cell activity. The upshot is a heightened mitogenic response, which means that there is an increase in the proliferation of these cells when foreign invaders arrive on the scene.

Free radicals, through their activity in the form of lipid peroxidation, are able to attack immune cell membranes. This has the effect of impeding normal membrane activity, such as the passage of nutrient and waste across it. Damage of this kind brings about an impediment to immune cell response, which is observed as a susceptibility to disease found in many aging mammals, including humans.

Besides impairing the normal flow of cell nutrient and waste, damage to immune cell membranes also interferes with crucial enzyme activity that involves the cell membrane. For example, in phagocytes, the proper employment of an enzyme called NADPH oxidase (which is triggered by another enzyme called protein kinase C) is adversely affected by membrane damage. This then manifests itself in a phagocyte's diminished capacity to battle foreign invaders. Ultimately, damage of this sort is reflected in the immunoincompetence associated with aging.

Further, it is on the outer membranes of immune cells that other molecular substances are employed which allow them to identify invaders by the molecular structures on the outside of the invaders, or by the structure of substances attached to these invaders by other components of the immune system. With membrane damage that results from lipid peroxidation, this aspect of the immune response is also compromised.

Some of the more telling evidence concerning the effects of free radical activity on the immune system comes from research employing various antioxidants in combating this free radical activity.

Antioxidants and the Immune System

We have seen that enzyme antioxidants such as superoxide dismutase (SOD), catalase (Cat), and glutathione peroxidase (GPx) make up the first line of defence against free radicals. That is because they are able to disrupt or defuse the chemical processes by which free radicals are formed, or they neutralize them at their formation, before they can cause harm.

Research by Umeki et al measured SOD concentrations and the concentrations of superoxide radicals in pneumonia patients with and without compromised immune systems, and compared them with comparable controls. Those with the disease who also exhibited a compromised immune system also had lower levels of SOD activity, and higher concentrations for the superoxide radical. The study suggests most strongly that decreased SOD activity may explain the depressed immune function that was also found in these patients

Other experiments involving bone marrow transplant patients also indicate that higher levels of catalase activity correlate with greater immune function.

Zinc

A predominant form of SOD (Cu/Zn SOD) has zinc as a constituent component. Serving in this function, and in a number of other ways, zinc has shown itself to be a critical player in healthy immune function. Since zinc competes directly with copper and iron, its presence tends to decrease the production of hydroxyl radicals resulting from the Fenton reaction, which is dependant upon the availability of free iron in the form of ions for its completion.

Zinc also protects sulfhydryl groups (as found in alpha lipoic acid and glutathione) from oxidation, which keeps more of them in play and combating free radicals.

There is substantial research indicative of zinc's widespread value in fortifying the immune system. Where zinc is in deficiency, as is frequently the case in the aged, other associated conditions are also found. These include lymphoid atrophy and a diminution in thymus hormone activity, affecting hormones such as thymulin, of which zinc is a constituent element.

As well, zinc likely plays a role in controlling the activity of numerous enzymes related to immune function, including NADPH (Nicotinamide Adenosine Diphosphate-H) oxidase.

Specific studies have produced a range of evidence supporting the role of zinc in bolstering the immune system.

Dardenne et al supplemented aging mice with zinc for 3-6 months, while a similar control group received none. The mice supplemented with zinc had the levels for this mineral restored almost to youthful mouse levels. Zinc supplementation also stimulated thymic growth, increased thymulin levels, and decreased the levels of thymulin inhibitors. It also improved epithelial structure and brought about the disappearance of epithelial cysts often present in the thymus glands of aging mice.

Studies on humans have also produced reports pointing up the improvements to immune function conferred by zinc. Duchateau et al treated a group of people over the age of seventy with zinc supplementation. In contrast with the control group, the supplemented group exhibited the following: an increase in circulating T-cells; increased immunoglobulin G antibody response to tetanus vaccine; improved lymphocyte mitogen response, meaning the lymphocytes tended to increase in number in response to antigenic stimulation; and an improved delayed hypersensitivity response to several proteins, indicating a diminished autoimmune response.

Other studies have produced results indicating similar beneficial results for zinc. One striking study (Beck et al) demonstrated that various immune cells and immune factors became depressed when suboptimal levels of zinc were induced. In the experiment a zinc deficiency was induced in young adult men by use of a low zinc diet along with substances that inhibited zinc absorption. The zinc deficiency produced a reduction in immune function as indicated by a reduction in interferon-gamma, interleukin-2, and tumor necrosis factor alpha.

From these, and a host of other studies, maintaining optimal zinc levels is a must in achieving a strong immune system.

Selenium

Selenium, as a constituent element of glutathione peroxidase, is also a must in maintaining a healthy immune system. Where low levels of selenium are found, accompanying low levels of glutathione peroxidase also tend to be found. The deleterious effects of low selenium levels has been reported in numerous studies.

Research by Meeker et al, for example, has shown that selenium deficiencies produced a diminished capacity in natural killer cells, which are the body's battlers against would-be cancer cells.

Mice that are normally resistant to a certain strain of virus have been shown to be highly susceptible when low levels of selenium are present (Beck et al).

Where selenium is in low supply, there is an attendant decrease in lymphocyte proliferation (Sun et al). As well, deficiencies in selenium have also been shown to play a role in apoptosis induced by oxidative stress, where the oxidative stress was the result of decreased intracellular glutathione peroxidase activity. And in selenium deficient cells, there was a diminished capacity for neutralizing intracellular hydrogen peroxide by scavenger antioxidants, when compared to cells that had been supplemented with selenium.

The ACEs and Immune Function

There is a large body of research indicating that the antioxidant vitamins A, C, and E are especially important in maintaining a vigorous immune system. Vitamin C is especially effective in a water based medium, while vitamin E excels in fatty structures, so it is not surprising that these vitamins play a significant role in strengthening immune function.

Penn et al studied the effect of supplementation with vitamins A, C, and E on elderly patients, with a matched control group receiving no supplements. In this experiment, those receiving the supplements exhibited a strengthening of the immune system. This was seen by way of an increase in various immune cells, including circulating T-cells, CD4 (helper) lymphocytes, and in the total number of lymphocytes.

Other studies using vitamin E alone have also produced striking results. Along with elevated levels of vitamin E both in plasma and in immune cells, a number of immune factors were enhanced. The improvements in the immune system from the higher vitamin E levels included: an increased positive antigen response; an increased proliferation of immune cells; an increased production of IL-2; a decreased production rate for prostaglandins; and a decreased level of lipid peroxides.

The research also indicates that vitamin C plays a strong role in fortifying the immune system. Vitamin C is normally found in high concentrations in circulating leukocytes. Thus, when cells such as phagocytes release quantities of free radicals in battling foreign invaders, vitamin C is on hand to neutralize the excess of free radicals that are present after the battle. However, where there is prolonged and intense phagocytic activity, such as occurs in the case of an ongoing infection, vitamin C (and other scavenger antioxidants) may become depleted – and the antioxidant defence system may become overwhelmed. This is even more likely where adequate levels of these antioxidants have not been maintained to start with.

In vitro studies (Anderson, Lukey) have shown that the above description is a fair approximation of the roles played by immune cells, free radicals, and vitamin C, and how vitamin C may become depleted in circumstances such as prolonged infection. This same research also showed that vitamin C was particularly effective at enhancing the performance of neutrophils. This explains the rationale of vitamin megadoses during times of stress (increased oxidative stress) although there has been some recent concern about DNA damage from chronic, megadoses of ascorbic acid (vitamin C).

There are numerous studies pointing up the importance of vitamin C in maintaining an effective immune system. And the fact that vitamin C is able to restore vitamin E only adds to its importance in this regard.

The Carotenoids

The carotenoids, too, have demonstrated effectiveness in boosting the immune system. Studies on both humans and animals bring findings that underscore the value of the carotenoids – particularly beta-carotene – in this respect.

Daniel et al, using lymphocytes from cows, incubated them in vitro with beta-carotene. These cells showed an increased proliferation when compared to the control cells without beta-carotene.

Other experiments of this nature have also demonstrated the value of beta-carotene in improving immune function. This improved immune function was seen in the following: an increase in T-cell numbers; an increase in natural killer cell cytotoxicity or potency; and increased secretions of tumor necrosis factor alpha and IL-2.

In an extremely interesting experiment (Meydani et al) elderly women were supplemented with either beta-carotene or a placebo over a three week period. The plasma levels for various antioxidants were measured before and after the experiment. Those receiving the placebo experienced antioxidant depletion, with the drop in levels occurring in the following order: first the vitamin C levels, followed by those for bilirubin, alpha-tocopherol and gamma tocopherol (forms of vitamin E), uric acid, and finally beta-carotene. The authors of the study concluded that antioxidant levels in older women could be increased by beta-carotene supplementation.

Glutathione

Glutathione, working in concert with glutathione peroxidase, neutralizes hydrogen peroxide before it can be converted to the highly destructive hydroxyl radical. In addition to this crucial function, glutathione performs many other beneficial jobs in the body.

One of the most important of these functions involves its role in the immune system. In this role glutathione is essential for lymphocyte activation and proliferation. Where glutathione levels are altered, a corresponding alteration in T-cell performance is the result. This has been borne out by numerous studies, including that conducted by Fidelus and Tsan.

Using cultured spleen cells of mice, a rise in glutathione levels was effected in these cells by the use of substances such as N-acetylcysteine (NAC), which were known to bring about an elevation in glutathione levels. It was found that these elevated glutathione levels in turn brought about an enhanced proliferation in lymphocytes. Conversely, when the researchers effected a depletion of intracellular glutathione in these cells using a substance called buthionine sulfoximine, this glutathione depletion brought about a diminished proliferation in the lymphocytes.

Other studies (Smith, Yim, et al) have also demonstrated that inducing elevated levels of glutathione enhanced the proliferation of various T-cells, natural killer cells, and increased the production of IL-2.

Autoimmunity

The immune system is a war machine, where battles are carried out at the cellular and molecular level. The immune system prosecutes this war by seeking out foreign invaders, identifying them, and destroying them. It is able to do this because normally it is able to distinguish between the cells of the body it inhabits and protects, and cells that come from outside (or those that are potentially cancerous).

But in certain circumstances the identification process goes awry. It now begins to regard some cells of the body as it does antigens from without, and it develops autoantibodies to these cells, and autoantigen-specific T-cells. That is, it begins to attack some cells in its own body.

Where this autoimmunity is sufficiently pronounced, there is the incidence of autoimmune disease, which may take the form of systemic lupus erythematosis (SLE), and rheumatoid arthritis.

The Free Radical Factor

Research by Weisman and Weiser – and others – offers compelling evidence of free radical complicity in autoimmunity. These researchers demonstrated this by investigating the effects of antioxidants (vitamins A, C, E, and beta-carotene) in mice that had an autoimmune disorder resembling SLE. In the experiment antioxidant levels, and the levels for various immune factors, were measured at the outset for both the subject group and the control group. Their findings were as follows.

The supplemented mice had an increased mean survival of 26-28 weeks compared to 20-21 weeks for the control (unsupplemented) group. The control group developed some lymph node and spleen enlargement by 6-8 weeks, while the supplemented group did not. Immunoglobulin levels were markedly higher in the control group at 8 weeks of age, and at 20 weeks there was a reduction in the genetically driven antibody count. All of these results are indicative of a diminished autoantibody response in the supplemented mice, and the authors concluded that diets deficient in antioxidants can induce lupus-like syndromes.

Current research also indicts free radicals most strongly in cases of joint inflammation and rheumatoid arthritis.

Where immune complexes and bacterial products stimulate joint inflammation, they also activate neutrophils, and the resultant free radical production by the neutrophils. The free radicals generated then degrade components of the synovial fluid in the joint, which normally acts as a lubricant there. The free radicals are also able – albeit to a lesser extent – to degrade the collagen and elastin in the area of the affected joint.

There are other pathways as well that free radicals can use to cause tissue damage in the joints. The synovial fluid contains virtually no enzyme antioxidants (SOD, Cat, GPx), but it does have low levels of iron, where the iron is normally bound up and not harmful. However, in patients with rheumatoid arthritis, iron levels tend to be higher. Ischemia (impeded blood flow) resulting from the swelling in these joints may set in motion the production of superoxide radicals, which may then cause a release of iron from its bound up state. The iron, via the Fenton reaction, is then able to assist in the generation of hydroxyl radicals. This brings about further production of immune complexes, further neutrophil activation, and the entire process becomes a vicious cycle.

Nitric oxide, too, has been implicated in autoimmune disorders. Recent research by Weinberg et al produced results indicating most decidedly that increased nitric oxide production is a causative factor in the pathogenesis of autoimmunity.

Immune System Summary

The immune system is our defence against bacteria and viruses that come from the outside. It also defends us against cells that come from inside ourselves – the would-be cancer cells.

There are a number of organs and tissues that are a part of the immune system. The actual warriors are the leukocytes or white blood cells, and various proteins that serve as part of their weaponry. In addition, some immune cells produce free radicals as weapons against invaders such as bacteria. However, in addition to serving as weapons for some of the immune cells, free radicals also play a major role in the malfunctioning and decline of the immune system.

Besides damaging organs and tissues that produce the various immune warriors (and the proteins they employ in battling things like bacteria, viruses, and cancer cells), free radicals also damage the immune cells themselves, impairing their ability to defend us properly.

Free radicals also play a major role in autoimmunity, where immune cells end up attacking normal cells of the body as well as invaders from the outside. Where such autoimmunity is sufficiently pronounced, disorders such as lupus or rheumatoid arthritis are the result.

There is a substantial body of research detailing the many ways that antioxidants are able to counter free radical activity, and its damage to the immune system. Antioxidants prevent or reduce damage to parts of the immune system such as the thymus gland, and to the membranes of various immune cells as well. They also protect the glands of the endocrine system as well, slowing their decline as we approach middle age, which in turn slows the attendant decline of the immune system.

Numerous experiments with the vitamin antioxidants (A,C,E), as well as the carotenoids, have demonstrated the value of antioxidant supplementation in strengthening the immune system. Antioxidants will not only strengthen immune function in those who have not yet reached middle age, but will strengthen immune function when we need it the most – after middle age, when it tends to go into decline. Antioxidants have demonstrated that they can slow the decline in the immune system, and reduce its severity.

At a time when bacteria and viruses appear to be developing more and more virulent strains, maintaining a healthy and vigorous immune system would seem to be one of the best ways of holding them at bay.

The Ultimate Disease

There is one disease that is like no other. It is a disease which invariably predisposes us to other diseases, which inevitably weakens us and breaks us, and which drags us inexorably to the grave.

It takes our muscles and our sinews and it eats away at them and slackens them. It pumps us into bulges of fat. It sags our skin and scores it with wrinkles.

Where we were smooth it draws us into folds. Where we had lustre it makes us dull. Where we had vibrancy it leaves us slumped. Where we were warm it makes us cold, right to the bone. Where the bones were sturdy now they break. Where once we had life we are now brought to dying.

It is the ultimate disease. It is called aging.

It is the ultimate disease because it is irresistible. Against our will it tears us down, muscle by muscle and bone by bone. It is the ultimate disease because it comes to us all, big or small. There is no escaping it… or is there?

One Long Process

In a recent best seller "Tuesdays With Morrie", Morrie Schwartz – who is terminally ill – states that he wants to get out of bed for at least part of each day. It was his feeling that once you weren't able get out of bed, you were finished. Or as he put it, "When you're in bed, you're dead."

Samuel Butler put it this way: "Life is one long process of getting tired." We weaken and slow, and in the end we are too tired and too decrepit to get out of bed. And finally we succumb and pass into the eternal sleep.

Aging

The poet Shelley has said of it:

> The weariness, the fever, and the fret
> Here, where men sit and hear each other groan;

Where palsy shakes a few, sad, last grey hairs,
Where youth grows pale, and spectre-thin, and dies;
Where but to think is to be full of sorrow
And leaden-eyed despairs,
Where beauty cannot keep her lustrous eyes,
Or new love pine at them beyond tomorrow.

In times past, aging was not looked upon as a disease. But then, neither were the most conventional diseases. If we go back far enough, we find our forebears regarding diseases as evil spirits, or demons and the like.

But just as pioneers of a century or two back began to investigate conventional diseases, so too pioneers of today are investigating aging. And just as those early investigators were able to determine what gives rise to conventional diseases – at least to a considerable extent – so too are researchers of today coming to see what gives rise to aging. And just as many diseases of the past were brought under a fair measure of control, so too are the pioneers of today making solid headway in bringing the disease called aging under control. And just as early pioneers were able to defeat a number of the conventional diseases, so too the pioneers of today are striving to defeat this ultimate disease.

The Nature of the Beast

The research of the past two decades has shown that free radicals play a major role in the aging process. Free radicals can damage almost every part of a cell and almost every cell in the body.

Free radicals can attack the lipid (fatty) layers in the cell wall, setting in motion chain reactions where new radicals are formed to promote the chain reaction still further. Where left unchecked this can bring on the collapse and death of a cell, releasing this destructive mix to then go on and attack adjacent cells.

Free radicals can attack the lysosomes in cells, which are vacuoles or packets in which the cell stores enzymes. Where the enclosing membrane is breached, these enzymes are released and may easily cause enough damage to destroy a cell.

Free radicals are particularly active in the miniature power plants of cells, the mitochondria. In the production of energy, sugar is oxidized. In this stepwise process, electron transfers are involved, and occasionally an electron goes astray. These errant electrons are often snapped up by oxygen molecules that are on hand, giving rise to superoxide radicals, which are then armed and dangerous. And which are then ready to wreak havoc on the place of their birth, the mitochondria. With the accumulation of such damage, there is less energy produced in the cells, and less available for our daily activities. Inevitably comes the easy chair.

Some of the damage in the mitochondria may also be visited upon the mitochondrial DNA. In that circumstance, the message carried in the DNA may become scrambled, providing poor or garbled instructions as to the chemical workings in this part of the cell.

Perhaps the most insidious damage that free radicals can inflict upon us is that which they cause to the nucleus of a cell, and the precious DNA contained within. The DNA in the nucleus is the blueprint which encodes all the information necessary for the cell to function normally, and which also directs the crucial task of cell division. Where the DNA becomes damaged, it is as though a bottle of ink has been splashed over a page of the blueprints. In this circumstance, the information contained in the blueprint has now become unreadable. Where this happens all manner of incorrect information may be given to various chemical production lines in the cell.

One of these fouled transmissions may result in the construction of abnormal proteins. This will then give rise to faulty cell construction. In a worst case scenario, cell division itself is affected, and a cell may begin dividing out of control, passing on its maniacal message to each newly formed cell. And they too will continue dividing out of control, passing on still further the same destructive message. The end results here are diseases like cancer.

Protein Damage

Free radical activity, which impacts negatively on sugar metabolism, is also conducive to the formation of damaged proteins. These damaged proteins, called advance glycation end products or AGEs, are the result of sugar (glucose) reacting with proteins, producing damaged proteins. These damaged proteins in turn may undergo a cross-linkage, which then provides a faulty, less flexible structure in various tissues. Where this occurs in connective tissue such as collagen or elastin in the skin, it makes the skin more brittle, less supple. More seriously, where this increasing rigidity occurs in tissues of the heart, a loss of elasticity will also mean a loss of function.

AGEs also contribute to the formation of cataracts, and the formation of plaque on arterial walls. In addition, they have also been cited as a factor in joint problems, such as arthritis, and even in some of the brain deterioration that occurs in Alzheimer's disease. And all of these effects are part and parcel of aging. And remember as organs like skin become impaired through the buildup of lipofuscin (protein and lipid oxidized "age spots"), the aging process becomes further accelerated.

In very broad strokes, these are some of the ways free radicals damage our cells. And when they damage our cells, they damage ourselves. And through this damage they accelerate the aging process.

Second Nature

If inflicting various kinds of cellular damage is the nature of the beast, rendering this damage cumulative is second nature. Because this damage does not just happen and then disappear. It accumulates, especially later in life.

In our younger years free radicals are at lower levels generally, and antioxidants at higher levels. Anabolism outstrips catabolism and the body's repair faculties are capable of effecting considerable damage control. We heal more easily.

But all of this changes as we get into our thirties and beyond. Now free radicals come into ascendancy, and antioxidants begin to decline. And where the cellular damage was once insignificant and easily repaired by the body, now it is not.

Now the damage begins to accumulate. What was once microscopic is now macroscopic. What was once unnoticeable is now unmistakable: that first grey hair; the hint of a wrinkle around the eyes; that little roll around the abdomen that persists and seems to be taking up permanent residence there; and so on. The imperceptible has now become all too perceptible

At this point the tide has turned, and we now find ourselves being carried off beyond our will, slipping away on the ebbing tide of our youth, swept along on the flow of the ultimate disease. We are being drawn out to the sea of old age, and once we are out there, we know we can never make it back.

A Quantum Leap

These are some of the ways in which heightened free radical activity can age us, taking us along the "normal" pathways of aging, one molecule at a time, one cell at a time, one wrinkle at a time, one day at a time. And for a number of years we hardly notice it. But free radicals have another way of aging us, one which bumps us along into aging by a quantum leap. And it does this by promoting the occurrence of other diseases.

Most of us, often during childhood, have seen a grandparent (or an aunt or uncle) who has just got out of hospital. And we were shocked. For they now looked so thin and slow, so ashen and weak

It may have been only a matter of weeks or months since we had seen them last, but now they looked a decade older. Or more. And although they may have recovered from the disease and were back at home, they looked ghastly. And where they may have recovered a little further at home, they still never came close to how they were before. The disease had taken its toll. It had bumped them along the aging curve by a quantum leap.

And that is often the way aging proceeds: minuscule changes at the cellular and sub-cellular level through our thirties and forties, where we only gradually see the slight indications telling us that we are no longer young. But it is where these small changes lead to disease that the aging process is thrown into fast forward. Where free radical activity brings about plaque-lined arteries, for example, we have an increasingly impeded blood flow as time slips by. This impeded blood flow will then have its own impact on other organs and tissues, gradually impairing their function, each in its own way inching us along the aging curve.

And then at some point these small changes induce a

larger change, one wherein the aging process takes a quantum leap.

In the case of a heart attack, for instance, we may be going about our daily activities as usual, and then slowly awaken to the hum of a large building, and when we open our eyes we find we are in a white room, and we have a number of tubes sticking into us.

After the surgery, or whatever other treatments we have had administered unto us, we are eventually well enough to go home. But from that point on we are rarely the same. Often we move more slowly, we react more slowly. But there is one thing that has moved more quickly, and that is time. When we look in the mirror we see that we have aged by a quantum leap.

That is the way it works. And not just for heart disease, but for many diseases. Some, like diabetes, will age us more quickly, but at a gradual pace, robbing us of our vision, our mobility, our freedom from pain by degrees. And then somewhere along the way it can hit us with a quantum leap, where we are forced to have a limb amputated, for example.

Afflictions like stroke are another example, because a stroke may also slam us into a quantum leap along the aging process from out of the blue, like an unseen uppercut. And virtually all of these conditions will accelerate us into old age. And virtually all are aided and abetted by free radical activity.

It is a merciless cycle. Aging promotes disease. Disease promotes aging. And free radical activity promotes them both.

Expressway to Old Age

So it is that from middle age onward, due in considerable measure to the damage inflicted by free radicals, we begin the acceleration towards old age.

By then many of our organs have sustained a certain amount of damage and our repair systems are beginning to fail. Even our immune defences are now beginning to weaken, leaving us ever more vulnerable. And it is around this point that the antioxidant levels tend to decline, while free radical activity – given even more of a free hand – propels us ever more quickly toward the cane, the walker, and the home.

We are now picking up speed, approaching full throttle along the expressway to old age.

Getting Off the Expressway

There are a number of things we can do to get off the expressway to old age. We can steer ourselves to an off ramp. Once off the expressway we may not come to a complete stop toward the old age destination, but at least we will be on a slower road – something of a back road, providing a much happier and healthier ride. And this road is the antioxidant highway.

There are literally thousands of studies attesting to the involvement of free radicals in promoting both disease and aging, and to the effectiveness of antioxidants in their prevention or amelioration. When we increase our antioxidants we will reduce the chances of contracting disease, and we will greatly reduce the free radical damage that hastens our arrival into old age.

Preventive Maintenance

Allowing free radicals free reign to inflict their damage, and allowing the damage to accumulate, is something like never tending to your car's engine. Where oil changes are never done, or done too infrequently, sludge and grit begin to build up. The oil becomes dirty and thinner, and less capable of properly lubricating the moving parts. And where the engine is never given a tune-up, things like the fuel filter become clogged, and the spark plugs become coated and don't fire as well. Over time the engine begins missing and running rough. It loses its zip, it creeps away from the stop sign, often lurching and bucking. And when you are in a car like this it feels like you are in one of the old test planes buffeting and battling through the sound barrier – and you are doing all of twenty miles per hour.

If left without oil changes or tune-ups for too long, the problems in the engine become severe. The valves wear, the piston rings wear, everything wears. After a time the car is burning oil, billowing dark smoke. The engine is knocking and passengers jokingly ask why you don't answer it. And soon it is prone to stalling altogether.

If the lack of preventive maintenance goes on indefinitely the engine eventually dies, and it has to go into the shop for a complete motor overhaul. At this point the mechanics have to remove the motor from the car – a major job in itself – take it apart, and then completely rebuild the inner components. Welcome to the field of surgery.

The Owner's Manual

Had the owner's of the above car followed the owner's manual they would have taken the car in for regular oil changes and tune-ups. The engine would have lasted twice or three times as long before needing serious work. And it would likely have had a lifespan that also was twice or three times as long.

In human terms, allowing free radicals to damage the body means that we allow a certain "biosludge" to build up in it. We allow the oxidative processes to produce excesses of "biorust". We allow parts of the body to become worn more quickly. So that in places like the joints, for example, then the insulating sacs or bursa become worn down, and we get bone scraping against bone – the "biogrind".

The power plants of the cells also become impaired – something along the lines of the spark plugs in the car becoming coated – and we find we have much less energy.

Over time all this cellular and sub-cellular damage accumulates, and it ages us much sooner than need be. And then finally we have a heart attack or stroke, or come down with liver disease or lung disease, and we have to go into the shop. Only we are not going in for a tune-up, we are going in for a major overhaul.

When we get out of the shop we will not likely be capable of the performance we formerly had. And we will now likely need considerable maintenance just to get along. And our chances of reaching a normal lifespan – and enjoying a number of vigorous decades more – is drastically reduced.

Like the car engine that was allowed to go to ruin, we will now be limited to lurching and poking along – for as long as we can. And then it's off to the crusher. Many of us may be too busy to properly care for our cars but we must care for our cells.

Extending The Lifespan

During these halting, shuffle-along years, we will almost certainly lament not having taken better care of ourselves, of not following the owner's manual. And for many, there will not even be the awareness that there is an owner's manual.

But there is an owner's manual. And in the concluding chapters of this book we will provide the equivalence of an owner's manual for human beings – a manual for health, life, and longevity.

And a significant part of this manual will deal with antioxidants. We cannot promise that a healthy intake of antioxidants will allow you to live forever. But maintaining optimal levels of antioxidants will, we are confident, add a good decade or two to your life – decades of greater health and vigor. And if other parts of the manual are followed as well, another twenty or thirty years of healthy living should also be possible. With this extra time a further payoff comes about. Because now these extra decades allow another factor to come into play – that of future discoveries.

In North America we have seen the human lifespan almost double in the past hundred years. And the discoveries of the past two or three decades are nothing short of remarkable, both in the field of anti-aging, and in others. From looking at what is on the horizon, we are certain that even more amazing discoveries lie in wait for us. Research on hormone replacement, on telomeres (the tips on the ends of chromosomes), on the chromosomes and genes themselves – all hark to breakthroughs that will extend our lives still further, in some cases perhaps by even greater lengths of time. Which will then allow us to continue on still further with our lives, and to avail ourselves of even more outguessed-at discoveries taking place in the intermediate future. And beyond that? Well, it certainly tempts one to tantalizing contemplations.

And to reach that point all we have to do is follow the owner's manual. It will allow us to get off the road to ruin, off the expressway to old age, and to meander into the new pathway of antioxidant supplementation.

SECTION VI

Total Health

"There is overwhelming scientific evidence demonstrating that those of us who eat a diet rich in antioxidants and take antioxidant supplements will live longer, healthier lives."

–Dr. Lester Packer

"Every day you do one of two things: build health or produce disease in yourself."

–Adelle Davis

"Our remedies oft in ourselves do lie Which we ascribe to heaven."

–Shakespeare (All's Well That Ends Well)

"Rule youth well, for old age will rule itself."

–An Old Adage

"You're never too old to become younger."

–Mae West

"No matter how well we eat, it's not possible to get adequate nutrition."

–Toronto Globe and Mail, (July 2002)

Total Health

DIET AND EXERCISE

The word "diet" may be a four letter word, but then so are the words "food" or "love". And for all of the negative associations with the word "diet", its principle meaning merely indicates a particular regime of foodstuffs being consumed. So, where individuals are regularly consuming gobs of suet and other saturated fats, and are regularly taking in 4,000 calories per day, that is still their diet.

But the word has also assumed a different connotation, and now has an additional meaning. As is implied in the dreaded phrase "on a diet". In this usage the word implies a regime of food intake that is acutely restricted as to calories, foodstuffs, or both. And in this usage, the word strikes fear into the most intrepid of hearts.

FATal

The reason the "diet" word is so dreaded is because many North Americans are overweight, and constantly feel that they should be on a diet (in the second sense of the word). And the reasons they feel that they should be dieting are twofold: esthetics and health. They know they will look better if they drop those extra pounds. And they know they will be healthier. Because fat is fatal. Or ultimately it can be.

Fat is especially bad where it accumulates around the abdomen, because fat stored here carries the greatest health risks. It is this fat that tends to give one the shape of Tweedledum. And since it is dangerous and dumb to allow fat to accumulate here we have come to refer to it as Tweedledumb fat.

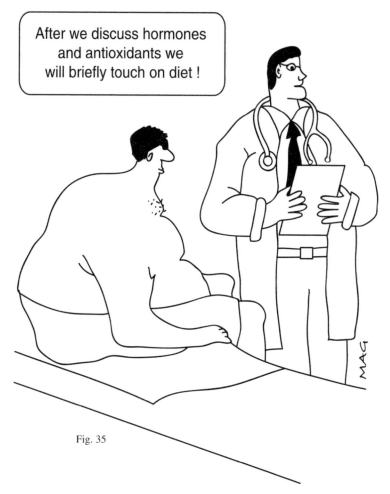

Fig. 35

Obesity tends to correlate with an increased risk for numerous health problems including cardiovascular disease, breast cancer, colorectal cancer, diabetes, etc.. Most people today are acutely – or at least vaguely – aware of the risks associated with obesity. Also, they want to look good in a swim suit or jeans. And in battling obesity they are constantly trying the latest fad diet.

Stopping The Yo-Yo

A common course for many overweight individuals is to overeat and to eat unwisely. And then to diet severely for a short period. And to repeat this kind of cycle endlessly .

The pounds go up, the pounds go down, over and over again. The yo-yo effect. With the yo-yo effect a person is forever trying to catch up, to make it to their ideal weight. Unfortunately, with each upswing the overweight condition tends to accentuate. The upper limit tends to become higher and higher, making it that much more discouraging through the dieting phase of the cycle.

Far better results have been obtained where, instead of forever trying to catch up, overweight individuals change their eating habits, and then try to maintain the improved habits indefinitely. They change their patterns to something they can live with on a daily basis, and the pattern becomes ongoing. Through these new patterns they lose the weight more slowly, but eventually they do arrive at their ideal weight. From then on it is simply a matter of maintaining that weight, of keeping up instead of forever trying to catch up.

They have stopped the yo-yo.

Habits

A habit is a behavioral pattern that is formed by frequent repetition. Once a habit is well established, the behavior involved often takes place with hardly a thought. This applies to good habits as well as to bad habits.

We tend to associate this kind of pattern more often with bad habits. We see it where people reach for a cigarette without even thinking about it. Or where someone orders a burger simply as a matter of course. And it's because they are so accustomed to doing so.

But it is equally possible to develop good habits, good behavioral patterns, where we can do something positive without giving it a thought. Almost all of us who drive cars have at one time or another been at the wheel thinking about something, and suddenly realize that we have been driving for miles without paying any attention to the actual driving. And only an occurrance out of the ordinary has returned our attention to the road once more, and to the matter of driving. We both discourage the use of cell phones while driving.

The point here is that if a pattern of desired behavior can be developed so that eventually it occurs almost without a thought, then it is worth the effort in establishing such a behavioral pattern. Because once established, the beneficial behavior will take place without effort or discomfort. Or very little, anyway. Because once the good habit is established it is like we are on automatic pilot.

Two Birds With One Stone

We began this section with a mention about obesity because obesity is often the obvious and most visible sign of poor eating patterns. Another aspect of poor eating patterns does not advertise itself so openly, and this aspect has to do with the inadequate intake of antioxidants. However, the two often go hand in hand. Because frequently, the two are a result of a less than ideal diet.

As a result we are often able to kill two birds with one stone. If we alter our eating patterns intelligently so as to lose weight, we will usually increase our intake of antioxidants as well. Conversely, if we adopt a diet that increases our antioxidant intake, we may also use it to lose weight, or to maintain an ideal weight.

However, a person does not have to be overweight to have less than optimal levels of antioxidants. In fact, most

North Americans, including those who are lean, tend to have an insufficient intake of antioxidants, and it shows in their antioxidant profiles that we do in our clinics. It also shows in the diseases to which they are prone.

Very often, the low antioxidant profile will be indicative of a less than ideal diet, whether a person is overweight or not. As a consequence, improving the antioxidant levels for anyone through the foods they eat will almost certainly improve their diet in other ways. Pursuant to that, at the end of this section we will include a list of the antioxidants we have looked at in this book, and some of the better sources for them.

But before looking at ways of improving our antioxidant intake specifically, it will be helpful in taking a cursory look at nutrition in general.

Nutritional Overview

It is rare that any person's diet in North America will be lacking in carbohydrates. However, carbohydrates do come in different guises, and we would do well to eschew those of little value, such as candy or sugar. These are "empty" calories and provide little else besides calories. And the added sugar in our bodies is conducive to the production of advanced glycation end products, or AGEs.

However when we ingest carbohydrates in the form of whole grains and whole grain products, as well as in fruits and vegetables, along with the calories we get the other nutritional benefits these foods confer, including vitamins, phytonutrients, fiber, protein, and antioxidants.

Protein is another essential component to an ideal diet. Here again, for the average North American, protein deficiency in the diet is not a frequent occurrence. And where it does occur, it is often less the consequence of need, but of choice: too many sweets or too much junk food, and no cottage cheese, meat, or suitable vegetables.

Protein is made up of amino acids, and like carbohydrates, protein also comes in varying guises. There are amino acids which our bodies cannot produce and which are essential for good health. Fittingly, they are called the essential amino acids. Protein sources such as meat, tofu, and cottage cheese supply all the essential amino acids, and are referred to as complete proteins, while those sources that do not are called incomplete proteins.

For those who do not eat meat or dairy products, the essential amino acids must be obtained from plant sources, which in proper combination are able to supply all the essential amino acids. By combining such complementary sources such as certain beans, nuts and grains, all the essential amino acids may be obtained and the protein needs of vegetarians may thus be met.

In North America getting too much protein may be a greater problem than not getting enough. There is evidence that getting too much protein may be harmful to both joints and kidneys. By too much we mean greater than 45% for some.

Once protein needs are met the next consideration is that of source. Where we obtain our protein then becomes the important question. There is a difference between the protein in a fried hamburger and that in a lean grilled steak. And the difference is fat. To be sure, the protein in both meats is of similar composition, but a fried hamburger will usually come with a great deal more fat than is found in a similar weight of lean steak. Obviously, choosing our protein sources wisely so that we get all the essential amino acids, while at the same time minimizing the animal fat intake, is of signal importance.

There is much controversy about the amount of protein,

carbohydrate and fat the ideal diet should contain. The Barry Sears "Zone Diet" had everyone arguing over percentages to stay in the "Zone". With the heart problems experienced recently by Dr. Robert Atkins, the champion of the high fat, high protein "Dr. Atkin's Diet", the rival diet gurus are jockeying for position on the best seller list. The Mediterranean diet is gaining ground again with the American public promoting more fruit, vegetables, olive oils (hormonally neutral) and light on the meat and possibly wine with meals.

Paleo (Stone Age) Diet

More than 60 % of Americans are overweight and there seems to be no end in sight to this dilemma. Centuries ago, only the wealthy could attain the overweight status by eating more than their share of food. Most doctors now agree on the importance of diet and are referring more of their patients to dieticians for a variety of disorders now, not just the usual diabetes and bowel disorders. Unfortunately there is a wide range of opinion regarding the proper diet for the future. I have had many an argument about the benefits of high protein diets with the establishment. Pushing the idea of "glycemic index" of carbohydrates (sugars) was a difficult task but is now recognized as an important tool for controlling diabetes and obesity. The information flies into the face of the food processors and bucks the trend of Western fast food market. It certainly is difficult to provide fresh fruit, vegetables and low fat wild meat to our population but we will have to do our best. Brad King has done an excellent job in his book "Fat Wars" of explaining the rationale of the "Paleo Diet" which essentially is a diet similar to what our relatives of 5000 years ago would eat. Our genetics that evolved over millions of years did not prepare us for the quick drastic changes that we have made to our diets and subsequently we are having trouble coping with our obesity and

Insulin resistant Type 2 Diabetes that is endemic in America.

Our diet today is deficient in protein, with the average American getting about 15% protein, 35 % fat and 50% carbohydrates as a daily source. Some of you ask and say that since we eat so many calories, do we not get enough protein by eating more. The answer is partially true but the type of protein that we take in is unhealthy. The high glycemic carbohydrates (quickly digesting sugars) interfere by causing obesity by Insulin overproduction and the scarcity of good omega 3 fats in our meat causes more problems by elevating low density cholesterols. It has been estimated that 5000 years ago, the ideal diet would be made up of 30% calories from protein, 35% from fat and 35% from carbohydrate but different forms of each. And this is what has caused the confusion with dieting. It may not matter what percentages we choose of the typical foods available to us, the change will have to be in our new selection of foods.

The Secret of Fish

In the Diet and Reinfarction Trial (DART) it was shown that eating fish in 3 meals per week improved survival in post heart attack patients when compared to controls in Britain. Thus the British paradox involving fish and chips and English tea showing favorable health benefits. The fatty acids in fish are linolenic acids, eicosapentaenoic acid (EPA) and docosahexaenoic acid (DHA). North Americans eat more saturated fats from meat and linoleic acid from corn and safflower oil which is converted to arachidonic acid. Arachidonic acid converts by the enzyme COX (cyclo-oxygenase) into inflammatory eicosanoids (locally acting hormones) that promote clotting. If the COX is activated in the blood vessels by damage, then EPA and DHA if they are present will convert to good eicosanoids and prevent clotting and further blockage in the arteries.

Essential Fatty Acids

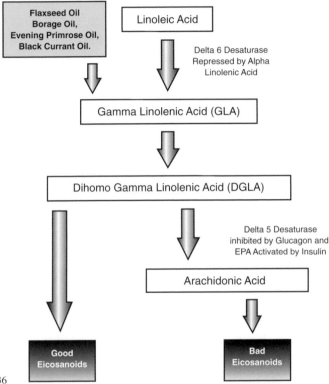

Fig. 36

Fish oils will provide the good eicosanoids this way and this is why the Japanese and Scandinavians do well with fish diets. The fish oils also reduce the levels of triglycerides, relax coronary arteries, reduce the cytokines (inflammatory mediators) in the blood vessels and reduce irregular heart rhythms. The National Institute of Health recommends 650 mg of EPA per day and that is equal to a small fish each day! In a Danish study, fish providing omega-3 fatty acids conferred protection from preterm delivery and low birth weight when 8,729 women were followed in pregnancy. But remember the dangers of mercury present in some seafoods and a study from the University of Illinois in June 2001 presented the concern about Great Lake's fish with high PCBs impairing memory in elderly subjects.

The essential fatty acids (EFAs) are not produced by humans and therefore omega-6 and omega-3 fatty acids must be taken in the diet. Too much omega-6 (common in our diet) may lead to cell proliferation and increase the chance of cancer. Decreased levels of omega-3 fatty acids can lead to less dopamine synthesis and altered serotonin function progressing to depression. One study by Adams in Lipids 1996, 31 showed a correlation of severity of depression to lower omega-3/omega-6 ratios.

Eschew, Less Chew

From this brief overview, two points are apparent. The first is that since foodstuffs come in various forms, we are well advised to choose not the dismal but the optimal – complex carbohydrates like whole grains, fruits, and vegetables, instead of sugar, sugar, sugar; lean protein instead of fatty protein; and unsaturated fat instead of saturated fat.

The second point is that we would do well to choose carefully our fat and oils in general, and if we are overweight, take in less calories than we have been. Eschew means less chew. If we eschew certain foods and cut back on the total, we will not only be on the road to greater health in general, we will also be exploring the miracle of antioxidants.

Refuse, Rechoose, Revitalize

An old proverb says: "Enough is as good as a feast." In actuality, enough is probably better than a feast, for there is another proverb that says: "Gluttony kills more than does the sword." The implication is that we will almost certainly be healthier if we eat only enough, and not too much.

In the matter of cutting down on the garbage and waste we produce, and by reconfiguring the ways in which we deal with our wastes, our society has adopted the motto: Reduce, Reuse, Recycle. If we wish to reconfigure our eating habits we might adopt a similar motto: Refuse, Rechoose, Revitalize.

Refuse

Where any foodstuff offers little by way of nutrition and much by way of potential harm, we would do well to refuse it – refuse it at the supermarket, at restaurants, and at home.

We would not guzzle down a pint of palm oil for lunch, and yet we do just that when we order fatty foods. It may take a few lunches rather than just one, but the result is not appreciably different – we pack on more Tweedledumb fat. We provide the raw material for plaque to form and line our arteries. And after such meals we tend to feel heavy, sluggish, and lethargic.

Certainly, some proper fat will not harm us, and neither will some sugar or salt – especially if we are keeping active physically, where we burn the sugar and fat away through exercise, and sweat the salt out. But for the most part, these are foods we should frequently and regularly refuse because they are overabundant in our society. And it is much easier to do if we employ the second part of our new motto. The 11th European Congress on Obesity held in Vienna May 2001 stated that 30-40% of all cancers stem from excessive weight, not to mention leading to diabetes and cardiovascular disease.

Rechoose

In refusing certain foods on a regular basis it is not necessary to leave their place on our plate empty. We can fill this space with something better. We can rechoose.

We can cook with oils like canola oil or olive oil instead of butter or lard. We can rechoose our meats for leaner cuts, and grill them rather than fry them. We can more often choose lean chicken or fish rather than red fatty meat, and choose fish that give us the omega 3 fatty acids. And we can even rechoose our menus so that some of the time we have no meat at all, using cottage cheese, yogurt, tofu, and the like instead. Try it again!

Such rechoosing need not compromise taste. There are thousands of cookbooks out there, with many thousands of delicious recipes. It is now eminently possible to have the words healthy and tasty go together.

We can rechoose our carbohydrates, cooking wild rice rather than white or brown. Or have whole grain cereals or oatmeal rather than those with stripped down grains. Because, in many of the stripped down products, components like the germ or bran have been removed, and in their place dyes, preservatives, and other additives have been substituted. Recently there has been concern about the cancer causing substance acrylamide, found in carbohydrates baked at high temperatures. Foods like crackers, puffed rice cereals, potato fries, crisps and potato chips have high levels of acrylamide and the World Health Organization has appointed a committee to study the effects of this known carcinogen on all of us.

We can also rechoose our grains from time to time, exploring the possibilities of using grains like barley, rye, oats or quinoa in recipes. We can try new recipes using pulses such as peas, beans, or lentils.

Most particularly we can rechoose the emphasis placed on certain foods in our diet, increasing the quantity and variety of fruits and vegetables. More and more, the research is showing that we obtain a host of benefits by taking this simple step alone.

In rechoosing a diet based on some of the above considerations, we will at the same time be increasing greatly our intake of those marvelous antioxidants. In a word, we will revitalize our diet.

Revitalize

By refusing certain foods, and by rechoosing our foods, we will at the same time revitalize our diet. We will enjoy foods that have a greater vitality to them, and they will bring a greater vitality to our lives. Much of this vitality will derive from the many nutritious aspects of the foods themselves. But a great deal of this vitality will also derive from the added antioxidants they give us.

Reducing the fat intake will revitalize us by cutting down on calories, and by cutting down on the bad cholesterol that tends to choke the artery walls. Limiting our caloric intake may increase the lifespan. Such a step will also cut down on the Tweedledumb fat that accumulates around the midsection, as well as that which pads the posterior. Over time, this simple step will have us looking better, feeling lighter, and moving about with a greater ease.

When we substitute some of the animal fats with omega 3 fats such as are found in various fish or flax seed oil, we will increase our vitality still further by reducing the bad cholesterol and triglycerides in our system.

By replacing starchy foods with lower glycemic carbohydrates like whole grain foods, we will take in more vitamins and minerals, some of which will also do double duty as antioxidants. Also, these will better supply the body with nutrients needed in its general physiological needs, including manufacturing glutathione and the enzyme antioxidants.

Such will also be the case where we have increased the quantity and variety of fruits and vegetables in our diet. This, along with cutting down on saturated fats, will do more to revitalize our diet, and ourselves, than all the fad diets put together.

Vegetarians

Most of us, at one time or another, have known or been acquainted with a vegetarian. (They are not as rare as they used to be.) And we may have been struck with the lightness and gentleness they possess. True vegans avoid all food of animal origin; Lacto-ovo-vegetarians may eat eggs and dairy but Ovo-vegetarians eat eggs but not dairy products. Fruitarianism, raw foodism, pesco and pollo vegans are some of the new diet variants.

Many of us will also have observed the radiant glow frequently seen in pregnant women and that comes from hormone change of pregnancy. Now vegetarians have to be experts in the diet business to maintain all their nutrients. Many will be deficient in iron, coenzyme Q-10, folic acid, zinc and vitamin B12.

Now, by vegetarian we are not talking about dilettantes – like the Haight-Ashbury hippies of the sixties, or others – who made claims like having lived on nothing but peanut butter for a month, or subscribed to other fad diets of this sort. What we are talking about are those who have educated themselves about nutrition, and have embarked upon a sensible dietary regime. And often it shows in their calmness, in their leaness, and frequently in the very lightness of their being. And hopefully with a diet rich in spinach, seeds, nuts, prunes and whole grains with flaxseed oil there will be little chance of deficiencies but a low cholesterol and low blood sugar.

With much less dedication, and much less detailed knowledge, we can achieve virtually the same healthy results by adding a few supplements like folate and CoQ-10. That is, like the vegetarians, we will incorporate more fruits and vegetables into our diet. Unlike the vegetarians, we will still allow ourselves a certain amount of meat protein – in quantities not excessive, and in cuts well chosen.

Fruits and Vegetables

The traditional Chinese or Japanese diet of a hundred years ago is probably very close to what we would recommend today: only a little of the dairy products; a little lean meat; a certain amount of fish; and a preponderance of whole grains, fruits, and vegetables. And in keeping with the traditional Japanese diet, we would recommend a certain amount of cooked tofu as well.

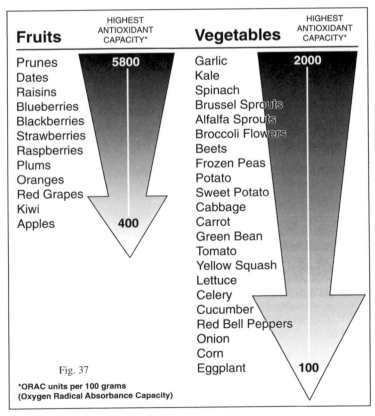

Fruits	HIGHEST ANTIOXIDANT CAPACITY*	Vegetables	HIGHEST ANTIOXIDANT CAPACITY*
Prunes	5800	Garlic	2000
Dates		Kale	
Raisins		Spinach	
Blueberries		Brussel Sprouts	
Blackberries		Alfalfa Sprouts	
Strawberries		Broccoli Flowers	
Raspberries		Beets	
Plums		Frozen Peas	
Oranges		Potato	
Red Grapes		Sweet Potato	
Kiwi		Cabbage	
Apples	400	Carrot	
		Green Bean	
		Tomato	
		Yellow Squash	
		Lettuce	
		Celery	
		Cucumber	
		Red Bell Peppers	
		Onion	
		Corn	
Fig. 37		Eggplant	100

*ORAC units per 100 grams
(Oxygen Radical Absorbance Capacity)

Antioxidant Capacity of Fruits and Vegetables

Even today, out in the countryside in China and Japan, where the traditional diet is adhered to, there is a greatly diminished incidence of the cardiovascular diseases and cancers that are so prevalent in North America. And that is because such diets provide the many nutritional benefits that confer health and longevity – including a host of antioxidants that are part of it.

The antioxidant capacity of fruit and vegetables has traditionally been measured in ORAC units (Oxygen Radical Absorbance Capacity) per 100 grams of the food. As seen from our table of ORAC units for common fruits and vegetables, the fruits are more powerful as antioxidants but don't be discouraged by your lack of garlic in your diet because 1 ounce of carrots will equal 1 clove of garlic for antioxidant capacity (minus the odor). Americans on average eat up to 1 lb. of garlic per year while the Asians eat up to 25 lbs. of garlic per year.

Although the meat, fish, and grains all bring their own nutritional benefits, it is in the fruits and vegetables that the broad range of vitality is to be found. And the broad range of antioxidants. Their life giving vitality of fruits and vegetables can almost be seen in the sheen of their skins, in their peels, and in their vibrant colors. Besides being a feast for the eyes, they are a banquet for the body as a whole.

In addition to all of their nutritive qualities, fruits and vegetables also provide us with roughage. Roughage is a factor that is little thought of as a dietary benefit, and yet it is of great value. It is roughage that keeps the muscles of the digestive tract well toned, for it gives these muscles something to work on. Just by being there, roughage reduces the transit time of food through the digestive tract. This allows the body to more quickly clear some of the potentially harmful by-products of digestion. The consequence of this is a reduced risk for disease like diverticulosis and perhaps colorectal cancer by future studies.

Although fruits and vegetables provide us with vitamins, minerals, enzymes, phytonutrients, and roughage – as well as a wealth of antioxidants – they do have one negative aspect – their reputation. At worst they may be remembered from childhood as those terrible things that mother made us eat, and at best as simply being dull. Yet nothing could be further from the truth. And in coming to enjoy them, and more of them, sometimes all we have to do is re-educate our taste buds.

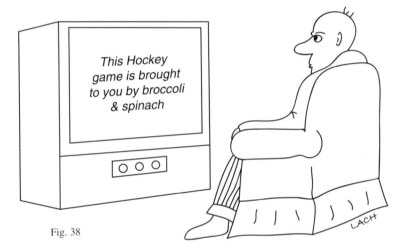

This Hockey game is brought to you by broccoli & spinach

Fig. 38

A sponsor unlikely to be seen!

For The First Time

Altering our diet does not have to be regarded as some kind of insurmountable challenge, or a life sentence. Rather, we might wish to look upon it as the start of a wonderful journey – a journey filled with new taste sensations and new culinary discoveries.

Incorporating health giving foods into our diet does not have to put us in mind of meals served in a dungeon, devoid of flavor and leaving us perpetually hungry. In fact the complete opposite is true.

There was a commercial on TV some years back for a particular kind of cereal flakes that enjoined us to taste them again for the first time. We might want to try this sort of approach for incorporating more fruits and vegetables (and whole grains) into our diet. Most fruits and vegetables are rich with flavor – all we have to do is taste them again for the first time – to re-educate our taste buds.

Re-educating The Taste Buds

For instance, if you have not tried biting into a red or green pepper by itself, we suggest you do so, just as a trial. They are crispy, succulent, and tangy, and you may find that you actually like them. You may find that to be the case for a great many other fruits and vegetables as well.

Give them a tryout, raw or cooked, as is appropriate. There are thousands of ways of incorporating them into a meal so that they add their own wonderful flavors to a harmonic whole. The same can be done with various cereal grains such as rice, barley, bulgar, and the like.

There are a great many herbs and spices – all waiting to add their intriguing flavors to your taste buds. And there are literally thousands of cookbooks out there too, all waiting to guide you in the use of herbs, spices, and other flavoring agents. Ask around, experiment, find which recipes tickle your taste buds. There is an entire universe to be discovered – and its right there in your kitchen.

One important consideration to keep in mind is freshness. Fresh fruits and vegetables are best, and home grown are best of all. Those succulent, juicy tomatoes grown in the back yard have so much more flavor than do those that have been bred for their ability to withstand shipping. And the research has shown that they are far more nutritious. That will be most likely be the case for other vegetables as well.

There has recently been released, the top 10 foods for health and longevity:

1) Broccoli-contains sulphoraphane, indole-3-carbinol, vitamin C, carotenes

2) Spinach-loaded with iron, folate, lutein and zeaxanthin

3) Nuts-antioxidant ellagic acid, vitamin E, polyunsaturated fats

4) Tomatoes-corotenoid lycopene released when cooked and with olive oil

5) Oats-contain tocotrienols, fibre and beta-glucan to bind fats in bowel

6) Green tea-full of polyphenols like catechins (less cancer in the East)

7) Blueberries-flavonoids like anthocyanins like huckleberry and bilberry

8) Garlic-allyl sulfide and other phytochemicals decrease fats and clots

9) Salmon-omega-3 fatty acids decrease inflammation joints and brain

10) Red wine-polyphenols (resveratrol) raises HDL and inhibits endothelin 1

A Rule of Thumb

It is a simple rule of thumb: a varied and healthy diet along the lines of what we have described above will also provide a veritable feast of antioxidants. So it is that when we fill our table with a wide variety of fresh, unprocessed food-stuffs, we will provide ourselves with a wide variety of antioxidants as well. And in providing our bodies with elevated levels of antioxidants, we will also provide them with the means of countering the destructive activity of free radicals within.

There is a mountain of research showing that free radicals play an important role in predisposing us to many serious diseases, and are complicit in their development. The research also shows that antioxidants, in combating and neutralizing free radicals, play a major role in preventing these diseases. And for those who have already contracted the diseases, antioxidants are often able to limit the severity of their impact and ameliorate the intensity of their symptoms.

The role played by antioxidants in keeping us healthy has a wonderful spillover into another important area of our lives: they help keep us young. Antioxidants are able to hold back the gnarled grip of the aging process, thereby deferring and delaying it. Perhaps as important, antioxidants have the potential of making our latter decades much less burdened with the infirmities common to those later years. They have the capacity of helping us live longer and live stronger.

Supplements

In attaining an optimal level of antioxidants in the body, there are many who may only achieve this through the use of supplements

For instance, some antioxidants – such as vitamin E or lipoic acid – would require that we consume inordinate quantities of butter or oils or meats in obtaining optimal levels of them. In such instances, dietary means alone are not practical and may not suffice.

Certainly, we may take in sufficient quantities of such antioxidants to keep us going. But most of us are seeking more than that. We would like to attain optimal quantities of antioxidants so as to keep ourselves disease free and youthful.

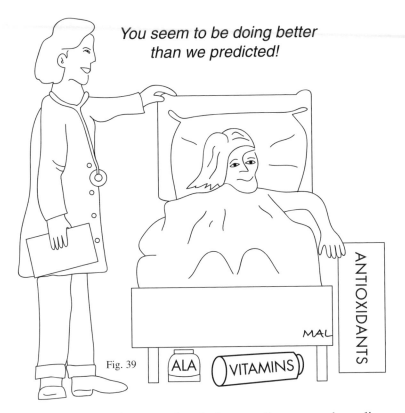

Fig. 39

For those who may already have a disease, such as diabetes or arthritis, the need for antioxidants may be quite pronounced. People in this circumstance will want to maximize certain antioxidants that have been shown to have positive benefits in helping them battle their conditions. So here too supplements will be of strong benefit.

There are also those approaching middle age, who typically exhibit decreased levels of antioxidants, and higher levels of free radical activity. They too may desire supplements to help nature correct this imbalance.

Those who are getting along in years often do not absorb nutrients as well as they used to. (The digestive tract ages along with the rest of us.) They too are candidates for antioxidant supplementation.

For those who cut back on their food intake in order to lose weight, there will also be an accompanying reduction in antioxidants, so these people too may wish to consider taking supplements during their period of dieting, and perhaps afterwards.

There are other ways as well in which people may be coming up short of an ideal antioxidant intake. Those whose diet has a large proportion of processed foods may fall into this category, since processed foods often have much of their nutritional richness stripped away. Busy people who are always on the run and who eat out a lot will often fall short of the mark in their antioxidant intake. Or those who eat the same foods week in and week out – their antioxidant consumption will likely be limited both as to quantity and diversity.

Canned food, fast food, junk food – where these make up a significant part of the diet, there will likely be a corresponding shortfall in antioxidants.

Another circumstance where supplements should be considered has to do with elevated levels of free radical activity. We have mentioned how aging and disease are often accompanied by increased levels of free radicals. Another source lies in the environment.

Those who work in or live near factories or industrial sites where the air quality is poor, and where pollutants foul the air – these are candidates for higher levels of free radical activity, and the damage they cause. The same for those who spend a lot of time in traffic fumes. Others may be subjected to a greater load of free radicals because of their water supply.

Smokers present an especially urgent case. They inflict countless free radicals (and other toxins) upon themselves with every puff.

All of these are people who would almost certainly benefit from antioxidant supplements. Such supplements will compensate for both an inadequate level of antioxidants supplied in the diet, and for the heightened levels of free radical activity coming from the environment or other sources. In either case, antioxidant supplements will neutralize much of the free radical activity, and the tissue damage they bring about.

And finally we come to a group who will almost certainly have increased levels of free radicals and who least deserve them. These individuals too will benefit from antioxidant supplements to counteract their higher load of free radicals. These are the people who get a lot of exercise.

Exercise

In his poem "Abel Melveny", Edgar Lee Masters creates a character inappropriatly named Abel, who does nothing with his life. In the poem Abel speaks of the machinery and equipment he acquired early in life, and the grand ambitions he had for it, and for himself. But instead of using the machinery in any useful way, he just let it sit there, as he did himself. And now, in his later years, he sees his unused machinery rusted and decaying. And in a parallel fashion, because he has not put himself to work over those years, Abel, too, is a decaying shell of a man. He has gone to rust.

In a way, human beings are like machines. We need to be maintained and we need to be used – we need to be worked physically. We need regular exercise. That is how we developed and evolved over the ages, and that is how we are today. Without regular exercise we fall into decay long before our time. We don't wear out, we rust out.

Aerobic and Resistance

There are two broad categories of exercise – aerobic and resistance.

In aerobic exercise we carry out lighter physical exertions over an extended period of time. This brings about an increased oxygen uptake and an elevated heart rate over a protracted period of time, giving both the lungs and the cardiovascular system a good workout. Examples of this sort of exercise are jogging, brisk walking, distance swimming, and the like.

This kind of exercise does not build up a large muscle mass, but it does keep the muscles very well toned. And it does strengthen them and give them endurance. It also burns up energy and helps keep the body lean. Most importantly, it strengthens the heart and lungs.

Resistance exercise involves a more vigorous workout, where weights or other devices are used in supplying the resistance. These exercises provide an ever increasing resistance to our muscles during exercise sessions, causing them to grow larger and bulk up over time. Although resistance exercise does work the heart and lungs to a certain extent, its principle result lies in producing an increase in muscle mass – on the macroscopic level. On the physiological level, another result of intense exercise is that it is conducive to increased secretions of human growth hormone, the levels of which have a strong bearing on aging.

Both forms of exercise are of value to us. Whether we go for a brisk thirty minute walk, or hit the gym for a workout with the weights, both will confer their own benefits. Both help set the body chemistry in motion to burn calories rather than store them as fat. And both keep the body chemistry working rather than rusting.

The drawback is that exercise also produces free radicals

but resistance exercises produce less of the damaging free radicals. Have you ever seen an old looking body builder? (Put your hand down Ben Weider)

Draw Back on the Drawback

When we burn sugar to produce energy, the transfer of electrons in the process often results in some of them going astray, and latching onto oxygen molecules that are present. This produces an added load of free radicals.

Notwithstanding this drawback, we are always better off if we get a certain amount of exercise, even with the increased load of free radicals it brings. The way around this problem is not to curtail exercise, but rather, to curtail free radical activity. This way we are able to draw back on the drawback.

We can appreciably limit both the production of free radicals and the extent of their damage by increasing our antioxidant intake. And we can do this in two ways – by increasing foods in our diet that provide antioxidants, and through the use of supplements. Supplements are particularly handy here, because they can be taken a half hour or an hour before exercising, which will have them available in the body to neutralize the added free radicals that the exercise will produce. This then gives us a win-win situation. Further, it will provide us with heightened levels of antioxidants throughout the day, and counter the action of additional free radicals that may try to assault us, whatever their source.

Shoes or Sheets?

There is an old adage that says: "It is better to wear out shoes than sheets."

Even centuries ago, when this adage first surfaced, people realized the benefits of exercise. We look better and feel better when we exercise. And we do better.

Although exercise uses up energy, it also provides more energy. It gets our chemical cycles working to provide energy throughout the rest of the day, long after we have finished exercising. This means that we continue to burn up more calories long afterwards. So if we are dieting to get into shape, or to keep in shape, exercise is a natural complement to our dietary efforts.

For those who, for one reason or another, cannot do heavy or prolonged physical workouts, there is always isometrics. Or yoga. Or tai-chi. Or a simple walk around the neighborhood. All of these can be done at a relatively gentle level, accommodating almost anyone who has a limited physical capacity. And all of these forms of exercise will provide their own physical benefits.

Perhaps even more important than the physical benefits are the psychological benefits. When we are physically active we invariably feel better, we feel more positive. And there is a good physiological reason for this. When we exercise the brain produces more endorphins, which are chemicals related to morphine, but which do not have the corresponding negative effects.

If we wish to improve our lives, one of the simplest and least expensive ways is to get enough exercise. It is simply a matter of making a choice: do we want to wear out sheets or shoes?

A Divinity That Shapes Our Ends

Shakespeare wrote: "There is a divinity that shapes our ends, rough hew them how we will."

Most of us believe in a higher power in the universe. For Christians it is God; for Jews it is Jehovah; for Muslims it is

Allah. Every cultural group has its own recognition of this higher power. And yet all to often many of us, as individuals, do not call upon this higher power in times of challenge or endeavor. And that is a major oversight or shortcoming. For in this oversight we neglect a magnificent source of strength and inspiration. We waste this source of heat and light that can be called upon to kindle a fire within us, that can empower us to meet our challenges, that can steady our resolve in times of wavering.

All too often when we embark on a quest, seeking to achieve certain ends – rough hewing them how we will – we do not invoke the divinity underlying all things to shape them with us.

Yet when we do, an uncanny thing seems to happen. Invariably we find ourselves strengthened and inspired. We feel ourselves working in union with something greater than ourselves. The fear of failure evaporates, and an almost joyous acceptance of the path we have chosen comes to pervade us. And things begin to change. People seem to be that much more inclined to encourage or assist us in our quest. We become imbued with a quiet confidence. Small details tend to fall into place, almost of their own accord. And with every passing day we then find ourselves moving steadily and every more confidently toward our desired ends.

And it all begins by first invoking the inspiration and strength of the "divinity that shapes our ends."

Antioxidants And Their Sources

The Front Four

The three enzyme antioxidants – superoxide dismutase (SOD), Catalase (Cat), and glutathione peroxidase (GPx) – are all produced by the body, as is glutathione.

There are no particular foodstuffs that appreciably elevate their levels, but a good healthy diet will generally provide the body with the nutrients needed for their production in the body.

However, where the diet is lacking, their levels will be diminished. This also tends to occur during times when we are weakened by disease or other stresses, and their levels in the body also diminish as we approach middle age. In all of these circumstances supplements will be of particular benefit. Supplements will also be of benefit in the case of certain minerals that are essential components of the enzyme antioxidants.

SOD, for example, has zinc, copper, and manganese as components in its various forms. For GPx, selenium is a crucial component. Diet may be used to supply these minerals, although for most people, supplements will increase the likelihood of attaining optimal levels in the body.

For many years researchers have studied the Hunzas of West Pakistan, renowned for their longevity and health. Dr. Flanagan relates that possibly the silica in the glacial water may have some antioxidant properties. This brings us to a silica molecule (Microhydrin) that may act as a non-organic cage effective as a quencher of superoxide free radicals.

Food Sources

Zinc: meats, fish, egg yolks, and milk.

Copper: organ meats, shellfish, nuts, fruit, legumes, raisins, mushrooms.

Manganese: bran, coffee, tea, nuts, peas, beans.

Selenium: seafood, egg yolk, chicken, milk, whole grain products. (Variable in the water supply from region to region, and therefore, variable in the foods produced in these regions)

Supplements

Supplements for the enzyme antioxidants are becoming more comonly available, and multi-antioxidants will have combinations that will often include SOD and Cat.

The mineral antioxidants associated with these enzymes may be found in a superior multi-vitamin. Some of these minerals will also be available as individual preparations, as is the case for zinc, which is commonly available in the form of lozenges.

Glutathione

Glutathione is a special case. It consists of three peptides joined together, which are normally split apart during digestion. However, the body can use these components in its production of glutathione. Therefore, it is of benefit to include foods in our diet that contain glutathione.

Food Sources

Fruits, vegetables, freshly cooked meats (but the glutathione in them will be broken down during digestion).

Supplements

Because glutathione is broken down in the stomach during digestion, there have been problems in producing a glutathione supplement that has proven effective, one which survives this breakdown. One way around this is to take supplements that provide building blocks used by the body in the production of glutathione. One of the foremost of these is N-acetylcysteine or NAC. NAC is an antioxidant in its own right, and it provides the crucial, sulfur-containing peptide so necessary in the production of glutathione.

More recently, a process has been implemented whereby glutathione is compressed into the center of a pill. This allows it to pass through the stomach without being broken down. For those who do not have absorption or digestive difficulties, the glutathione may then be absorbed into the body through the small intestine.

The Antioxidant Vitamins

Vitamins A, C, and E (the ACEs) are those which also act as antioxidants. They may be obtained from the diet and by supplements.

Food Sources

Vitamin A: liver, butter, whole milk, cheese, egg yolk.

Vitamin C: citrus fruits, strawberries, tomato, broccoli, peppers, collard greens, brussels sprouts, kale, papaya, mango, potato, spinach.

Vitamin E: vegetable oil, butter, margarine, egg yolk, liver, green leafy vegetables, wheat germ, whole grain products.

Supplements

All of the vitamin antioxidants may be obtained from individual preparations, as well as in multi-vitamins.

Alpha Lipoic Acid

Lipoic acid is another special case in our list of antioxidants. Lipoic acid is produced by the human body, but only in extremely small amounts. It also occurs in other animals and plants, in equally small amounts. It is estimated that it would take seven pounds of spinach to produce one mg of lipoic acid. (Lester Packer, one of the foremost authorities on lipoic acid, recommends 100 mg of lipoic acid per day by way of supplementation.) Clearly, a good balanced diet will maximize the amount of lipoic acid that we may derive from our food. Equally clearly, supplements of lipoic acid are called for if we are to maintain optimal levels in the body. And for those with diabetes or other diseases where lipoic acid is of particular benefit, supplements should definitely be considered. Side effects of skin rash are rare and hypoglycemia in diabetics has been reported.

The Carotenoids

The principal carotenoids may be obtained from a variety of brightly colored fruits and vegetables. This is one group of antioxidants where diet is strongly emphasized as a source for them.

Food Sources

Beta-carotene: sweet potatoes, carrots, apricots,spinach, collard greens, canned pumpkin, beet greens, cantalope.

Alpha-carotene: canned pumpkin, carrots, yellow corn, red peppers.

Lycopene: tomato juice, watermelon, guava, pink grapefruit, tomatoes, tomato sauces.

Lutein: kale, collard greens, spinach, broccoli, mustard greens, red pepper, Romaine lettuce.

Zeaxanthine: Swiss chard, water cress, okra, beet greens.

Cryptoxanthin: papaya, peach, tangerine, oranges.

Supplements

Supplements are available for most of the carotenoids listed above.

The Flavonoids

The flavonoids make up another group of antioxidants that have a similar chemical arrangement. Although there are hundreds of them, they can be grouped into less than a dozen families. Only a few of the flavonoids are found in commonly available foods, while the majority are available in supplemental form. That being the case, we will include both food and supplemental sources on one list, and we will use the flavonoid name(s) that we believe will be most recognizable.

Sources

Proanthocyanidins (The Pros): maritime pine bark preparations, grape seed extracts, huckleberry (bilberry) leaves, gingko biloba leaves, birch leaves.

Flavonols: green tea, grape seed, pine bark.

Flavones (quercetin): green tea, garlic, onions, cayenne pepper.

Biflavones: gingko biloba.

Flavonones (hesperidin): citrus peels.

Flavononoles: milk thistle, pine bark.

Anthocyanins: red grapes, wine, huckleberries.

Flavonolignans (silymarin): milk thistle, artichokes.

Isoflavones (genistein and diadzein): soy beans, tofu.

Coenzyme Q-10

Ubiquinone or CoQ-10 is produced by the body as a coenzyme for at least 3 mitochondrial enzymes (complexes I, II and III) for the production of energy via ATP, but occurs in very small amounts. Research has shown that it is beneficial to maintain higher levels than are normally found in the body. Here again, supplements are recommended in attaining optimal levels, since CoQ-10 is found only at low levels in most foods. For example, it is estimated that to attain optimal levels we would have to eat three pounds of liver, or one pound of sardines, or three pounds of peanuts each day. Supplements are particularly recommended for those at risk for heart disease, stroke, for vegetarians and for those taking statin cholesterol lowering medicines. It may act as an immunomodulating agent. CoQ-10 is structurally similar to Vitamin K and may interfere with blood thinners like warfarin (Coumadin) so these patients should receive guidance from their doctors before taking CoQ-10.

Food Sources

seafood, organ meats like beef hearts, peanuts.

Supplements

CoQ-10 is available at most health food stores, usually as a supplement on its own. Synthetic near copies that claim to be better are appearing on the market.

Cheaper sources are on the horizon so put up with the cost for now.

Total Health

In his recent translation of the ancient Chinese text, "Sun-Tzu: The Art of War", Dr. Roger T. Ames provides a masterful interpretation and commentary on this timeless subject. Since its publication, the work has been adopted by the business community for the insights it provides that also apply to the realm of business. For many in the field of commerce, the feeling is that the competition and struggle found in the marketplace make it not unlike a low grade war, in which the casualties are recorded in red ink rather than blood.

There are also those who regard life in general as a low grade war, where – in a Darwinian sense – we struggle to survive and succeed. And part of this involves keeping ourselves alive and healthy. Which brings us to the hidden war from which none of us can escape: the war inside our bodies.

"Medical decisions should never be based on chronological age; only biological age"
–Donald McLeod M.D. CLA4

The Hidden War

Every day of our lives bacteria, viruses, and other microbes are laying in wait to invade us, to infect us, to take us down. Through the immune system, and other means, the body fights back against these foreign invaders.

The body is also under attack from the activity of free radicals that we take in through the air we breathe, the water we drink, and the food we eat. More insidiously, there are those free radicals that are akin to fifth columnists, since they are produced in the body and are part of the body. They, too, will weaken us and help take us down.

Perhaps the ultimate enemy working on us is the aging

process itself, a process in which free radicals play a substantial role. We are pre-programmed to age, and eventually, to succumb. Aided by free radicals, the body's defences decline over time.

A great deal of this decline also has to do with the decline of our hormonal levels as we come up to middle age. As they go into decline, much of the body chemistry that keeps us youthful also goes into decline.

It is at this time of life that we are hit with this formidable triple whammy. The levels of free radicals in the body tend to increase. The antioxidants which fight against and neutralize free radicals go into steady decline. And the hormones that keep the body functioning with a youthful physiology also go into decline.

In the past there was little we could do in this war against the aging process, now there is much. As Dr. Ames puts it in his explication of the timeless Chinese text: "All determinate situations can be turned to advantage."

Being Ready

"Do not depend on the enemy not coming; depend rather on being ready for him." This advice from the Sun-Tzu is as relevant today as when it was set forth centuries ago.

In the context of total health, we can make the body ready for the assaults of the aging process that will be coming at us as we hit middle age. And we can ready ourselves and fortify ourselves on several fronts.

Battling Free Radicals

We have seen that by following healthy and intelligent eating patterns that we can reduce our free radical intake. Even more advantageous, through diet we can greatly increase antioxidant levels in the body, both in variety and in quantity. The levels of antioxidants can be further augmented by a judicious use of antioxidant supplements. Such supplements will also be of benefit for those fighting various diseases, or who are at risk for disease.

Hormones and Antioxidants Affecting
The Cell via Receptors and Actions

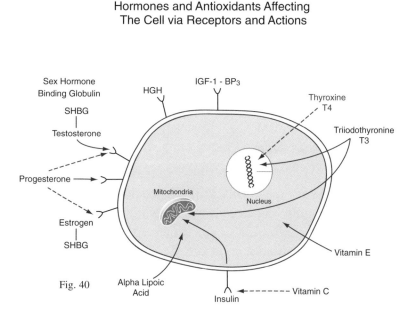

Fig. 40

Through exercise we can tone the body, building up muscle while burning off fat. And although exercise does increase the production of free radicals, these can be offset by increasing the antioxidants in us, through diet and supplements.

By maintaining optimal levels of antioxidants we will also decrease the risk for many diseases, most of which will also weaken and age us.

By such simple means as diet, exercise, and supplements, we ready the body in the battle against the aging process in two important ways: we bring ideal antioxidant levels in the body with us as we approach middle age; and we also bring healthy patterns that will continue to combat and forestall the aging process as we go through it.

Battling Hormonal Decline

In our previous book, "Doctors' Secrets: The Road to Longevity", we have described in detail how the levels of most hormones tend to decline as we approach middle age. These hormones are the body's messengers, and are somewhat like stage directors, working behind the scenes in regulating so much of our body chemistry.

Foremost among them, particularly with regard to keeping us young, is human growth hormone, or HGH. HGH has been called the master hormone because it has such a far reaching effect on the body as a whole, and on the performance of other hormones as well. Its effects are reinforced by restoring the sex hormones and thyroid in a balanced fashion.

Human Growth Hormone

HGH has provided some of the most remarkable results in the battle against aging. In lab experiments on animals, HGH has consistently extended their lifespans. Study after study on humans has shown that HGH replacement therapy can bring about the following improvements:

- increased muscle mass

- fat loss

- increased sexual potency and pleasure

- a reversal in graying hair, and new hair growth

- menstrual cycle regulation

- higher energy levels

- improved sleep patterns

- an improved mental outlook.

The amazing thing is that all of the changes brought about by HGH were obtained without changes in diet or exercise patterns. Further, from the many animal and human studies, it is easy to see why researchers have concluded that in humans, HGH may well be able to add an extra two or three decades of strong, healthy years to our lives. More research is looking at the importance of the IGF-1 binding proteins and their relationship to health.

Hard, vigorous exercise may help offset the decline in HGH levels that invariably come with middle age. But we cannot all be olympic class weightlifters. Fasting, too, may increase HGH levels. But we cannot fast indefinitely. Injections may be the most efficient way of replacing HGH to its youthful levels. But such a regime requires health professionals to administer the injections, and to provide the ongoing monitoring they require. In addition, injections are expensive, and to some, painful.

But there is another way to restore fading HGH to its youthful levels: by means of secretogogues.

Secretogogues

A secretogogue is a substance designed to induce a particular gland in the body to release a hormone. In the case of HGH, secretogogues provide the simplest, safest, and least expensive means by which we may recapture the levels of this hormone that we had in our younger years.

Secretogogues are simpler than injection, since they merely consist of amino acid formulations in pill form that may be self-administered. This means that we do not need a health professional on hand for this.

Secretogogues are safer because they stimulate the pituitary gland to release more HGH, rather than just adding it to the body as do injections. This means that there is no chance in attaining overly high levels, since the pituitary is subject to regulation by a feedback loop. It will stop releasing HGH when normal levels are reached, and will not exceed them.

Secretogogues are also much cheaper than injections.

When taken before bed, secretogogues do their work during the night, after we have fallen asleep. They stimulate the pituitary, which then releases more HGH than it had been releasing in previous months and years, bringing the levels of this hormone to where they were in our younger days. These youthful levels of HGH then work throughout the day inducing a corresponding change in the rest of our body chemistry, making it more youthful as well. In turn, this youthful body chemistry proceeds to halt and in some cases, to even reverse the aging process – to turn back the clock.

Reversing the aging process in this manner is better than face lifts, liposuction, tummy tucks, or hair dyes and such – because this restored body chemistry works from the inside out. It rebuilds muscles, eases wrinkles, melts away fat, etc. in the way our body chemistry did when we were younger. It keeps us young where it counts most, on the inside. Because when our body chemistry is younger on the inside, that will keep us younger on the outside.

Not only will we look better, and move about better – we will feel better. And healthier. And these effects will continue to be felt over the years, as our younger HGH levels work inside us to limit and forestall the aging process.

Other Hormones (Melatonin)

Replacement therapy is also possible with many other hormones that tend to drop off as we come up to middle age, each conferring its own beneficial results. Melatonin is a simple molecule produced in our pineal gland and serves a variety of functions. It is available in foods like brown rice, oats,

corn, bananas and tomatoes. Dr. Russel Reiter of the
University of Texas showed in 1993 that melatonin quenches
hydroxyl free radical better than glutathione and quenches
peroxyl free radical better than vitamin C and E. After the age
of 18 years, melatonin production plummets to very low levels by the age of 50 years when we need it most to help with
our sleep patterns, promote Human Growth Hormone production and quench the ever increasing free radicals. Even
primitive one celled organisms, dinoflagellates, contain
melatonin which implies that this antioxidant has been present for billions of years and serves a useful purpose.

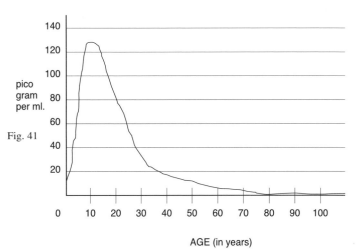

MELATONIN LEVELS WITH AGING

Fig. 41

pico gram per ml.

AGE (in years)

Hormones such as melatonin, DHEA, estrogen, proges-
terone, testosterone – all confer their own special benefits
when restored to youthful levels.

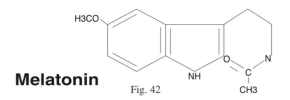

Melatonin

Fig. 42

Hormone replacement therapy should only be carried out under the care of a qualified physician.

Smoking

There is but one thing to be said about smoking: DON'T.

And if you are smoking, stop.

If you cannot stop immediately, make a solid plan to stop in the near future. And in the meantime, be careful of antioxidant overload causing problems as pointed out with the cadmium in cigarette smoke forming a deadly mix with vitamin C.

A noted researcher, C. Borek, has estimated that there are billions of free radicals in each puff of cigarette smoke.

The free radicals and toxins in cigarette smoke are extremely harmful to the body. If you do not stop smoking, smoking will stop you. End of discussion.

For those of you seeking further discussion, we refer you to the section on disease, with particular emphasis on those chapters dealing with cancer and heart disease.

Alcohol

Alcohol is different from smoking in that a little bit – for most people – may be a good thing. People who have one or two glasses of beer each day, or one or two glasses of wine, generally tend to live longer than those who do not.

Red wine, when limited to a glass or two each day may be particularly beneficial. Red wine is blessed with antioxidants from the flavonoid group called procyanidins. These antioxidants have demonstrated a particular effectiveness in preventing cardiovascular disease. The emphasis here is on

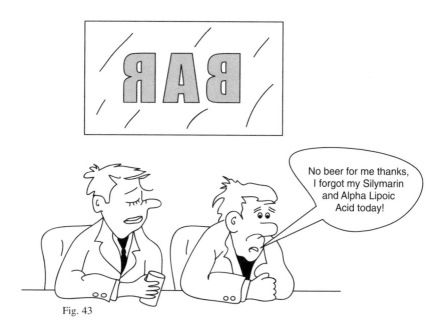

Fig. 43

one or two glasses a day. Anything beyond that and the negative effects begin to outweigh the positive, and the negative
effects increase with each additional drink. A study done in
Finland by Dr. Karhunen showed that at autopsy, 1-3 drinks
per day had no effect on the lipids in the coronary artery
walls but there was less risk of heart attack and less narrowing of the arteries. More than 3 drinks per day had less heart
attacks again but more fatty livers with cirrhosis and more
violence related deaths. Not the best way to reduce atherosclerosis. With a family history of colon cancer, an analysis
of the Nurse's Health Study showed that more than 2 hard
drinks per day increased the risk of colon cancer 4 times
compared to nondrinkers. But folic acid supplement could
reduce the risk by 50% of developing colon cancer.

Light beer and spirits may be as good for your health as
drinking wine says a study in the Journal of Epidemiology
and Community Health. The most important factor seemed to
be the quantity of alcohol and not the type when studying

19,000 Spanish adults. There were less health related complaints with more alcohol consumed up to a certain point.

Alcohol for some is ultimately a poison. Those who become addicted to alcohol eventually hijack their normal body chemistry. They harm their kidneys and ruin their livers. In short, they shorten their lives, sometimes by decades. And from the stress they often cause to loved ones around them, they very likely shorten their lives as well. In this sort of scenario, alcohol can be even more ruinous than cigarettes.

One particular case that underscores the deadly effects of alcohol concerns teen-agers. Alcohol is the number one factor in teen-age deaths. For it is alcohol that is involved in so many of their accidents and mishaps.

Alcohol should always be treated as an acquaintance – enjoyed in brief encounters. Alcohol can become a friend in moderation, but it can easily become a deadly enemy. In summary, alcohol can be enjoyed in moderation with some antioxidant benefits but the ethanol component could ultimately become a toxin if overdone.

Sleep

Of sleep, Shakespeare wrote:

"Sleep that knits up the ravelled sleeve of care,
The death of each day's life, sore labour's bath,
Balm of hurt minds, great nature's second course,
Chief nourisher in life's feast."

Sleep is as necessary as food, water, or exercise. Sleep does all that Shakespeare describes above, and more.

Sleep allows the body to rest and regenerate. It is during sleep that most of the HGH is released from the pituitary. Much of the rebuilding and repair occurs in the body while we are asleep.

Perhaps as important, sleep allows the mind to rest, to put itself away for a time – at least the conscious part. And then it brings out our dreams, a phenomenon which appears to be equally important.

Dreaming, as part of sleep, is acutely necessary for our psychological well being. Why this is so is beyond our present understanding. But experiments have shown that when people are kept from dreaming, they very soon slip into unhealthy psychological patterns. In one experiment, where the subjects were allowed to get enough sleep, but were awakened when they began to dream, the people in these experiments eventually began to hallucinate, to exhibit symptoms of paranoia.

Other research has shown that insufficient sleep – over time – brings about a shortened lifespan. In other words, if we save an hour or two each day of our lives, we will likely lose that time saved at the end because our lives will be cut short.

Insufficient sleep also robs us of our abilities. We lose our mental sharpness and we diminish our physical capacity and coordination. This has been demonstrated in research and has shown up as a factor in late night automobile accidents.

For those not getting enough sleep, a few simple measures may be tried.

– Avoid stimulants such as tea or coffee in the evening.

– Try getting to bed around the same time each night.

– Don't bring your problems to bed with you.

– Don't oversleep in the mornings.

– Avoid heavy smoking or use of alcohol, especially during the evenings.

– Look into melatonin supplement therapy.

– Get enough exercise during the day.

Emphasizing the last point, the Bible says: "The sleep of a labouring man is sweet." Or as Shakespeare put it: "Weariness can snore upon flint, when resty sloth finds the pillow hard."

Also, it will always be more difficult to sleep at night if we sleep the day away. As Nietchze put it: "Sleeping is no mean art. For its sake one must stay awake all day."

Besides, if we are active during the day, solving the problems of the day, we will not be taking them to bed with us, when we can do nothing to solve them except to toss and turn.

Insufficient sleep can detract from our total health as readily as poor eating habits or lack of exercise. Getting enough sleep, therefore, should be as eagerly sought after as is a good meal. If proper sleep is proving elusive, a visit to the family physician might be in order. Remember, studies have shown the maximum longevity occurs in the population that can sleep 6-8 hours maintaining proper Human Growth Hormone and antioxidant status.

Stress

Only a block of wood does not feel stress. And if it has just been cut from the tree, perhaps even a block of wood can feel something like a lingering stress. Because all living things experience stress.

Experiencing stress is necessary for our survival. If we never feel stress, we will never feel motivated to escape from that which is stressing us. And if that happens to be a charging lion, it can be deadly.

Equally deadly is to experience too much stress – to be too highly stressed for too much of the time.

We are animals, animals that evolved and developed

over countless thousands of years. We became adapted to a simple life of eat or be eaten. The stresses may have been great, but they were likely infrequent, and short lived. In an encounter with a wild animal, either we were victorious and had dinner, or we were not and were dinner.

Our body chemistry, in adaptation to such circumstances, goes into a fight or flight response when we are stressed. Our hearts beat faster, the adrenalin flows, the cortisol flows, blood is pumped to the skeletal muscles, digestion stops. We are then ready to battle the tiger or to flee from him.

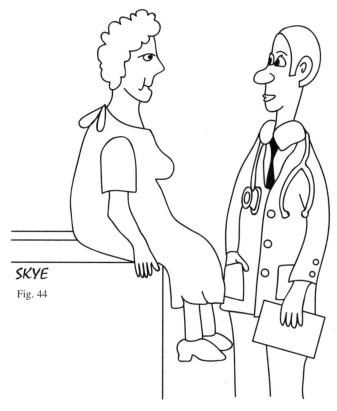

SKYE

Fig. 44

You have family stress and financial stress, but the most serious is your oxidative stress !

In today's world, the tiger never comes. The stresses are usually of a different kind, where we cannot go into a physical battle and we cannot escape them. Things like: we are caught in a traffic jam and are about to miss an important business meeting; or the flight has been cancelled and we cannot make our daughter's wedding; or we find that the bills at the end of the month far exceed the family income. The stresses in the modern world tend to be frequent and ongoing, and most of the time they cannot be solved by strong physical action. We cannot battle and we cannot skedaddle. Instead we just get rattled.

We get all pumped up but we can do little but sit and stew, with the acids pooling in the stomach and the cortisol eating at the brain. Frequent and ongoing stress is harmful to the body. It was not designed to handle it.

We have all heard of the data indicating that people who have had two or three major stresses over a few months or a year are much more susceptible to disease. A death in the family, divorce, bankruptcy – any of the major stresses of modern life coming one upon the other tends to weaken us.

Similarly, a life full of lesser stresses also tends to weaken us. And although most of these stresses do not kill us at the moment they are upon us, they do add up, and they do kill us over time. Early research by Hans Seyle by has shown that prolonged stress in animals will eventually lead to exhaustion, and ultimately to death.

The reason for this is that stress brings about elevated levels of hormones such as cortisol, epinephrine, adrenalin, and testosterone. Heightened levels of cortisol tend to raise our levels of cholesterol and triglycerides. Associated with the physiological response to prolonged stress are atherosclerosis, a weakening of the immune system, and an increased risk for many diseases.

When we contract a disease, this also weakens and ages us. Which then sets up a vicious cycle, since disease tends to induce stresses of its own.

In the end, such boxed-in stresses eventually put us in a box, years before our time.

We may take steps to avoid or alleviate stress in a number of ways. We can set aside some time each day for relaxation. Exercise again comes to the fore as a health benefit, since it is marvelous at dissipating stress. We can take up yoga, or practice self-hypnosis, or undergo biofeedback training. We can cut back on stimulants, and on drugs and alcohol, since all of these can affect stress levels.

For those who feel they are particularly stressed, there are books available that deal solely with stress management. Such individuals may want to seek out their family physician or other health professional for advice or further counselling. If stress is a major problem it should be dealt with and alleviated.

Hans Seyle wrote: "No living organism can exist continuously in a state of alarm."

Anti-Aging Centres: Putting It All Together

We may embark on a program of good health, and try putting it all together on our own. And this approach can be very effective.

But in striving for total health, in striving for those extra decades and more of youthful vigor, we may want to look into the services of an anti-aging center. Furtunately, such centers are now beginning to spring up all over North America.

Such centers have usually been founded by pioneers in the field, by doctors who have made anti-aging therapies their specialty, and who have been part of the anti-aging movement in medicine. They have apprised themselves of the data available in the field, and often have contributed to this data through experience and studies of their own. They regard aging as a disease which can be effectively treated, and forestalled, and perhaps in time, defeated.

At such anti-aging centers, assessments can be made of various factors for aging. These include measuring for levels of advanced glycation end products (AGEs), declining hormonal levels, declining antioxidant levels, and so on. An individual's genetic material may also be stored at some of these centers, making it available for analysis for their offspring and future generations. Risks for genetically based diseases may also be assessed.

At the end of such assessments, a program designed specifically for a particular individual can be drawn up, one which addresses the unique needs of the individual. These may involve the replacement of specific hormones, or the use of secretogogues. The anti-aging health professionals may suggest supplementation of particular antioxidants to compensate for their decline in the body, or to offset risks for certain diseases. We like to use the term Maximal Antioxidant Protection (MAP-ing) for the treatment plan we provide for the liver, heart, kidney, brain and gut. Some have referred to this as detoxifying and then applying an antioxidant protocol. The full armamentarium in the field of anti-aging can be brought to bear, the latest discoveries offered, all tailored to the individual's own unique body chemistry. Such an approach will likely provide the surest route to attaining total health. And to enjoying those extra decades of strong, healthy life.

Measurement of Antioxidant Status

The days of guessing at health status by clinical observation are coming to an end. As physicians, we certainly don't wish to become obsolete as far as our clinical exams are concerned but we must accept that as we treat the body at the cellular level, then we need information that is impossible to find except with the newer sophisticated tests. We have discussed the importance of antioxidants, how they save our cells and tissues from free radical damage. We don't want to wait for that damage to occur before we notice something is wrong with us and we are aging with decay. We want to be proactive and preventative so tests for each one of our antioxidant systems is important for monitoring one's health and so important for our research. Some of the antioxidant parameters that we feel are important are levels of selenium, superoxide dismutase, glutathione reductase and a total antioxidant status. At present, a Biological Terrain Assessment (BTA) is popular to measure oxidation-reduction potential of body fluids like urine, blood and saliva. Other routine tests are important for albumin, bilirubin, ferritin, uric acid, total iron binding capacity (TIBC) and transferrin.

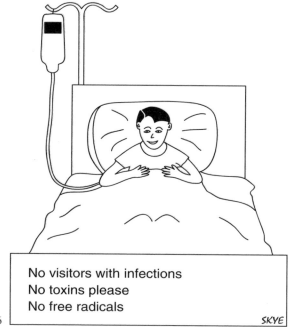

Fig. 46

Glutathione peroxidase measurements are so important since this is one of our most important intracellular antioxidants. Cumene hydroperoxide = ROOH in this reaction and rising levels of NADP[1] will decrease the absorption of 340 nm light passing through this reacting solution.

$2GSH + ROOH \rightarrow$Glutathione Peroxidase$\rightarrow GSSG + ROH + H_2O$

$GSSG + NADPH + H^+ \rightarrow$Glutathione Reductase$\rightarrow 2GSH + NADP^+$

This reaction also allows a calculation of the activity of Glutathione Reductase, which reduces the glutathione allowing it to once more act as an antioxidant.

Superoxide Dismutase is one of our most important intracellular antioxidants as previously explained. An easy way to amylase SOD status is to look at red blood cells. First superoxide free radicals are produced with xanthine.

XANTHINE $\rightarrow$XanthineOxidase$\rightarrow$ URIC ACID $+ O_2^{\cdot-}$

Then p-iodonitrotetrazolium salts $+ O_2^{\cdot-} \rightarrow \rightarrow \rightarrow$ RED FORMAZYN DYE

The SOD from the red blood cells will compete with the salts for the superoxide free radicals ($O_2^{\cdot-}$) and the level of SOD will prevent formation of this red dye.

Total Antioxidant Status is important for looking at the overall picture of an individual's nutrition, supplement status, risk for disease and to assess therapy for illness. The easiest method is to measure:

methmyoglobin + hydrogen peroxide to produce ferrylmyoglobin (free radical)

$HX-Fe^{3+} + H_2O_2^{\cdot} \rightarrow \rightarrow \rightarrow \cdot X-(Fe^{4+}=O)$ then add a chemical that changes color when it is oxidized. The more antioxidant in the fluid sampled, then less color change seen.

Many of the progressive labs will do these tests as the public demands more information to assess their real status to prepare for future oxidative damage.

Oldest Persons File

It is interesting that our previous record holder for longevity, Eva Morris, attributed her good health to whisky and boiled onions at 115 years. Recently, Maud Farris-Luse of Michigan at 115 years, passed on leaving the title to Kamato Hongo of Kagoshima on the island of Kyushu, Japan. She attributes her health to rice wine (sake), black salt, sashimi, green tea and eliminating stress. She is 114 years and counting.

John McMorran celebrated his 113th birthday in Lakeland, Florida 2002 as the oldest man in the US.

The U.S. based Population Reference Bureau has reported that the developed countries will increase their population by nearly 50 million by 2050 but the underdeveloped countries (Latin American, African, Asian) will increase the population by nearly 3,000 million.

Parting Thoughts

For all sad words of tongue or pen
The saddest of all: "It might have been."

–John Greenleaf Whittier

There are no such things as incurables, there are only
things for which man has not found a cure.

–Bernard M. Baruch

So teach us to number our days, that we may
apply our hearts unto wisdom.

–The Holy Bible (5,12)

Research And Study Summary

85,000 Nurses Health Study – 1993 showed an 8 year major coronary disease (CAD) reduction in risk by 43% for vitamin E users.

Health Professional Follow Up Study – (HPFS) 39,000 males for 4 years by Rimm et al showed vitamin E and beta-carotene benefits and reduction in smoker's CAD.

NHANES I study showed 11,000 adults taking vitamin C had lower death rates from all causes and less CAD risk.

Alpha-Tochopherol, Beta-Carotene Cancer Prevention Study (ATBC) – 29,000 male smokers in 5-8 years showed no less heart disease and more lung cancer with ATBC

Beta-Carotene and Retinol Efficacy Trial (CARET) – 18,000 smokers or asbestos history showed increase in heart disease and lung cancer with the supplement.

Physicians' Health Study – 22,071 male MD's took 50 mg beta-carotene and 325 mg ASA for 12 years and showed no change for risk of cancer or CAD.

National Cancer Institute 1998 showed 30,000 poor Chinese (Linxian) benefit from selenium, beta-carotene and vitamin E by reducing cancer by 13%.

Cambridge Heart Anti Oxidant Study (CHAOS)- 400 or 800 IU of alpha tochopherol (vitamin E) for CAD patients had 47% and 77% less heart attacks and cardio vascular events but the same overall death rates.

ATBC Study showed that heart attack patients had 38% less recurrence of heart attack if taking alpha-tocopheral.

Cholesterol Lowering Atherosclerosis Study (CLAS)- suggested that vitamins slowed progression or growth of atherosclerosis plaque.

1,795 Nurses in 1998 had 33% less heart attack and 71%

less stroke if they ate a quota of spinach and carrots each week.

JAMA Study 2001 – 352,000 women were followed 6-15 years for breast cancer showed only 7% reduction if ate a high fruit, vegetable diet (not significant).

Iowa Women's Study – 34,000 postmenopausal women followed 7 years showed diet rich in vitamin E foods decreased risk from heart attack death.

Zutphen Elderly Study over 10 years showed flavonols (quercetin) ingestion had an inverse relation to death rate for males (less risk for dying).

Microhope by Dr. Eva Lon as part of the larger Hope study of 3,654 diabetics getting 400 IU of vitamin E or placebo. After 4.5 years the incidence of heart attack, stroke, death (17.5%) or diabetic complication was the same.

Indian Experiment of Infarct Survival Study showed reperfusion oxidative injury (heart attack size) was less with antioxidant supplement.

Multivitamin and Probucol Study (MVP) – and angioplasty restenosis trial (PART) showed probucol had less stenosis but there was no benefit from vitamin C, E or beta-carotene.

Heart Outcomes Prevention (Hope) Study showed decreased cancer risk but no improved cardiovascular risk for vitamin E users. But the blood pressure medicine, ramapril, showed unexpected benefits as an antioxidant.

Dr. Shaheen Study King's College showed that people that ate 2 apples per day or high selenium diet (also wine, tea, onions) had reduced incidence of asthma.

University of Bergen 4,766 men and women 65-67 years in 1993 studied showed that those with the highest homocysteine levels died 49% more for each 5 umol/L increase in serum homocysteine.

US Department of Agriculture found rats and humans had improved diabetes when supplemented with chromium picolinate.

New England Journal of Medicine 2001 – Patients taking Simvastatin and niacin received no benefit for cholesterol regression or heart attack by adding a simple combination of vitamin antioxidants.

Dr. R. Chandra of Memorial University, St. John's studied 96 patients over 65 years and found antioxidants given every day for one year improved memory, abstract thinking, problem solving and attention span in 40% of elderly.

National Institute of Aging Study by Losonczy showed long term users of vitamin E out of 11,000 elderly people were 60% less likely to die from heart disease and 59% less likely to die from cancer.

JAMA reported 75,000 middle aged women had 43% less stroke if they ate at least 2.7 servings of whole grain foods versus controls when adjusted for smoking.

Japan Study of 2,000 patients over age 40 studied for 20 years showed the lowest quartile of vitamin C levels had 70% more stroke risk.

87,245 Nurses followed for 14 years showed 50% reduction in heart disease when supplemented with 4 times the recommended government dose of B6 and folate.

Harvard Medical School 6 year study on 48,000 male health professionals found that tomato products served twice per week reduced prostate cancer by 35%.

MIRACL Study of interest 3,000 patients showed 16% improvement in complications after heart attack if cholesterol lowering statin was started soon.

Heart Protection Study of 15,000 patients showed no benefit from alpha tocopherol, beta carotene and vitamin C for improving lipid profiles.

Clinical Chemistry 2000,vol 46 showed that 62 coronary patients had lower levels of standardized vitamin E levels than control patients.

Quebec Vitamin Users Study showed antioxidant benefits for 2,313 men for prevention of disease.

Massachusetts Residents Study with 747 men and Seven Countries Study with 12,763 men showed no benefit for supplementation of vitamins.

Finnish Healthy Population Study for both 5,133 men and women showed antioxidant benefits.

The Happy (Antioxidant) Highway

Into my heart an air that kills
From yon far country blows:
What are those blue remembered hills,
What spires, what farms are those?

That is the land of lost content,
I see it shining plain,
The happy highways where I went
And cannot come again.

In his poem "Into My Heart an Air That Kills" A. E. Housman sets forth images recalled from his youth, and his words are redolent with nostalgia. He realizes that he will never recapture these places of his youth, or for that matter, recapture those youthful days themselves. There is a poignancy that accompanies the realization that gone forever are "The happy highways where I went, and cannot come again."

The Shortness of Time

As we edge up to middle age, many of us encounter this feeling of nostalgia, this poignant pang of knowing that our youth is behind us.

In our bittersweet replaying of the past, we experience the sweet part through cherished memories – our good times, our friends and loved ones, our achievements. As for the bitter part of the bittersweet, we look back with a forlorn aching because we know that those times are gone now, that we cannot ever return to them. And besides our achievements, we also see the goals that have not been met, that in the shortness of time may never be met.. And we realize that now, as we move on into middle age that there are many dreams that will likely remain just that – dreams.

We find suddenly that our days of youth are fading. That the energy and zest of those days is fading too. The unbridled verve and vigor are in retreat. And at times when we are caught up in and transfixed by such moments, we may hear the breath go out of us in an audible sigh.

The Evitable

Fifty years ago, even twenty years ago, that's how it was. That's how it had to be. We came up to middle age and we went into rapid decline, with only creaking old age staring us in the face. And the face peering back at us in the mirror each morning looking more and more like a relief map of mars. Only there was no relief. Because that's how it was from time immemorial.

But it does not have to be that way – not any more, not today. When we hit forty or fifty, the downward spiral is no longer the inevitable course, with its empty plodding into the world of gray, marking time until we go into "the home". This is not the way we have to go. This does not have to be our lot. Not today.

There are so many new techniques that have come forward in medicine, so many new discoveries, especially in the past couple of decades. And nowhere have these discoveries been more exciting than in the field of anti-aging.

With all the new discoveries we no longer have to view the part of our lives that continues on past middle age as a sagging slump into decrepitude. That this is our inevitable lot. Because it is evitable. And there is – and the word is "evitable". So much of the aging process today is evitable, is avoidable. And that which is not totally avoidable is certainly postponable.

All of it: the procession into hobbling and pain; the reflection in the mirror of sags and folds; the eyesight not even able to properly see the sags and folds, although it can vaguely make out the bulges; and the hair graying or going; the energy going, going, gone; and the sex drive.... But it is all evitable, it is avoidable.

With all the new discoveries in the field of anti-aging we can avoid so much of it. We can slow it down, and in some ways even halt or reverse it. We can lessen it and defer it, and we can gain ourselves an extra twenty, thirty years, and probably even more. But we can only do so if we avail ourselves of the recent discoveries, if we pursue a program of total health.

At the rate new discoveries are surging forth, it is eminently possible that some of the discoveries of the next ten or twenty years will be able to extend our time and our health for a further few decades still. And the new discoveries that are made in those further decades? Well, at this point we move somewhat beyond prognostication and deeper into speculation. But the speculations at this point are tantalizing.

New discoveries in hormone replacement therapy are coming forth every few months. Work on telomeres – the tips on our chromosomes – show a definite promise in deferring the aging process by a quantum leap. And in genetics it is certainly possible that scientists will one day strike the mother lode, and through genetic manipulation shut down the aging process altogether. All of these areas are burgeoning with promise, as are others. So who can say?

Certainly there have been marvelous gains made in the past decade or so, gains which have been highly instrumental in slowing the aging process. And current research bodes well for even more striking gains to come in the near future. If we take advantage of the discoveries already upon us, we will at least be around to take advantage of the discoveries yet to come. And so on down the line.

In any case, where we pursue a total health program we will give ourselves a good twenty or thirty years longer to live than we would have had otherwise, maybe even more. With the emphasis on good. For those years will be healthier as well. Not only will we have superior health, but we will have all that goes with it: well oiled joints; greater musculature and strength; trimmer physique; improved appearance; improved eyesight with which to enjoy our spouse's improved appearance; and when such a sight moves us, the power and ardor to renew our love.

We will not only live longer, we will live stronger.

The Perfect Day

We awaken softly, and even before we are fully conscious we do a lazy stretch. It feels good. When we are fully awake we slip effortlessly out of bed.

Before we shower we do a little yoga, perhaps followed by a few minutes of calisthenics, or other light exercises. They are a tonic to the muscles, a balm to the joints. We have been doing this morning routine for some time now and it feels good. The joints feel especially good.

After our morning ablutions we head for the kitchen and set an aromatic pot of tea steeping. While it does so we have a glass of fruit juice, and then perhaps a succulent grapefruit. After that, with our tea, we indulge ourselves with a coddled egg and some whole wheat toast, followed by a multi-vitamin.

And then, feeling well fueled but with a lightness in our steps, it's off to work.

At morning break we have juice and a protein snack. At lunch perhaps a large bowl of soup.

Still feeling energized and yet easy of movement, we whip through the afternoon, filling it with accomplishment

After work we take a multi-antioxidant and then head over to the gym, where we run through our routine in the weight room, or perhaps do a dozen or two vigorous laps in the pool, or play a hard fought game of squash.

And then to home, feeling relaxed and refreshed.

While we get dinner on the go we put our favorite music on the stereo. For the evening meal we begin with a gorgeous salad and a whole wheat panini roll, accompanied by a glass of red wine. This is followed by the main course, which is a full bodied serving of spinach lasagna with a side dish of stir fried vegetables, and perhaps a second glass of wine. To finish up a bowl of low fat spumoni ice cream, and maybe a clump of grapes as well. And then linger over a cup of black or white tea.

Throughout the evening we work on whatever we wish, perhaps that special project we are in the middle of. Or take in a movie, or go for a walk – whatever we wish.

If we feel like a snack through the evening we might have a bowl of popcorn, very lightly buttered, along with a glass of our favorite juice.

A little before bed we might do a few minutes of gentle

stretches, and then take our HGH secretogogue.

As we crawl cozy under the covers we feel the satisfaction of a well nigh perfect day, and then drift off into a peaceful, restful sleep, preparing us for another perfect day.

All Perfect Days

What we have described above is just one of what can be an endless succession of perfect days. They do not have to be exact replicas of the one we have described. We all have different family configurations, different schedules, different tastes, different needs, different limitations. But within our own parameters they can all still be perfect.

The main thing is that we strive to follow a total health routine that includes the same healthy components found in our example of a perfect day. The crucial thing is that we make these patterns enjoyable.

Healthy food choices will cease to be healthy if we don't enjoy them, because we will soon cease to bother. The same for exercise and the rest. There are countless foods that are good for us, and countless recipes. The most important thing is to choose the ones we enjoy. If we choose the healthy foods that we enjoy, if we involve ourselves in exercises that we like, there is a greater likelihood that we will be continue with them throughout our lives. As for other total health measures, such as hormone replacement and antioxidant supplements – that is the easy part. An anti-aging clinic can arrange a tailor-made program, and often this program may require little more than taking appropriate supplements and the like each day, just like we take our vitamins.

But the key word is enjoyable. By making your total health program enjoyable you will ensure yourself of not only a perfect day, but an endless succession of perfect days.

An Invitation

By way of encouragement to all who would seek an endless succession of perfect days, we would like to set forth the words of Lord Alfred Tennyson, taken from his poem, Ulysses.

The passage is from the end of the poem, where Ulysses and his crew are no longer young, and their many voyages are behind them. But with the boat nearby and the sea beckoning, Ulysses will not accept that all their voyages and accomplishments are behind them. And he urges his men – exhorts them – to join with him in one more magnificent voyage, and his own words, too, are magnificent:

Come my friends,

'Tis not too late to seek a newer world.

Push off, and sitting well in order smite

The sounding furrows; for my purpose holds

To sail beyond the sunset, and the baths

Of all the western stars, until I die...

Though much is taken, much abides; and though

We are not now that strength which in old days

Moved earth and heaven, that which we are, we are–

One equal temper of heroic hearts,

Made weak by time and fate, but strong in will

To strive, to seek, to find, and not to yield.

As we, the authors, finish up a perfect day of our own, dining out at the patio restaurant of a lovely estate winery in celebrating the completion of this book, we will raise our wine glasses to you in a toast to your commitment to total health. And we hope that the sound of our glasses clinking together will reverberate across space and time, beckoning you to join us as we proceed to toast the miracle of antioxidants, and that you will hear the faint echo of our voices as we say: "Come my friends!"

References & Bibliography

Section I: Introduction

Ames, BN, Shigenago Mk, Hagen TM. Oxidants, antioxidants, and the degenerative diseases of aging. Proc. Natl Acad Sci USA, 1993; 90:7915-7922.

Balch JF, Balch PA. Prescription For Nutritional Healing. New York: Avery Publishing, 1990.

Balch JF. The Super Antioxidants. New York: M. Evans and Company, Inc, 1998.

Binger CAL, Faulkner JM, Moore RL. Oxygen poisoning in mammals. J Exp Med 1927; 45: 849-864.

Borek C. Antioxidants and cancer. Sci & Med 1997;November/December:52-61.

Borg DC. In: Pryor WA, ed. Free Radicals in Biology, Vol3. New York:Academic Press;1977:69-147.

Cadenas E, Packer L. Antioxidants in health and disease. Handbook of Antioxidants. 1996;3.

Comro JH Jr, Dripps RD, Dumke PR, Deming M. Oxygen toxicity. J Am Med Assoc 1945;128:710-717.

Dormandy TL. Biological rancidification. Lancet 1969;2:684-688.

Fenton HJH. Oxidation of tartaric acid in presence of iron. J Chem Soc 1894;65:899-910.

Floyd RA, Warson JJ, Wong PK, Miller DH, Richard RC. Hydroxyl free radical adduct of deoxyguanosine: Sensitive detection and mechanism of formation. Free Radical Res Commun 186;1:163-172.

Frei G. Ascorbic acid protects lipids in human plasma and low density lipoprotein against oxidative damage. Am J Clin Nutr 1991;54:1113S-1118S.

Gamache PH, McCabe DR, Parvez H, et al. The measurement of markers of oxidative damage, antioxidants and related compounds using HPLC and coulometric array analysis. Prog HPLC-HPCE 1997;6:99-126.

Gomberg M. An instance of trivalen carbon: Triphenylmethyl. J Am Chem Soc 1900;22:757-771.

Gjorup T, Hendriksen C, Lund E, Stromgard E. Is growing old a disease? A study of the attitudes of elderly people to physical symptoms. J Chron Dis 1987;40:1095-1098.

Harman D. Aging: A theory based on free radical and radiation chemistry. J Gerontol 1956;11:298-300.

Harman D. The aging process. Proc Natl Acad Sci 1981;78:7124-7128.

Harvey AM, McKusick VA, eds. Osler's Textbook Revisited. New York:Appleton-Century-Crofts; 1967:103.

Halliwell F, Gutteridge JMC. Free Radicals in Biology and Medicine. Oxford:Clarendon Press, 1998.

Hine J. Physical Organic Chimistry. New York:McGraw-Hill;1956:377.

Kellogg EW, Fridovitch I. Superoxide dismutase in the rat and mouse as a function of age and longevity. J gerontol 1976;31:405-408.

Knight JA, Pieper Rk, Smith SE, Crockett HH. Increased urinary lipoperoxides in drug abusers. Ann Clin Lab Sci 1988;18:374-377.

Knight JA. Free Radicals, Antioxidants, Aging, And Disease. Washington: AACC Press, 1999.

Lohman PHM, Sankaranarayanan K, Ashby J. Choosing the limits of life. Nature 1992;357:185-186.

Nash G, Blennerhassett JB, Pontoppidan H. Pulmonary lesions associated with oxygen therapy and artificial ventilation. N Engl J Med 1967;276:368-374.

National Center for Health Statistics. Vital Statistics of the United States, 1987. Washington, DC: US Public Health Service; 1990.

Olshansky SJ, Carnes GA, Cassel CK. The aging of the human species. Sci Am 1993;April:46-52.

Packer JE, Slater TF, Wilson Rl. Direct observation of a free radical interaction between vitamin E and vitamin C. Nature 1979;278:737-738.

Packer L, Colman C. The Antioxidant Miracle. New York: John Wiley & Sons, Inc, 1999.

Packer L. Oxygen radicals in biological systems. Methods in enzymology, 1994;233.

Packer L. Oxidants and antioxidants. Methods in enzymology, 1998;299.

Slater TF. Free radical mechanisms in tissue injury. Biochem J 1984;222:1-15.

Smith JL. Pathological effects due to increase of oxygen tension in air breathed. J Physiol 1899;24:19-35.

Steinberg D, Parthasarathy S, Carew TE, et al. Beyond cholesterol:

Modification of low density lipoprotein that increases its atherogenicity. N Engl J Med 1989;320:915-924.

Steinberg D. Modified forms of low density lipoprotein and atherosclerosis. J Intern Met 1993;233:227-233.

Tolmasoff JM, Ono T, Cutler RG. Superoxide dismutase correlation with lifespan and specific metabolic rate in primate species. Proc Natl Acad Sci USA 1980;77:2777-2781.

Section II: Free Radicals

Angier N. Free radicals: The price we pay for breathing. New York Times 1993;April 25.

Anggard E. Nitric oxide: Mediator, murder, and medicine. Lancet 1994;343:199-206.

Beckman KB, Ames BN. The free radical theory of aging matures. Physiol Rev 1998;78: 547-581.

Beckman JS, Koppenol WH. Nitric oxide, superoxide, and peroxynitrite: The good, the bad, and the ugly. Am J Physiol 1996;271 (Cell Physiol, 40):C1424-1427.

Binger Cal, Faulkner JM, Moore Rl. Oxygen poisoning in mammals. J Exp Med 1927;45:849-864.

Borek C. Antioxidants and cancer. Sci & Med 1997;November/December:52-61.

Borg DC. In: Pryor WA, ed. Free Radicals in Biology, vol3. New York: Academic Press; 1977:69-147.

Church, DF, Pryor WA. Free-radical chemistry of cigarette smoke and its toxicological implications. Environmental Health Perspectives 64:111-126.

Cohen S, Tyrrell DAJ, Smith AP. Psychological stress and susceptibility to the common cold. N Engl J Med 1991;325:606-612.

Diaz J, Serrano E, Acosta F, Carbonell LF. Reference intervals for four biochemistry analytes in plasma for evaluating oxidative stress and lipid peroxidation in human plasma. Clin Chem 1998;44:2215-2217.

Diechle F, Malinski T. Indirect detection of nitric oxide effects: A review. Ann Clin Lab Sci 1996;26:501-511.

Emerit L, Chance B, eds. Free radicals and aging. Basel, Switzerland: Berkhauser Verlag.

Fenton HJH. Oxidation of tartaric acid in presence of iron. J Chem Soc 1894;65:899-110.

Finkel T. Oxygen radicals and signalling. Current Opinion in Cell Biology

1998;(2):248-253.

Frage CG, Shigenage MK, Park J-W, et al. Oxidative damage to DNA during aging: 8-Hydroxy-2-deoxyguanosine in rat organ DNA and urine. Proc Natl Acad Sci USA 1990;87:4533-4537.

Gamache PH, McCabe Dr, ParvesH, et al. The measurement of markers of oxidative damage, antioxidants and related compounds using HPLC and coulometric array analysis. Prog HGLC-HPCE 1997;6:99-126.

Gomberg M. An instance of trivalent carbon: Triphenylmethyl. J Am Chem Soc 1900;22:757-771.

Halliwell B Antioxidants in human health and disease. Annual Review of Nutrition 1996;16:33-50.

Halliwell B, Gutteridge JMC. Oxygen toxicity, oxygen radicals, transition metals and disease (Review). Biochem J 1984;219:1-14.

Halliwell F, Gutteridge JMC, eds. Free radicals in biology and medicine. 3d ed. Oxford, England: Clarendon Press.

Halliwell B, Gutteridge JMC. Oxygen toxicity, oxygen radicals, transition metals and disease. Biochem J 1984;219:1-14.

Harman D. Aging: A theory based on free radical and radiation chemistry. J Gerontol 1956;11:298-300.

Hippel s, Elstner EF. Biological and biochemical effects of air pollutants: Synergistic effects of sulphite. In: Free radicals and oxidative stress: Environment, drugs and food additives. Rice-Evans C, Halliwell B, Lunt GG, eds. London: Portland Press; 1995:153-61.

Kanofsky JR, Hoogland H, Wever R, Weiss SJ. Singlet oxygen production by human eosinophils. J Biol Chem 1988;263:9692-9696.

Kanofsky JR, Sima P. Singlet oxygen production from the reactions of ozone with biological molecules. J Biol Chem 1991;266:9039-42.

Kedziora J. Journal of Free Radical Biology and Medicine 1984.

Kloss MW, Rosen GM, Rauckman EJ. Evidence of enhanced in vivo lipid peroxidation after acute cocaine administration. Toxical Lett 1983;15:65-70.

Lloyd RV, Hanna Pm, Mason RP. The origin of the hydroxyl radical oxygen in the Fenton reaction. Free Radical Biol Med 1997;22:885-888.

Loscalzo J. Nitric oxide and vascular disease. N Engl J Med 1995;333:251-253.

Lunec J. Oxygen radicals: Their measurement and role in major disease. JIFCC 1992;4:58-63.

Martin WJ II, Dachel DL. Oxygen-mediated impairment of human pulmonary endothelial cell growth. Evidence for a specific threshold of toxicity. J Lab

Clin Med 1989;113:413-421.

Packer L, ed.1984. Oxygen radicals in biological systems. In Methods in enzymology. Vol 105. Orlando, Fla: Academic Press.

Packer L. 1998. Oxidants and Antioxidants. In Methods in enzymology. Vol 299. San Diego: Academic Press.

Packer L, Ong A, eds. 1998. Biological oxidants and antioxidanta: Molecular mechanisms and health effects. Champaign, Ill:AOCS Press.

Packer JE, Slater TF, Wilson RL. Direct observation of a free radical interaction between vitamin E and vitamin C. Nature 1979;278:737-738.

Richter C, Park J-W, Ames BN. Normal oxidative damage to mitochondrial and nuclear DNA is extensive. Proc Natl Acad Sci USA 1988;85:6465-6467.

Slater TF. Free radical mechanisms in tissue injury. Biochem J 1984;222:1-15.

Smith JL. Pathological effects due to increase of oxygen tension in air breathed. J Physiol 1899;24:19-35.

Stadman ER. Protein oxidation and aging. Science 1992;257:1220-1224.

Teixeira HD, Schumacher RI, Meneghini R. Lower intracellular hydrogen peroxide levels in cells overexpressing CUZn-superoxide dismutase. Proc Natl Acad Sci USA 1988;95:7872-7875.

Thiele JJ, Traber MG, Tsang K, et al. In vivo exposure to ozone depletes vitamins C and E and induces lipid peroxidation in epidermal layers of murine skin. Free Radical Biol Med 1997;23:385-91.

Wagner JR, Hu C-C, Ames Bn. Endogenous oxidative damage of deoxycytidine in DNA. Proc Natl Acad Sci USA 1992;89:3380-3384.

Wennberg PO, Hanisco TF, Jaegle L, et al. Hydrogen radicals, nitrogen radicals and the production of O3 in the upper troposphere. Science 1998;279:49-53.

Section III: Aging

Ames BN, Shigenaga MK. Oxidants and aging. Ann NY Acad Sci 1992;663:85-96.

Beckman KB, Ames BN. The free radical theory of aging matures. Physiol Rev 1998;78:547-581.

Bezlepkin VG, Sirota NP, Gaziev AI. The prolongation of survival in mice by dietary antioxidants depends on their age by the start of feeding this diet. Mech Ageing Dev 1996;92:227-34.

Bodnar AG, Ouellette M, Frolkis M, et al. Extension of life-span by introduction of telomerase into normal human cells. Science 1998;279:349-352.

Borek, C. Antioxidants and cancer. Sci Med 1997;Nov/Dec:53-61.

Brack C, Bechter-Thruing E, Labuhn M. N-Acetylcysteine slows down ageing and increased the life span of Drosophila melanogaster. Cell Mol Life Sci 1997;53:960-66.

Brown WT. Genetic diseases of premature aging as models of senescence. Annu Rev Gerontol Geriatr 1990;10:23-42.

Brownlee M. Cerami A, Vlassara H. Advanced glycosylation: Chemistry, biology, and implications for diabetes and aging. Adv Pharmacol 1992;23:1-33.

Brunk Ut, Jones CB, Sohal R. A novel hypothesis of lipofuscinogenesis and cellular aging based on interactions between oxidative stress and autophagocytosis. Mutat Res 1992;275:395-403.

Busciglio J, Yankner BA. Apoptosis and increased generation of reactive oxygen species in Down's syndrome neurons in vitro. Nature 1995;378:776-779.

Ceballow-Picot I, Nicole A, Briand P, et al. Neuronal-specific expression of human copper-zinc superoxide dismutase gene in transgenic mice: Animal model of gene dosage effects in Down's syndrome. Brain Res 1991;552:198-214.

Cerami A, Vlassara H, Brownlee M. Glucose and aging. Sci Am 1987;256:90-96.

Counter CM, Hirte HW, Bacchetti S, et al. Telomerase activity in human ovarian carcinoma. Proc Natl Acad Sci USA 1994;91:2900-2904.

Cutler RG. Peroxide-producing potential of tissues: Inverse correlation with longevity of mammalian species. Proc Natl Acad Sci USA 1985;82:4798-4802.

Daynes RA, Araneo BA. Prevention and reversal of some age-associated changes in immunologic responses by supplemental dehydroepiandrosterone sulfate therapy. Aging: Immunol Infect Dis 1992;3:135-154.

deGrey ADNJ. A mechanism proposed to explain the rise in oxidative stress during aging. J Anti-age Med 1998;1:53-65.

Di Guiseppi J, Fridovich I. The toxicology of molecular oxygen. CRC Crit Rev Toxicol 1984;12:315-42.

Dimri GP, Lee X, Basile G, et al. A biomarker that identifies scenescent human cells in culture and in aging skin in vitro. Proc Natl Acad Sci USA 199r;92:9363-9367.

Farber JL, Kyle ME, Coleman JB. Mechanisms of cell injury by activated oxygen species. Lab Invest 1990;62:670-79.

Finch CE, Tanzi RE. Genetics of aging. Science 1997;278:407-411.

Friedman DB, Johnson TE. A mutation in the age-1 gene in Caenorhabditis elegans lengthens life and reduces hermaphrodite fertility. Genetics 1988;118:75-86.

Fu MX, Knecht KJW, Blackledge JA, et al. Glycation, glycoxidation and crosslinking of collagen by glucose. Kinetics, Mechanisms, and inhibition of late stages of the Maillard reaction. Diabetes 1994;43:676-683.

Esterbaur H, Schaur RJ, Zollner H. Chemistry and biochemistry of 4-hydroxynonenal, malondialdehyde and related aldehydes. Free Radical Biol Med 1991;11:81-128.

Goldstein S. Lifespan of cultured cells in progeria. Lancet 1969;1:424.
Gota M, Rubenstein M, Wever J, et al. Genetic linkage of Werner's syndrome to five markers of chromosome 8. Nature 1992;355:735-738.

Halliwell B. Oxygen radicals: A commonsense look at their nature and medical importance. Med Biol 1984;62:71-77.

Halliwell B, Gutteridge JMC. Oxygen toxicity, oxygen radicals, transition metals and disease. Biochem J 1984;219:1-14.

Hari R, Burde V, Arking R. Immunologica confirmation of elevated levels of CUZn superoxide dismutase protein in an artificially selected long-lived strain of Drosophila melanogaster. Exp Gerontol 1998;33:227-237.

Harley CB, Futcher AB, Greider CW. Telomeres shorten during ageing of human fibroblasts. Nature 1990;345:458-460.

Harman D. Prolongation of the normal lifespan and inhibition of spontaneous cancer by antioxidants. J Gerontol 1961:16:247-254.

Hartnell JM, Morley JE, Mooradian AD. Reduction of alkali-induced white blood cell DNA unwinding rate: A potential biomarker of aging. J Gerontol 1989;44:B125-B130.

Harman D. Prolongation of the normal lifespan by raidation protection chemicals. J Gerontol 1957;12:257-263.

Harman D. The aging process. Proc Natl Acad Sci USA 1981;78: 7124-7128.

Harman D. Free radicals in aging. Mol Cell Biochem 1988;84:155-161.

Hart RW, Setlow RB. Correlation between deoxribonucleic acid excision-repair and life span in a number of mammalian species. Proc Natl Acad Sci USA 1974;71:2169-2173.

Hayflick L. The limited in vitro lifetime of human diploid cells. Exp Cell Res 1965;37:614-636.

Horan MA, Fox RA. Ageing and the immune response – A unifying hypothesis? Mech Ageing Dev 1984;26:165-181.

Horton AA, Fairhurst S. Lipid peroxidation and mechanisms of toxicity. CRC Crit Rev Toxicol 1987;18:27-79.

Hunt JV, Smith CCT, Wolff SP. Autoxidative glycosylation and possible involvement of peroxides and free radicals in LDL modification by glucose. Diabetes 1990;39:1420-24.

Jacobson Md, Weil M, Raff MC. Programmed cell death in animal development. Cell 1997;88:3470354.

Jazwinski SM. Longevity, genes, and aging. Science 1996;273:54-59.

Kaiser FE, Silver AJ, Morley JE. The effect of recombinant growth hormone on malnourished older individuals. J Am Geriatr Soc 1991;29:235-240.

Kay M, Makinodan T. Immunobiology of aging: Evaluation of current status. Clin Immunol Immunopathol 1976;6:394-413.

Kedziora J, Bartosz G, Gromadzinska J,m et al. Lipid peroxides in blood plasma and enzymatic antioxidative defence of erythrocytes in Down's syndrome. Clin Chim Acta 1986;154:191-194.

Kim NW, Piatyszck MA, Prowse KR, et al. Specific association of human telomerase activity with immortal cells and cancer. Science 1994;266:2011-2015..

Kirkwood TBL. DNA, mutations, and aging. Mutat Res 1989;219:1-7.

Knight JA. Laboratory Medicine and the Aging Process. Chicago: ASCP Press: 1996:89-143.

Koizumi A, Weindruch R, Walford RL. Influences of dietary ristriction and age on liver enzyme activities and lipid peroxidation in mice. J Nutr 1987;117:361-367.

Lakowski B, Hekimi S. Determination of life-span in Caenorhabditis elegans by four clock genes. Science 1996;272:1010-1013.

Lang CA, Naryshkin S, Schneider DL, et al. Low blood glutathione levels in healthy aging adults. J Lab Clin Med 1992;120:720-725.

Larsen PL. Aging and resistance to oxidative damage in Caenorhabditis elegans. Proc Nat'l Acad Sci USA 1993;90:8905-8909.

Lindahl T. Instability and decay of the primary structure of DNA. Nature 1993;362:709-715.

Linnane AW, Marzuki S, Ozawa T, Tanaka M. Mitochondrial DNA mutations as an important contributor to ageing and degenerative diseases. Lancet 1989;1:642-645.

Loschen G, Flohe L, Chance B. Respiratory chain linked H_2O_2 production in pigeon heart mitochondria. FEFS Lett 1971;18:261-264.

Marklund S, Nordensson I, Back O. Normal CuZn superoxide dismutase, Mn superoxide dismutase, catalase and glutathione peroxidase in Werner's syndrome. J Gerontol 1981;36:4-5--409.

Martin GM, Sprague CA, Epstein CJ. Replicative life span of cultivated human cells: Effects of donor's age, tissue, and genotype. Lab Invest 1970;23:86-92.

McCord JM, Fridovich I. Superoxide dismutase. An enzymatic function for erythrocuprein (hemocuprein). J Biol Chem 1969;244:6049-6055.

Melov S, Lithgow DR, Fischer DR, et al. Increased frequency of deletions in the mitochondrial genome with age of Caenorhabditis elegans. Nucleic Acids Res 1995;23:1419-1425.

Melov S, Shoffner JM, Kaufman A, Wallace DC. Marked increase in the number and variety of mitochondrial DNA rearrangements in aging human skeletal muscle. Nucleic Acids Res 1995;23:4122-4126.

Nohl H, Hegner D. Do mitochondria produce oxygen radicals in vivo? Eur J Biochem 1978;82:563-567.

Oliver CN, Ahn BW, Moerman EJ, et al. Age related changes in oxidized proteins J Biol Chem 1987;262:5488-5491

Orr WC, Sohal RS. Extension of life-span by overexpression of superoxide dismutase and catalase in Drosophila melanogaster. Science 1994;263:1128-1130.

Poot M. Oxidants and antioxidants in proliferative senescence. Mutat Res 1991;256:177-189.

Orgel LE. The maintainance of the accuracy of protein synthesis and its relevance to aging. Proc Natl Acad Sci USA 1963;49:517-521.

Oshima J, Brown WT, Martin GM. No detectable mutations at Werner helicase locus in progeria. Lancet 1996;348:1106 (Letter).

Pacifici RE, Davies KJA. Protein, lipid and DNA repair systems in oxidative stress: The free-radical theory of aging revisited. Gerontology 1990;37:166-180.

Pearl R. The Rate of Living. New York:Knopf;1928.

Reiter RJ. Pineal function during aging: Attenuation of the melatonin rhythm and its neurobiological consequences. Acta Neurobiol Exp 1994;54 (Suppl.):31-39.

Richter C. Reactive oxygen and DNA damage in mitochondria. Mutat Res 1992;275:249-255.

Richter C. Oxidative damage to mitochondrial DNA and its relationship to ageing. Int J Biochem Cell Biol 1995;27:645-653.

Rothstein M. Biochemical Approaches to Aging. New York: Academic press;1982:2.

Rozenscwaig R, Grad BR, Ochoa, J. The role of melatonin and serotonin in aging. Med Hypoth 1987;23:337-352.

Rudman D, Feller AG, Nagraj HS, et al. Effects of human growth factor in men over 60 years old. N Engl J Med 1990;323:1-6.

Rusting RL. Why do we age? Sci Am 1992;267:130-144.

Salganik RI, Solovyova NA, Dikalov SI, et al. Inherited enhancement of hydroxyl radical generation and lipid peroxidation in the S strain rats results in DNA rearrangements, degenerative diseases, and premature aging. Biochem Biophys Res Commun 1994;199:726-733.

Sajathal GB, Chithra P, Chandrakasan G. The role of metal-catalyzed oxidation in the formation of advanced glycation end products. An in vitro study on collagen. Free Radical Biol Med 1998;25:265-69.

Schachter F, Cohen D, Kirkwood T. Prospects for the genetics of human longevity. Hum Genet 1993;91:519-526.

Schleicher ED, Wagner E, Nerlich AG. Increased accumulation of the glycoxidation product N(epsilon)-(carboxymethyl) lysine in human tissues in diabetes and aging. J Clin Invest 1997;99:457-468.

Schnider S, Kohn RR. Glycosylation of human collagen in aging and diabetes mellitus. J Clin Invest 1980;66:1179-91.

Sell DR, Monnier VM. Structure elucidation of a lysine-arginine crosslink from aging human extracellular matrix: Implication of ribose in the aging process. J Biol Chem 1989; 264:21597-21602.

Shigenaga MD, Hagen TM, Ames BN. Oxidative damage and mitochondrial decay in aging. Proc Natl Acad Sci USA 1994;91:10771-10778.

Shigenaga MK, Gimeno CJ, Ames BN. Urinary 8-hydroxy-2-deoxyguanosine as a biological marker of in vivo oxidative DNA damage. Proc Natl Acad Sci USA 1989;86:9697-9701.

Sohal RS, Allen RG. Oxidative stress as a causal factor in differentiation and aging: A unifying hypothesis. Exp Gerontol 1990;25:499-522.

Sohal RS, Agarwal S, Dubey A, Orr WC. Protein oxidative damage is associated with life expectancy of houseflies. Proc Natl Acad Sci USA 1993;90:7255-7259.

Sohal RS, Agarwal A, Agarwal S, Orr WC. Simultaneous overexpression of copper- and zinc- containing superoxide dismutase and catalase retards age-related oxidative damage and increases metabolic potential in Drosophila melanogaster. J Biol Chem 1995;270:15671-15674.

Sohal RS, Weindruch R. Oxidative stress, caloric restriction, and aging. Science 1996;273:59-63.

Stadtman ER. Protein oxidation and aging. Science 1992;257:1220-1224.

Starke-Reed PE, Oliver CN. Protein oxidation and proteolysis during aging and oxidative stress. Arch Biochem Biophys 1989;275:559-567.

Strehler B, North D. Cell-type specific codon usage and differentiation. Mech Ageing Dev 1982;18:285-313.

Strehler BL. A critique of the theories of biological aging. In: Dietz AA (Ed), Aging – Its Chimistry. Washington, DC: American Association of Clinical Chimistry; 198025-45.

Strehler BL. A critique of theories of biological aging. In: Aging – Its Chemistry, AA Dietz (Ed), Washington, DC: American Association of Clinical Chemistry;1980:25-45.

Thiele JJ, Traber MG, Tsang K, et al. In vivo exposure to ozone depletes vitamins C and E and induces lipid peroxidation in epidermal layers of murine skin. Free Radical Biol Med 1997;23:385-91.

Tolmasoff JM, Ono T, Cutler RG. Superoxide dismutase: Correlation with life-span and specific metabolic rate in primate species. Proc Natl Acad Sci USA 1980;77:2777-81.

Vanfleteren JR. Oxidative stress and ageing in Caenorhadditis elegans. Biochem J 1993;292:605-608.

Viner RI, Ferrington DA, Huhmer AFR, et al. Accumulation of nitrotyrosine on the SERCA2a isoform of SR Ca-ATPase of rat skeletal muscle during aging: A peroxynitrite-mediated process? FEBS Lett 1996;379:286-290.

Walford L. The immunologic Theory of Aging. Baltimore: Williams & Wilkins; 1969.

Wallace DC. Mitochrondrial DNA in aging and disease. Sci Am 1997;August:40-47.

Wallace DC. Mitochondrial genetics: A paradigm for aging and degenerative diseases? Science 1992;256:628-632

Weindruch R, Sohal RS. Caloric intake and aging. N Engl J Med 1997;337:986-994.

Weindruch R, Walford RL. Dietary restriction in mice beginning at 1 year of age: Effect on life-span and spontaneous cancer incidence. Science 1982;215:1415-1418.

Ying W. Deleterious network hypothesis of aging. Med Hypoth 1997;48:143-148.

Zadik A, Chalew SA, McCarter JF, et al. The influence of age on 24-hour integrated concentrations of growth hormone in normal individuals. J Clin Endocrinol Metab 1985;60:513-516.

Zemlam F, Thienhaus OJ, Bosman HB. Superoxide dismutase activity in Alzheimer's disease: A possible mechanism for paired helical filament formation. Brain Res 1989;476:160-162.

Section IV: Antioxidants

Acuff, RV, Thedford SS, Hidiroglou NN, et al. Bioavailability of RRR- and

All-Rac-Alpha-Tocopherol Acetate in humans: Deuterated Compounds. Am J Clin Nutr 1994;60:397-402.

Advanced glycation end product-induced activation of NF-kappaB is suppressed by alpha-lipoic acid in cultured endothelial cells.

Alpha-lipoic acid in the treatment of diabetic peripheral and cardiac autonomic neuropathy. Diabetes, 25(4):562-6. 1997 Sep.

The Alpha-Tocopherol, Beta Carotene Cancer prevention Study Group. The effect of vitamin E and beta carotene on the incidence of lung cancer and other cancers in male smokers. New Engl J Med. 1994;330(15):1029-35.

Allard JP. Am J Clin Nutr. Apr 1994.

Ames BN, Shienago MK, Hagen Tm. Oxidants, antioxidants, and the degenerative diseases of aging. Proc Natl Acad Sci USA 1993;90: 7915-7922.

Anderson JW, Breecher MM. Dr. Anderson's Antioxidant, Antiaging Health Program. New York: Carroll& Graf Publishers Inc, 1996.

Anderson ME. Glutathione and glutathione delivery compounds. Adv Pharmacol 1997;38:65-78.

Aw TY, Wierzbicka G, Jones DP. Oral glutathione increases tissue glutathione levels. Chem Biol Interact 1991;80:89-97.

Balch JF. The Super Antioxidants. New York: M Evans and Company, Inc, 1998.

Balijepalli S, Boyd Mr, Ravindranth V. Inhibition of mitochondrial complex 1 by haloperidol: the role of thiol oxidation. Neuropharmacology 1999; Apr;38(4):567-577.

Bendich A, Langseth L. The health effects of vitamin C supplementation: A review. J Am College of Nutr. 1995;14:124-136.

Berkson BM. A conservative triple antioxidant approach to the treatment of hepatitis C. Combination of alpha oipoic acid (thioctic acid), silymarin, and selenium: three case histories. Med Clin 1999; Oct 15;94 Suppl 3:84-89.

Berkson BM. Nutrient herb synergy: Silybum marianum (Milk Thistle) and Selenium. Med Klin 1999 Oct 15; 94 Suppl 3:84-89.

Berkson B. The Alpha Lipoic Acid Breakthrough. 1998;Rockland, CA: Prima Publishing.

Biaglow JE, Varnes Me, Epp ER, et al. Role of glutathione and other thiols in cellular response to radiation and drugs. Drug Metab Rev 1989;20:1-12.

Bierbaum M, Watkins TR, Gapor, A, Geller M, Tomco AC. Antioxidant effects of tocotrienols in patients with hyperlipidemia and carotid stenosis. Lipids. 1995;30:1179-1183.

Block G, Patterson B, Subar A. Friut, vegetables, and cancer prevention: A review of the epidemiological evidence. Nutr and Cancer 1992; 18 (1):1-29.

Block G. Vitamin C and cancer prevention: The epidemiologic evidence. Am J Clin Nutr. 1997;66(5):1165-71.

Blot WJ, Li JY, Taylor PR, Guo W, Dawsey S, Wang GQ, Yang CS, Zheng SF, Gail M, Li GY, Yu Y, Liu B, Tangrea J, Sun Y, Liu F, Fraumeni JF, Zhang YH, Li B. Nutrition intervention trials in Linxian, China: supplementation with specific vitamin/mineral combinations, cancer incidence, and disease-specific mortality in the general population. J Nat Cancer Inst 1993;85(18):1483-92.

Brack C, Bechter-Thuring E, Labuhn M. N-acetylcysteine slows down aging and increases the life span of Drosophila melanogaster. Cell and Mol Life Sci 1997;53 (11-12):960-66.

Bray TM, Bettger WJ. The physiologic role of zinc as an antioxidant. Free Radical Biol Med 1990;8:281-291.

Brown AJ. Acute effects of smoking cessation on antioxidant status. Exp J of Nutr Biochem. 1996;7:29-39.

Brown DJ. Herbs for Health. Sept-Oct; 1997.

Bunnell E, Pacht ER. Oxidized glutathione is increased in alveolar fluid of patients with adult respiratory distress syndrome. Am Rev Resp Dis 1993;148:1174-78.

Bustamante J, Lodge JK, Marcocci L, Tritschler HJ, Packer L, Rihn BH. a-lipoic acid in liver metabolism and disease. Free Rad Biol & Med 1998;24:1023-1039.

Buzzelli G, et al. A pilot study on the liver: protective effect of Silybin-Phosphatidylcholine Complex (IdB1016) in chronic active hepatitis. Int J Clin Pharm Therapeutics and Toxicology. 1993; 31:456-60.

Cambridge Heart Antioxidant Study. Lancet 1996;347:781-786.

Caragay AB. Cancer-preventive foods and ingredients. Food Tech 1992: 65-68.

Carroll, KK, Chambers AF, Gapor A, Guthrie N. Inhibition of proliferation of estrogen-receptor-negative MDA-MB-435 and -positive MCF-7 human breast cancer cells by palm ocotrienols and Tamosifen, alone and in combination. J Nutr 1997;127:544S-48S.

Cenacci T, et al. Journal of Aging 1993;5:123-33.

Cheshier JE, Ardestani-Kaboudanian S, Liang B, Araghiniknam M, Chung S, Lane L, Castro A, Watson RR. Immunomodulation by Pycnogenol in retrovirus-infected or ethanol-fed mice. Life Sci 1996;(5):PL 87-96.

Christen S, Woodall AA, Shigenaga MD, Southwell-Keely PT, Duncan MW, Ames BN. g-tocopherol traps mutagenic electrophiles such as NOX and complements a-tocopherol : Physiological implications. Proc Nat Acad Sci

1997;94:3217-22.

Clark LC et al. Decreased incidence of prostate cancer with selenium supplementation: Result of a double-blind cancer prevention trial. Brit J Urol
1998;81 (5):730-34.

Clark LC et al. Effects of selenium supplementation for cancer prevention in
patients with carcinoma of the skin. A randomized controlled trial.
Nutritional Prevention of Cancer Study Group. J Am Med Ass
1996;276(240:1957-63.

Clinton SK. Lycopene: Chemistry, biology and implications for human health
and disease. Nutr Rev 1998;56 (2):35-51.

Coassin M, Ursini F, Bindoli A. Antioxidant effect of manganese. Arch
Biochem Biophys 1992;299:330-333.

Conlon BJ, Aran JM, Erre JP, Smith Dw. Attenuation of aminoglycoside-
induced chochlear damage with the metabolic antioxidant alpha-lipoic acid.
Hear Res 1999; Feb;128(1-2):40-44.

Cooney RV, Franke AA, Harwood PJ, Hatch-Piggot V, Custer LJ, Mordan L.
G-tocopherol detoxification of nitrogen dioxide: Superiority to a-tocopherol.
Proc Nat Acad Sci 1993;90:1771-75.

Corcoran GB, Wong BK. Role of glutathione in prevention of acetaminophen-
induced hepatotoxicity by N-acetyl-cysteine in vivo. J Pharmacol Exp Ther
1986;238:54-61.

Crayhon R. Robert Crayhon's Nutrition Made Simple. M. Evans and
Company: New York, 1994.

Cross CE, Halliwell B, Borish ET, et al. Oxygen radicals and human disease
(proceedings of a conference), Ann Intern Med 1987;107:526-45.

Deleve LD, Kaplowitz N. Importance and regulation of hepatic glutathione.
Seminars Liver Dis 1990;10:251-66.

Differential effects of lipoic acid stereoisomers on glucose metabolism in
insulin-resistant skeletal muscle. Am J Physiol. Jul 1997;25(4):E185-91.

Diplock A, Machlin L, Packer L, Pryor WA. eds, Vitamin E: Biochemistry and
health implication. Annals of the New York Academy of Sciences. 1989; Vol
570.

Dormandy TL. Biological rancidification. Lancet 1969;2:684-88.

Drehsen, G. From ancient pine bark uses to Pycnogenol. In Antioxidant Food
Supplements in Human Health. 1999; edited by L. Packer, T. Yoshikawa, and
M Hiramatsu. 1999; San Diego: Academic Press.

Droge W, Schulze-Osthoff K, Mihm S, et al. Functions of glutathione and glutathione disulfide in immunology and immunopathology. FASEB J
1994;8:1131-38.

Edmomds SE, et al. Putative analgesic activity of repeated oral doses of vitamin E in the treatment of rheumatoid arthritis. Results of a prospective placebo-controlled double-blind trial. Annals of Rheumatic Diseases 1997;56(11):649-55.

Egan KM. J Biochemica et Biophysica Acta. June 1992.

Enhancement of glucose disposal in patients with type 2 diabetes by alphalipoic acid. Arzneimittelforschung. Aug 1995;25(4):872-4.

Enstrom JE. Vitamin C in prospective epidemiological studies. Vitamin C in Health and Disease 1997; edited by L. Packer and J. Fuchs. New York: Marcel Dekker.

Ernster L, Dallner G. Biochemical, physiological, and medical aspects of ubiquinone function. Biochimica et Biophysica Acta 1995;1271:195-204.

Esterbauer H, Gebicki J, Puhl G, Jurgens G. The role of lipid peroxidation and antioxidants in oxidative modification of LDL. Free Radical Biology & Medicine1992;13(4);341-90.

Farooqui MYH, Day ww, Zamorano DM. Glutathione and lipid peroxidation in the aging rat. Comp Biochem Physiol 1987;88B:177-180.

Firshein R. The Neutraceutical Revolution. New York: Riverhead Books, 1998.

Francheschi S, Bidoli E, La Vecchia C, et al. Tomatoes and risk of digestive tract cancers. Int J Cancer 1994;59:181-84.

Frie B, Kim MC, Ames BN. Ubiquinol-10 is an effective lipid-soluble antioxidant at physiological concentrations. Proc Nat Acad Sci 1994;87:4879-83.

Galland L. The Four Pillars of Healing. Random House: New York, 1997.

Garland, M, Stampfer MJ, Willett WC, Hunter DJ. The epidemiology of selenium and human cancer. In Natural Antioxidants in Human Health and Disease. 1994; edited by B. Frei. New York: Academic Press.

Gazeiano JM. J Arteriosclerosis, Thrombosis & Vascular Biol. June 1995.

Gershoff SN. Vitamin C (ascorbic acid): New roles, new requirements: Nutr Rev 1993;51:313-26.

Ghiselli A, Serafini M, et al. A fluorescence-based method for measuring total plasma antioxidant capability. Free Radical Biol Med 1994;18:29-36.

Giovannucci E, Clinton SK. Tomatoes, lycopene, and prostate cancer. Proc Soc Exp Biol and Med. 1998; 218(2):129-39.

Giovannucci E, et al. Intake of carotenoids and retinol in relation to risk of prostate cancer. J Nat Cancer Inst. 1995; Vol 87, No. 23.

Goh SH, Hew NF, Norhanom AW, Yadav M. Inhibition of tumor promotion by various palm-oil tocotrienols. International J Cancer 1994;57:529-31.

Gohil K, Rothfuss L, Lang J, Packer L. Effect of exercise training on tissue vitamin E and ubiquinone content. Journal of Applied Physiology 1987; 63(4):1638-41.

Gould MN, Haag JD, Kennan WS, Tanner MA, Elson CE. A comparison of tocopherol and tocotrienol for the chemoprevention of chemically induced rat mammary tumors. Am J Clin Nutr 1991;53:1068S-70S.

Guthrie N, Gapor A, Chambers AF, Carrol KK. Palm oil tocotrienols and plant flavonoids act with each other and with Tamoxifen in inhibiting proliferation and growth of estrogen receptor-negative MDA-MB-435 and -positive MCF-7 human breast cancer cells in culture. Asia Pacific J Clin Nutr 1997;6:42-45.

Halliwell B. Free Radicals and antioxidants: A personal view. Nutr Rev 1994;53:253-65.

Hanioka T, Tanaka M, Ojima M, Shizukuishi S, Folkers K. Effect of topical application of coenzyme Q10 on adult periodontitis. Molecular Aspects of Medicine1994;15 (Suppl):241-48.

Hankinson SE, Stampfer MJ. All that glitters is not beta carotene. (Editorial) J Am Med ASS. Nov 9, 1994.

Hara Y. Prophylactic functions of antioxidant tea polyphenols. In Food Factors for Chemistry and Cancer Prevention, edited by H ohigashi, T. Osawa, J Tero, S Watanabe, and T. Yoshikaw. Tokyo: Springer-Verlag.

Haramaki N, Packer L, Droy-Lefaix MT, Christen T. Antioxidant actions and health implications of ginkgo biloba extract. Handbood of Antioxidants 1996; edited by E Cadenas and L Packer. New York: Marcel Dekker.

Hari R, Burde V, Arking R. Immunological confirmation of elevated levels of CuZn superoxide dismutase protein in an artificially selected long-lived strain of Drosohpila melanogaster. Exp Gerontol 1998;33:227-37.

Harman D. Prolongation of the normal lifespan and inhibition of spontaneous cancer by antioxidants. J Gerontol 1961;16:247-54.

Henderson BE, Kolonel LN et al. Cancer incidence in the islands of the Pacific. Nat Cancer Institute Monograph 1986;69:73-81.

Hertog MG, et al. Dietary antioxidant flavonoids and risk of coronary heart disease: The Zutphen Elderly Study. 1993; Lancet 342 (887):1007-11.

Hidalgo J, Garvey JS, Armario A. On the mettallothienein, glutathione and cysteine relationship in rat liver. J Pharmacol Exptl Ther 1990;255:554-64.

Hikino H, et al. The antihepatotoxic actions of flavonolignans from Silybum marianum fruits. Planta Medica 1984;50:248-50.

Hinninger I, et al. European J Clin Nutr. 1997;51:01-606.

Hirahara F. Effects of d-a-tocopherol, d-g-tocopherol and d-a-tocotrienol on atherogenic diet fed rats after high-dose administration. Nutr Rep Int

1987;36:161-67.

Ho YS, Lee Hm, Mou TC Wang Yj, Lin JK. Suppression of nitric oxide-induced apaptosis by N-acetyl-cysteine through modulation of glutathione, bcl-2 protein levels. Mol Carcinog 1997;Jun; 19(2):101-13.

Hoyumpa AM, Schenker S. Drugs and the liver. In: Maddrey WC, ed. Gastroenterology and Hepatology: The Comprehensive Visual Reference. Philadelphia: Current Medicine; 1996:6.1-6.22.

Hughes D. J Nutr. Mar 1992.

Hughes D. J Lab & Clin Med. Mar 1997.

Hunjan MK, Evered DF. Absorption of glutathione from the gastrointestinal tract. Biochim Biophys Acta 1984;815:184-88.

Jacobs MM. Diet, nutrition, and cancer research: An overview. Nutrition Today 1993; 28 (3):19-23.

Jenner P. Oxidative damage in neurodegenerative disease. Lancet 1994 (Sep 17):796-98.

Johnson CS, Meyer CG, Srilakshmi JC. Vitamin C elevates red blood cell glutathione in healthy adults. Am J Clin Nutr 1993; 58 (1):103-05.

Jones DP. Glutathione distribution in natural products: Absorption and tissue distribution. Glutathione and Thioredoxin: Thiols in Signal Transduction and Gene Regulation. 1995; in Vol 252 of Biothiols, Methods in Enzymology, edited by L. Packer. San Diego: Academic Press.

Kagan, VE, Serbinova EA, Packer L. Antioxidant effects of ubiquinones in microsomes and mitochondria are mediated by tocopherol recycling. Biochem and Biophys Res Communications. 1990;169:851-57.

Kagan VE, Serbinova EA, Forte T, Scita G, Packer L. Recycling of vitamin E in human low density lipoproteins. J of Lipid Res 1992;33:385-97.

Kagan VE, Shvedova A, Serbinova E, Kahn S, Swanson C, Powell R, Packer L. Dihydrolipoic acid – a universal antioxidant both in the membrane and in the aqueous phase. Biochem Pharm 1992;44:1637-49.

Kalebic T, Kinter A, Poli G, Anderson ME, Meister A, Fauci AS. Suppression of human immunodeficiency virus expression in chronically infected monocytic cells by glutathione, glutathione ester, and N-acetylcysteine. Proc Nat Acad Sci 1991;88:986-90.

Kanetsky PA, Giammon MD, Mandelblatt J, et al. Dietary intake and blood levels of lycopene: association with cervical dysplasia among non-hispanic, black women. Nutr Cancer 1998;31:3140.

Keli SO, Hertog MG, Feskens EJ, Kromhout D. Diteary flavonoids, antioxidant vitamins, and incidence of stroke: The Zutphen study. Archives of Int Med 1996;156 (6):637-42.

Kelly FJ, et al. Respiratory Med 1995;89:647-56.

Ketterer B, Coles B, Meyer DJ. The role of glutathione in detoxication. Environ Health Perspect 1982;49:59-60.

Khor HT, Chieng DY, Ong KK. Tocotrienols inhibit liver HMG-CoA reductase activity in the guinea pig. Nutr Res 1995;15:537-44.

Kidd PM. Natural antioxidants Nfirst line of defense. In:Kidd PM, Huber W. Living with the AIDS Virus: A Strategy for Long-Term Survival. Albany, California: PMD Biomedical-Nutritional Consulting; 1991:115-142.

Kidd PM. Liver biotransformation of xenobiotics, foods, and drugs to free radical oxidants. In: Levine SA, Kidd PM. Antioxidant Adaptation in Its Role in Free Radical Pathology. San Leandro, CA: Biocurrents; 1985:222-281.

Kilic F Handleman GJ, Serbinova E, Packer L, Trevithick JR. Modelling cortical cataractogenesis 17: In vitro effect of a-lipoic acid on glucose-induced lens membrane damage, a model of diabetic cataractogenesis. Biochem and Mol Biol International 1995;37:361-70.

Kinscherf R, Fischbach T, Mihm S, et al. Effect of glutathione depletion and oral N-acetyl-cysteine treatment on CD4+ and CD8+ cells. FASEB J 1994;8:448-451.

Kinsella JE, Frankel E, German B, Kanner J. Possible mechanisms for the protective role of antioxidants in wine and plant foods. Food Technology 1993;47 (4):85-89.

Kleijnen J Knipschild P. Ginkgo biloba for cerebral insufficiency. Brit J Clin Pharm 1992;34 (4):352-58.

Knekt P. Vitamin E and cancer prevention: Methodological aspects of human studies. In Food Factors for Chemistry and Cancer Prevention, edited by H. Ohigashi, T. Osawa, J. Terao, S. Watanabe, and T. Yoshikaw. Tokyo: Springer-Verlag.

Knekt P, Jarvinen R, Reunanen A, Jaatela J. Flavonoid intake and coronary mortality in Finland: a cohort study. Brit Med J (Clin Research Ed.) 1996;312 (7029):478-81.

Knekt P, Marniemi J, Teppo L, Heliovaara M, Aromaa A. Is low selenium a risk factor of lung cancer? Am J Epidemiology 1998;148 (no. 10).

Knight JA. Free Radicals, Antioxidants, Aging, and Disease. Washington: AACC Press, 1999.

Kolonel LN, Marchand L, et al. Relation of nutrient intakes and smoking in relation to cancer incidence in Cook Islanders. Proc Am Ass for Cancer Res 1991;32:472.

Komiyama K, Iuzuka K, Yamaoka M, Watanabe H, Tsuchiya N, Umezawa I. Studies on the biological activity of tocotrienols. Chem Pharm Bulletin 1989;37:1369-71.

Kooyenga DK, Geller m, Watkins TR, Gapor A, Diakoumakis E, Bierenbaum ML. Palm oil antioxidants: Effects in patients with hyperlipidemia and carotid stenosis – 2 year experience. Asia Pacific Journal of Clin Nutr 1997;6:72-75.

Korver O. Tea components and cancer prevention. In Food Factors for Chemistry and Cancer Prevention, edited by H Ohigashi, T. Osawa, J Terao, S. Watanabe, and T. Yoshikaw. Todyo: Springer-Verlag.

Krinsky NL. Actions of carotenoids in biological systems. Ann Rev Nutr 1993;13:561-87.

Kumegaki. Am J Clin Nutr. Feb 1994.

Lang CA, Naryshkin S, Schneider DL, et al. Low blood glutathione levels in healthy aging adults. J Lab Clin Med 1992;120:720-225.

Langer S. Carotenoids may prevent cancer growths. Better Nutrition, March 1990.

Langsjoen PH, Folkers K, Lyson K, Muratsu K, Lyson T, Langjoen P. Pronounced increase of survival of pationts with cardiomyopathy when treated with coenzyme Q10 and conventional therapy. International J Tissue Reactions 1990;12 (3):163-68.

Larson RA. Phytochem. 1998.

Lass A, Agawal S, Sohal RS. Mitochondrial ubiquinone honologues, superoxide radical generation, and longevity in different mammalian species. J Biol Chem 1997;272:19199-204.

Lau B. Garlic and you: The modern medicine. 1997; Apple Publishing Co.

Le Bars PL, Katz MM, Berman N, et al. A placebo-controlled, double-blind, randomized trial of an extract of ginkgo biloba for dementia. North American Egb Study Group. J Am Med Assoc 1997;278 (16):1327-32.

Lee HP, Gorrley L, et al. Dietary effects on breast-cancer risk in Singapore. Lancet 1991; 28 (5):1197-200.

Leske MC, Chylack Jr. LT, He Q, Wu SY, Schoenfeld E, Friend J, Wolfe J. Antioxidant vitamins and nuclear opacities: The longitudinal study of cataract. 1997;105 (R):831-36.

Levine M, Conry-Cantilena C, Wang Y, Welch W, Washko PW, et al. Vitamin C pharmacokinetics in healthy volunteers: Evidence for a recommended dietary allowance. Proc Nat Acad Sci 1996; 93 (8):3704-09.

Lieber CS. Alcohol-induced liver disease. In: Maddrey WC, ed. Gastroenterology and Hepatology: The Comprehensive Visual Reference. Phaladelphia: Current Medicine; 1996:9.l-9.21.

Lipoic acid improves nerve blood flow, reduces oxidative stress, and improves distal nerve conduction in experimental diabetic neuropathy. Diabetes Care. Aug 1995;25(4):1160-7.

Lipoic acid increases de novo synthesis of cellular glutathione by improving cystine utilization. Biofactors. 1997;6(3):321-38.

Lipoic (thioctic) acid increases brain energy availability and skeletal muscle performance as shown by in vivo 31P-MRS in a patient with mitochondrial cytopathy. J Neurol. Jul 1995;25(4):472-7.

Lockwood K, Moesgarrd S, Hanioka T, Folkers K. Apparent partial remission of breast cancer in "High riskP patients supplemented with nutritional antioxidants, essential fatty acids and coenzyme Q10. Molecular Aspects of Medicine 1994;15 (suppl):S231-40.

Lomaestro BM, Malone M. Glutathione in health and disease: pharmacotherapeutic issues. Annals Pharmacother 1995;29: 1263-73.

Maitra L, Serbinova E, Tritschler HJ, Packer L. Alpha-lipoic acid prevents buthionine sulfoximine-induced cataract formation in newborn rats. Free Rad Biol & Med 1995;18:823-29.

Markesbery WR. Oxidative stress hypothesis in Alzheimer's disease. Am J Clin Nutr 1987;45:877-95.

Mayne ST. Beta-carotene, carotenoids and disease prevention in humans. The Federation of Am Soc for Exp Biol (FASEB) J 1996;10:690-701.

McCord JM, Fridovich Il Superoxide dismutase: An enzymic function for erythrocuprein (hemocuprein). J Biol Chem 1969;244:6049-55.

Meister A. Glutathione metabolism. Monothiols and Dithiols, Protein Thiols and Thiyl Radicals. 1995; in Vol. 251 of Biothiols, Methods in Enzymology, edited by L. Packer. San Diego: Academic Press.

Meister A. Minireview: Glutathione-ascorbic acid antioxidant system in animals. J Biol Chem 1994(April 1);269(13):9397-9400.

Meister A. Mitochondrial changes associated with glutathione deficiency. Biochim Biophys Acta 1995; 1271:35-42.

Meydani M, Evans WJ, Handelman G, Biddle L Fielding RA, Meydani SN, Bkurril J, Fiatarone MA, Blumberg JB, Cannon JG. Protective effect of vitamin E on exercise-induced oxidative damage in young and older adults. Am J Physiol 1993;264 (5pt. 2):R992-98.

Miller NJ, Rice-Evans C, et al. A novel method for measuring antioxidant capacity and its application to monitoring the antioxidant status in premature neonates. Clin Sci 1993;84:407-12.

Mills PK, et al. Cohort study of diet, lifestyle, and prostate cancer in Adventist men. Cancer 64:598-604.

Mindell E, Hopkins V. Dr. Earl Mindell's What You Should Know About the Super Antioxidant Miracle. Keats, 1996.

Mohr D, Bowry VW, Stocker R. Dietary supplementation with coenzyme Q10 within circulating lipoproteins and increased resistance of human low-density lipoprotein to the initiation of lipid peroxidation. Biochimica et Biophysica Acta 1992;1126:247-54.

Monks TJ, Lau SS. Glutathione conjugation as a mechanism for the transport of reactive metabolites. Adv Pharmacol 1994;27:183-206.

Morris DL. J Am Med Ass. Nov 1994.

Morris PE, Bernard GR. Significance of glutathione in lung disease and implications for therapy. Am J Med Sci 1994 Fef;307(2):119-27.

Mowrey DB. The Scientific Validation of Herbal Medicine. 1986.

Murakoshi M, et al. Inhibitory effects of alpha-carotene on proliferation of the human neuroblastoma cell line. J Nat Cancer Inst. 1989:81.

Murray M. Encyclopedia of Natural Med, revised second edition. Prima Publishers, 1998.

Murray MT. The Natural Way to Overcome Depression, Obesity, and Insomnia. Bantam Books: New York, 1998.

Nakamura R, Littarru GP, Folkers K, Wilkinson EG. Study of Co Q10 enzymes in gingiva from patients with periodontal disease and evidence for a deficiency of coenzyme Q10. Proc Nat Acad Sci 1974;71 (4):1456-60.

Nesaretnam, K, Guthrie N, Chambers AF, Carol KK. Effects of tocotrienols on the growth of a human breast cancer cell line in culture. Lipids 1995;30:1139-43.

Neuroprotection by the metabolic antioxidant alpha-lipoic acid. Free Radic Biol Med. 1997;25(4):359-78.

Ngah WW, Jarien,Z,San MM, Marznki A, Top GM, et al. Effect of tocotrienols on hepatocarcinogenesis induced by 2-acetylaminofluorene in rats. Am J Clin Nutr 1991;53:1076S-81S.

Noda Y, Anzai K, Mori A, Kohono M, Shinmei M, Packer L. Hydroxyl and superoxide anion radical scavenging activities of natural source antioxidants using the computerized JES-FR30ESR spectrometer system. Biochem and Mol Biol Int 1997;42:35-44.

Ochi H, Morita I, Murota S. Roles of glutathione and glutathione peroxidase in the protection against endothelial cell injury induced by 15-hydroperoxye-icosatetraenoic acid. Arch Biochem Biophys. 2992;294:407-11.

Omenn GS, Goodman GE, et al. Risk factors for lung cancer and for intervention effects in CARET, the Beta-Carotene and Retinol Efficacy Trial. J Nat Cancer Instute 1996; 88(21):1550-59.

Pacht ER, Timerman AP, Lykens MG, et al. Deficiency of alveolar fluid glutathione in patients with sepsis and the adult respiratory distress syndrome. Chest 1991;100:1397-1403.

Packer L, Colman C. The Antioxidant Miracle. New York: John Wiley & Sons, Inc, 1999.

Packer L. Antioxidant defenses in biological systems: An overview. In Proceedings of the International Symposium on Natural Antioxidants: Molecular Mechanisms and Health Effects, edited by L. Packer, M. Traber, and W. Xin. 1996; Champaign, Ill: Aocs Press.

Packer L. Prevention of free radical damage in the brain – protection by alpha-lipoic acid. In Free Radicals in Brain Physiology and Disorders, edited by L. Packer, M. Hiramatsu, and T. Yoshikawa. 1996; San Diego: Academic Press.

Packer L. Protective role of vitamin E in biological systems. Am J Clin Nutr 1991; 53 (suppl 4):1050-55.

Packer L. Oxidants, antioxidant nutrients and the athlete. J Sports Sci 1997;15:353-63.

Packer L, Saliou C, Droy-Lefaix MT, Christen Y. Ginkgo biloba extract Egb761: Biological actions, antioxidant activity, and regulation of nitric oxide synthase. In Vol 7 of Flavonoids in Health and Disease, edited by C. Rice-Evans and L. Packer. New York: Marcel Dekker.

Packer L, Smith JR, Extension of the lifespan od cultured normal human diploid cells by vitamin E. Proc Nat Acad Sci 1974; 71:4763-67.

Packer L, Sullivan JL. The promise of antioxidants. The Saturday Evening Post 1995; (January/February).

Packer L, Suzuki Y. Vitamin E and a-lipoate: Role in antioxidant recycling and activation of the NF-kB transcription factor. J Mol Aspects of Med 1993;14:229-39.

Packer L, Tritschler HJ. Alpha-lipoic acid – the metabolic antioxidant. Free Rad Biol & Med 1996;20:625-26.

Packer L, Witt EH, Tritschler HJ. Antioxidant properties and clinical implications of alpha-lipoic acid and dihydrolipoic acid. Handbook of Antioxidants, edited by E. Cadenas and L. Packer. New York: Marcel Dekker.

Packer L, Tritschler HJ, Wessel K. Neuroprotection by the metabolic antioxidant a-lipoic acid. Free Rad Biol & Med 1997;22 (1-2):359-78.

Panigrahi M, Sadguna Y, Shivakumar BR, Kolluri S, roy S, Packer L, Ravindranath V. Alpha-lipoic acid protects against reperfusion injury following cerbral ischemia in rats. Brain Research 1996;717:184-88.

Parker RA, Pearce BC, Clark RW, Gordon DA, Wright JK. Tocotrienols regulate cholesterol production in mammalian cells by post-transcriptional suppression of 3-hydroxy-3-methylglutaryl coenzyme A reductase. J Biol Chem 1993; 268:11230-38.

Passwater R. Important AIDS Discovery Explains the Importance of Selenium: An Interview with Will Taylor, PhD." Whole Foods Magazine.

Passwater R. Lipoic acid: The Metabolic Antioxidant. 1995; New Canaan (CT): Keats Publishing.

Pearce BC, Parker RA, Deason ME, Qureshi AA, Wright JK. Hypocholesterolemic activity of synthetic and natural tocotrienols. J Med Chem 1992;35:2595-606.

Phelps, S, Harris WS. Garlic supplementation and lipoprotein oxidation susceptibility. Lipids 1993; 28 (5):475-77.

Pinnell SR, Murad S, Darr D. Induction of collagen synthesis by ascorbic acid. Arch Derm 1987;123:1684-86.

Pressman A. The Glutathione Phenomenon. New York: St. Martin's Press, 1997.

Puglisi LL. J Fitother. 1994; p203-209.

Qureshi AA, Burger WC, Elson CE, Peterson DM. The structure of an inhibitor of cholesterol biosynthesis isolated from barley. J Biol Chem. 1986;261:10544-50.

Qureshi AA, Bradlow BA, Salser WA, Brace LD. Novel tocotrienols of rice bran modulate cardiovascular disease risk parameters of hypercholesterolemic humans. Nutr Biochem 1997;8:290-98.

Regnstrom JJ, Nilsson P, et al. Inverse relation between the concentration of low-density-lipoprotein vitamin E and severity of coronary artery disease. Am J Clin Nutr 1996;63 (2):277-85.

Renaud S. Flavonoids in red wine. J Epidemiology. Feb 1998.

Richie JB Jr, Mills BJ, Lang CA. Correction of a glutathione deficiency in the aging mosquito increases its longevity. Proc Soc Exp Biol Med 1987;184 (1):113-17.

Rimm EB, Stampfer MJ, et al. Vitamin E consumption and the risk of coronary heart disease in men. New Engl J Med 1993;328 (20):145-56.

Robertson JM, Donner AP, Trevithick JR. A possible role for vitamins C and E in cataract prevention. Am J Clin Nutr 1991; 53 (suppl 1):346-51.

Rock CL. Carotenoids: Biology and treatment. Pharm and Therapeutics 1997;75:185-97.

Rohdewald P. Pycnogenol. In Vol 7 of Flavonoids in Health and Disease, edited by C. Rice-Evans and L. Packer. New York: Marcel Dekker.

Rong Y, Li L, Shah V, Lau BH. Pycnogenol protects vascular endothelial cells from t-butyl hydroperoxide-induced oxidant injury. Biotechnology Therapeutics 1995; 5(3-4):117-26.

Rosen P, Packer L. Bitamin E and diabetes mellitus. Diabetes and Stoffwechsel 1997;6:2-3.

Saez G, Thornalley JP, Hill HAO, et al. The production of free radicals during the autoxidation of cystein and their effects on isolated rat hepatocytes. Biochim Piophys Acta 1982;719:24-31.

Salonen JT, et al. Increased risk of non insulin diabetes mellitus and low plasma vitamin E concentrations: A four year follow-up study in men. Brit Med J 1995;311:1124-27.

Salonen JT, Alfthen G, Huttunen JK, Puska P. Association between serum selenium and the risk of cancer. Am J Epidemiol 1984;120:343-345.

Sandhya P, Varalakshmi P. Effect of lipoic acid administration on gentamicin-induced lipid peroxidation in rats. J Appl Toxicol 1997; Nov-Dec;17(6):405-408.

Seddon JM et al. Dietary carotenoids, vitamins A, C, and E, and advanced age-related macular degeneration. J Am Med Ass 1994; Nov 9.

Sen CK, Roy S, Han D, Packer L. Regulation of cellular thiols in human lymphocytes by alpha-lipoic acid: A flow cytometric analysis. Free Rad Biol & Med 1997;22:1241-57.

Sen C, Roy S, Packer L. Therapeutic potential of the antioxidant and redox properties of a-lipoic acid. In Oxidative stress in cancer, AIDS, and neurodegenerative diseases, edited by L. Montagnier, R. Olivier, and C. Pasquier. New York: Marcel Dekker.

Serbinova E, Khwaja S, Reznick AZ, Packer L. Thioctic acid protects against ischemia-reperfusion injury in the isolated perfused Langendorff heart. Free Rad Res Comm 1992;17:49-58.

Serbinova E, Kagan V, Han D, Packer L. Free radical recycling and intramembrane mobility in the antioxidant properties of alpha-tocopherol and alpha-tocotrienol. Free Rad Biol & Med 1991;10:263-75.

Serbinova E, Khwaja S. Palm oil vitamin E protects against ishcemia/reperfusion injury in the isolated perfused Langendorff heart. Nutr Res 1992; 12 (suppl 1):203-13.

Sharoni Y, Levi J. Lycopene and the inhibition of cancer cell growth.

Sies H, Stahl W. Vitamins E and C, beta-carotene and other carotenoids as antioxidants. Am J Clin Nutr 1995;62:1315S-218.

Smith LJ, Houston M, Anderson J. Increased levels of glutathione in bronchoalveolar lavage from patients with asthma. Am Rev Resp Dis 1993;147:1461-64.

Sokal RJ Antioxidant defences in metal-induced liver damage. Sem Liver Dis 1996;16:34-46.

Soleas GJ, Diamandis EP, Goldberg DM. Wine as a biological fluid: History, production, and role in disease prevention. J Clin Lab Analysis 1997;11 (5):287-313.

Stahl W, Sies H. Lycopene: a biologically important carotenoid for humans: Arch Biochem Biophys. 1996;336:1-9.

Stamler JS, Slivka A. Biological chemistry of thiols in the vasculature and in vascular-related disease. Nutr Revs 1996;54:1-30.

Stampfer MJ, Hennekens CH, et al. Vitamin E consumption and the risk of coronary disease in women. New Engl J Med 1993;328 (20):1444-49.

Stephens NG, Parsons A, et al. Randomised controlled trial of vitamin E in patients with coronary disease: Cambridge Heart Antioxidant Study (CHAOS). Lancet 1996;347 (9004):781-86.

Sun Y, Oberley Lw. Redox regulation of transcriptional activation. Free Radical Biol Med 1996;21:335-48.

Suzuki YJ, Tsuchiva M, Packer L. Thioctic acid and dihydrolipoic acid are novel antioxidants which interact with reactive oxygen species. Published erratum appears in Free Rad Res Comm 1991;17 (2) (1992):155, Free Rad Res Comm 15:255-63.

Suzuki YJ, Tsuchiva M, Wassal SR, et al. Structural and dynamic membrane properties of alpha-tocopherol and alpha-tocotrienol: implications to the molecular mechanism of their antioxidant potency. Biochem 1993;32:10692-99.

Taming Oxygen's Wild Side: How Antioxidants Guard Your Health. Tapestry Press 1988; p9.

Tappel AL. Vitamin E as a biological lipid antioxidant. Inform 1997; 8 (4):293-95.

Tateishi N, Higashi T, Naruse A, et al. Relative contributions of sulfur atoms of dietary cysteine and methionine to rat liver glutathione and proteins. J Biochem 1981;90:1603-10.

Teixeira HD, Schumacher RI, Meneghini R. Lower intracellular hydrogen peroxide levels in cells overexpressing CuZn-superoxide dismutase. Proc Natl Acad Sci USA 1998;95:7872-75.

Traber MG. Podda N, Packer L, et al. Diet derived topically applied tocotrienols accumulate in skin and protect the tissue against UV light-induced oxidative stress. Asia Pacific J Clin Nutr 1997;6:63-67.

Treatment of symptomatic diabetic peripheral neuropathy with the antioxidant alpha-lipoic acid. A 3-week multicentre randomized controlled trial (ALADIN Study). Diabetologia. 1995; Dec 25(4):1425-33.

Truscott G. Lycopene twice as effective as beta-carotene in reducing ROS damage.

Valenzuela A, et al. Planta Medica. 1989; 50:420-22.

van den Brandt PA, Goldbohm RA, et al. A prospective cohort study on selenium status and the risk of lung cancer. Cancer Res 1993; 53 (20):4860-65.

van Poppel G, Kardinaal A, Princen H, Kok FJ. Antioxidants and coronary heart disease. Ann Med 1994; 26 (6):429-34.

van Zandwijk N. N-acetyl-cysteine (NAC) and glutathione (GSH): antioxidant and chemopreventive properties, with special reference to lung cancer. J Cell Biochem Suppl 1995;22:24-32.

Vinson JA, et al. In Vitro and In Vivo Reduction of Erythrocyte Sorbitol by Ascorbic Acid. Diabetes 1989;38:1036-41.

Virgil F, Kobuchi H, Noda Y, Cossins E, Packer L. Pro-cyanidins from Pinus maritima Bark: Antioxidants activity, effects on the immune system and modulation of nitrogen monoxide metabolism. In Antioxidant Food Supplements in Human Health, edited by L Packer, T. Yoshikaw, and M. Hiramatsu. San Diego: Academic Press.

Virgil F, Kobuchi H, Packer L. Nitrogen monoxide (NO) metabolism: Antioxidant properties and modulation of inducible NO synthase activity in activated macrophages by procyanidins extracted from Pinas maritima (Pycnogenol). Flavonoids in Health and Disease, edited by C. Rice-Evans and L Packer. New York: Marcel Dekker.

Watkins TR, Lenz P, Bierenbaum ML, et al. a-tocotrienol as a hypocholesterolemic and antioxidant agent in rats few atherogenic diets. Lipids 1993;28:1113-18.

Whei ZA, et al. Redox Report. 1997; Vol 3:219-24.

Wolfe G. Gap junctions. Nutr Rev. Sept 1992.

Woodall AA, Ames BN. Diet and oxidative damage to DNA: The importance of ascorbate as an antioxidant. Vitamin C in Health and Disease, edited by L. Packer and J. Fuchs. New York: Marcel Dekker.

Wu D, Meydani SN, Sastre J, Hayek M, Mdydani M. In vitro glutathione supplementation enhances interleukin-2 production and mitogenic response of periperal blood mononuclear cells from young and old subjects. J Nutr 1994;124 (r):655-63.

Yang CS, Wang ZY. Tea and cancer. J Nat Cancer Inst 1993; 85 (13):1038-49.

Ziegler D, Gries FA. Alpha-lipoic acid in the treatment of diabetic peripheral and cardiac autonomic neuropathy. Diabetes 46 (suppl 2):62-66.

Ziegler RG. Vegetables, fruits, and carotenoids and the risk of cancer. Am J Clin Nutr 1991;53 (suppl 1):251-59.

Section V: Disease

Cancer

Alabaster O, Tang Z, Frost A, Shivapurkar N. Effect of beta-carotene and wheat bran fiber on colonic aberrant crypt and tumor formation in rats exposed to azoxymethane and high dietary fat. Carcinogenesis 1995;91:125-32.

Alpha-Tocopherol, Beta-Caroten Cancer Prevention Study Group. The effect of vitamin E and beta-carotene on the incidence of lung cancer and other cancers in male smokers. N Engl J Med 1994;330:1029-35.

Ames BN, Gold LS, Willett WC. The causes and prevention of cancer. Proc Natl Acad Sci USA 1995;92:5258-65.

Ames BN, Shigenaga MK. Oxidants are a major contributor to cancer and aging. In: DNA and free radicals. Halliwell B, Aruoma O, eds. New York: Ellis Horwood; 1993:3-15.

Baker AM, Oberley LW, Cohen MB. Expression of antioxidant enzymes in human prostatic adenocarcinoma. Prostate 1997;32:229-33.

Beckman KB, Ames BN. Oxidative decay of DNA. J Biol Chem 1997;272:19633-36.

Bernstein L, Henderson BE, Hanisch R, et al. Physical exercise and reduced risk of breast cancer in young women. J Natl Cancer Inst 1994;86:1403-1408.

Block B, Patterson B, Subar A. Fruits, vegetables and cancer prevention: A review of the epidemiologic evidence. Nutr Cancer 1992;18:1-29.

Borek C. Antioxidants and cancer. Sci Med 1997;Nov/Dec52-61.

Blot WJ, Li J-Y, Taylor PR, et al. Nutrition intervention trials in Linxian, China: Supplementation with specific vitamin/mineral combinations, cancer incidence, and disease-specific mortality in the general population. JNCI 1993;85:1483-92.

Braun MM, Caporaso NE, Page WF, Hoover RN. Genetic component of lung cancer: Cohort study of twins. Lancet 1994;344:440-443.

Brewer DA, Bokey EL, Fung C, Chapuis PH. Heredity, molecular genetics and colorectal cancer: A review. Aust NZ J Surg 1992;63:87-94.

Burkitt DP. Epidemiology of cancer of the colon and rectum. Cancer 1971;28:3-13.

Carroll KK. Experimental evidence of dietary factors and hormone-dependent cancers. Cancer Res 1975;35:3374-83.

Cheeseman KH. Lipid peroxidation and cancer. In: DNA and free radicals. Halliwell B, Aruoma O, eds. New York Ellis Horwood; 1993:109-44.

Cerutti PA. Oxy-radicals and cancer. Lancet 1994;344:862-863.

Cheng KC, Cahill DS, Kasai H, et al. 8-Hydroxyguanine, an abundant form of oxidative DNA damage, causes G ® T and A ® C substitutions. J Biol Chem 1992;267:166-172.

Chinery R, Brockman JA, Peeler MO, et al. Antioxidants enhance the cytotoxicity of chemotherapeutic agents in colorectal cancer: A p53-independent induction of p21 WAF1/Cip1 via C/EBP beta. Nature Med 1997;2:1233-41.

Clinton SK, Emenhiser C, Schwartz SJ, et al. Cis-trans lycopene isomers, carotenoids, and retinol in the human Prostate. Cancer Epidemiol Biomarkers Prev 1996;823-33.

Cohen LA. Diet and cancer. Sci Am 1987;257:42-48.

Doll R, Peto R. The cause of cancer: Quantitative estimates of available risks of cancer in the United States today. J Natl Cancer Inst 1981;66:1191-1308.

Duthie GG, Arthur JR, James WPT. Effects of smoking and vitamin E on blood antioxidant status. Am J Clin Nutr 1991;53:1061S-63S.

Enstrom JE, Kanim LE, Klein MA. Vitamin C intake and mortality among a sample of the United States population. Epidemiology 1992;3:194-202.

Feig KI, Reid TM, Loeb LA. Reactive oxygen species in tumorogenesis. Cancer Res 1994;54(suppl):1890S-94S.

Floyd RA, Watson JJ, Harris J, et al. Formation of 8-hydroxy deoxyguanosine, hydroxyl free radical adduct of DNA in granulocytes exposed to tumor promoter, tetradecanoyl phorbolacetate. Biochem Biophys Res Commun 1986;137:841-46.

Ford D, Easton DF, Bishop DT, et al. Risks of cancer in BRCA1-mutation carriers. Breast Cancer Linkage Consortium. Lancet 1994;343:692-695.

Frank AL. The epidemiology and etiology of lung cancer. Clin Chest Med 1982;3:219-28.

Fredrikson M, Axelson O, Sun XF, et al. A pilot study on risk factors and p53 gene expression in colorectal cancer. BR J Cancer 1996;73:1428-30.

Frei B, Forte TM, Ames BN, Cross CE. Gas phase oxidants of cigarette smoke induce lipid peroxidation and changes in lipoprotein properties in human blood plasma: Protective effects of ascorbic acid. Biochem J 1991;277:133-38.

Fuchs CS, Giovannucci EL, Colditz GA, et al. A prospective study of family history and the risk of colorectal cancer. N Engl J Med 1994;331:1669-74.

Giovannucci E, Rimm EB, Colditz GA, et al. A prospective study of dietary fat and risk of prostate cancer. Cancer 1995;75:1766-77.

Giovannucci E. Epdemiologic characteristics of prostate cancer. Cancer 1995;75:1776-77.

Giovannucci E, Ascherio A, Rimm EB, et al. Intake of carotenoids and retinol in relation to risk of prostate cancer. J Natl Cancer Inst 1995;87:1767-76.

Giovannucci I Rimm EB, Stampfer MJ, et al. A prospective study of cigarette smoking and risk of colorectal adenoma and colorectal cancer in U.S. men. J

Natl Cancer Inst 1994;86:183-91.

Giovannucci E, Colditz GA, Stampfer MJ, et al. A prospective study of cigarette smoking and risk of colorectal adenoma and colorectal cancer in S.S. women. J Natl Cancer Inst 1994;86:192-99.

Gridley G, McLaughlin JK, Block G, et al. Vitamin supplement use and reduced risk of oral and pharyngeal cancer. JNCI 1988;80:1237-43.

Guyton KZ, Kensler TW. Oxidative mechanisms in carcinogenesis. Br Med Bull 1993;49:523-44.

Harman D. Dimethylbenzanthracene induced cancer: inhibiting effect of dietary vitamin E. Clin Res 1969;17:125 (abstr).

Heber D, Ashley JM, Leaf DA, Barnard RJ. Reduction of serum estradiol in post menopausal women given free access to low-fat high-carbohydrate diet. Nutrition 1991;7:120-128.

Henderson BE, Ross RK, Pike MC. Toward the primary prevention of cancer. Science 1991;254:1131-37.

Holt PR, Atillasoy EO, Gilman J, et al. Modulation of abnormal colonic epithelial cell proliferation and differentiation by low-fat dairy foods. JAMA 1998;280:1074-79.

Huang Z, Hankinson SE, Colditz GA, et al. Dual effects of weight and weight gain on breast cancer risk. JAMA 1997;278:1407-11.

Jick H, Walker AM, Watkins RN, et al. Replacement estrogens and breast cancer. Am J Epidemiol 1980;112:586-94.

Knekt P, Jarvinen R, Seppanen R, et al. Dietary flavonoids and the risk of lung cancer and other malignant neoplasms. Am J Epidemiol 1997;146:223-30.

Kvale G, Bjelke E, Gart JJ. Dietary habits and lung cancer risk. Int J Cancer. 1983;31:397-405.

Lynch HT, Krush AJ, Lemon HM, et al. Tumor variation in families with breast cancer. JAMA 1972;222:1631-35.

Malins DC, Polissar NL, Gunselman SJ. Progression of human breast cancers to metastatic state is linked to hydroxyl radical-induced DNA damage. Proc Natl Acad Sci USA 1996;93:2557-63.

Nakayama T, Kaneko M, Dodama M, Nagata C. Cigarette smoke induces DNA single-strand breaks in human cells. Nature 1985;314:462-64.

NCI, Annual Cancer Statistics Review Including Cancer Trends: 1950-1985. NI H Publ 88-2789. Betesda, MD: NIH;1988.

Paganini-Hill A, Chao A, Ross RK, Henderson BE. Vitamin A, beta-carotene and the risk of cancer: A prospective study. J Natl Cancer Inst 1987;79:443-48.

Parker SL, Tong T, Bolden S, Wingo PA. Cancer statistics, 1997. CA Cancer J Clin 1997;47:5-27.

Patterson BH, Block G, Rosenberger WF, et al. Fruit and vegetables in the American diet: Data from the NHANES 11 survey. Am J Public Health 1990;80:1443-49.

Peto R, Lopez AD, Boreham J, et al. Mortality from tobacco in developed countries: Indirect estimation from national vital statistics. Lancet 1992;330:1268-78.

Pryor WA, Stone K. Oxidants in cigarette smoke. Ann NY Acad Sci 1993;686:12-28.

Reddy BS, Sharma C, Simi B, et al. Metabolic epidemiology of colon cancer: Effect of dietary fiber on fecal mutagens and bile acids in healthy subjects. Cancer Res 1987;47:644-48.

Richter C, Park J-W, Ames BN. Normal oxidative damage to mitochondrial and nuclear DNA. Proc Natl Acad Sci USA. 1988;85:6465-67.

Salonen JT, Alfthen G, Huttunen JK, Puska P. Association between serum selenium and the risk of cancer. Am J Epidemiol 1984;120:343-49.

Sandler RS, Lyles Cm, McAuliff C, et al. Cigarette smoking, alcohol, and the risk of colorectaladenomas. Gastroenterology 1993;104:1445-51.

Schectman G, Burd JC, Hoffman R. Ascorbic acid requirments for smokers: Analysis of a population survey. Am J Clin Nutr 1991;53:1466-70.

Selikoff IJ, Lilis R, Nicholson WJ. Asbestos-associated disease in United States shipyards. Ann NY Acad Sci 1979;330:295-311.

Shivapurkar N, Tang Z, Frost A, Alabaster O. Inhibition of progression of aberrant crypt foci and colon tumor development by vitamin E and beta-carotene in rats on a high-risk diet. Cancer Lett 1995;91:125-32.

Silverberg E, Lubera UJ. Cancer statistics. CA 1988;38:2-22.

Simopoulos AP. Obesity and carcinogenesis: Historical perspective. Am J Clin Nutr 1987;45:271-76

Smoking and Health--A National Status Report. A Report to Congress. Publication NO. HHS/PHS/CDC 87-8396. Washington, DC: Department of Health and Human Services; 1987.

Statland BE. Nutrition and cancer. Clin Chem 1992;38:1587-94.

Vogelstein B, Fearon ER, Kern SE, et al. Alleotype of colorectal carcinomas. Science 1989:244:207-11.

Weber BL, Garber JE. Family history and breast cancer: probabilities and possibilities. JAMA 1992;270:1602-03.

Weisenberger JH. Nutritional approach to cancer prevention with emphasis on vitamins, antioxidants, and carotenoids. Am J Clin Nutr 1991;53:226S-37S.

Weitzman SA, Stossel TP. Effects of oxygen radical scavengers and antioxidants on phagocyte-induced mutagenesis. J Immunol 1982;128:2770-72.

Weitzman SA, Gordon LI. Inflammation and cancer: Role of phagocyte-generated oxidants in carcinogenesis. Blood 1990;76:655-663.

Willett WC. Diet, nutrition, and avoidable cancer. Environ Health perspect 1995;103(suppl 8):165-70.

Willett WC, Polk BF, Morris JS, et al. Prediagnostic serum selenium and risk of cancer. Lancet 1983;2:130-34.

Wooster R, Bignell G, Lancaster J, et al. Identification of the breast cancer susceptibility gene BRCA2. Nature 1995;375:789-92,

Wu AH, Paganini-Hill A, Ross RK, et al. Alcohol, physical activity and other risk factors for colorectal cancer: A prospective study. BR J Cancer 1987;55:687-94.

Yong L-C, Brown CC, Schatzkin A, et al. Intake of vitamins E, C, and A and risks of lung cancer. Am J Epidemiol 1997;146:231-43.

Zhuang JC, Lin C, Lin D, Wogan GN. Mutagenesis associated with nitric oxide production in macrophages. Proc Natl Acad Sci USA 1998;95:8286-91.

Ziegler RG. Vegetables, fruits, and carotenoids and the risk of cancer. Am J Clin Nutr 1991;53:251S-259S.

Cardiovascular Disease

Basha BJ, Sowers JR. Atherosclerosis: An update. Am Heart J 1995;131:1192-1202.

Belcher JD, Balla J, Balla G, et al. Vitamin E, LDL, and endothelium: Brief oral vitamin supplementation prevents oxidized LDL-mediated vascular injury in vitro. Arterioscler Thromb 1992;13:1779-89.

Boli R, Patel BS, Jeroudi MO, et al. Demonstration of free radical generation in "stunned" myocardium of intact dogs with the use of the spin trap alpha-phenyl N-tert-butyl nitrone. J Clin Invest 1988;82:476-85.

Boli R, McCay PB. Use of spin traps in intact animals undergoing myocardial ischemia/reperfusion: A new approach to assessing the role of oxygen free radicals in myocardial "stunning." Free Radical Res Comm 1990;9:169-80.

Braunwald E, Kloner RA. The stunned myocardium: Prolonged postischemic ventricular dysfunction. Circulation 1982;66:1146-49.

Buttery LDK, Springall Dr, Chester AH. Inducible nitric oxide synthase is present within human atherosclerotic lesions and promotes the formation and activity of peroxynitrite. Lab Invest 1996;75:77-85.

Dargel R. Lipid peroxidation – A common pathogenetic mechanism? Exp Toxic Pathol 1992;44:169-81.

Davies MJ, Thomas A. Thrombosis and acute coronary-artery lesions in sudden cardiac ischemic death. N Engl J Med 1984;310:1137-40.

Devaraj S, Li D, Jialal I. The effects of alpha-tocopherol supplementation on monocyte function. J Clin Invest 1996;98:756-63.

Diplock AT. Antioxidant nutrients and disease prevention: An overview. Am J Clin Nutr 1991;53:189S-193S.

DiMascio P, Kaiser S, Sies H. Lycopene is the most efficient biological carotenoid singlet oxygen quencher. Arch Biochem Biophys 1989;274:1-7.

Esterbaur H, Puhl H, Dieber-Rutheneder M, et al. Effect of antioxidants on oxidative modification of LDL. Ann Med 1991;23:573-81.

Frei B. Reactive oxygen species and antioxidant vitamins: Mechanisms of action. Am J Med 1994;97 (suppl 3A):5S-13S.

Frei B, England L, Ames BN. Ascorbate is an outstanding antioxidant in human blood plasma. Proc Natl Acad Sci USA 1988;85:9748-52.

Fuster V, Badimon I, Badimon JJ, Chesebro JH. The pathogenesis of coronary artery disease and the acute coronary syndrome. N Engl J Med 1992;326:242-50.

Goldstein JL, Ho Yk, Basu Sk, Brown MS. Binding site on macrohpages that mediate uptake and degradation of acetylated low density lipoprotein producing massive cholesterol deposition. Proc Natl Acad Sci USA 1979;76:333-37.

Gordon T, Castelli WP, Hjortland MC, et al. High density lipoprotein as a protective factor against coronary heart disease. Am J Med 1977;62:707-14.

Graham IM, Daly LE, Refsum HM, et al. Plasma homocysteine as a risk factor for vascular disease. JAMA 1997;277:1775-81.

Granger DN, Rutili G, McCord JM. Superoxide radicals in feline intestinal ischemia. Gasroenterology 1981;81:22-29.

Harats D, Chevion S, Hahir M, et al. Citrus fruit supplementation reduces lipoprotein oxidation in young men ingesting a diet high in saturated fat: Presumptive evidence for an interaction between vitamin C and E in vivo. Am J Clin Nutr 1998;57:240-45.

Henriksen T, Mahoney EM, Steinberg D. Enhanced macrophage degradation of low-density lipoprotein previously incubated with cultured endothelial cells. Recognition by receptors for acetylated low-density lipoproteins. Proc Natl Acad Sci USA 1981;78:6499-6503.

Hertog MGI, Feskins EJM, Hollman PC, et al. Dietary antioxidant flavonoids and risk of coronary artery disease: The Zutphen elderly study. Lancet 1993;342:1007-11.

Jialal I, Norkus EP, Cristol L, Grundy SM. Beta-carotene inhibits the oxidative modification of low density lipoprotein. Biochim Biophys Acta 1991;1086:134-38.

Jialal I, Fuller CJ, Huer B. The effect of alpha-tocopherol supplementation on LDL oxidation. Arterioscler Thromb Vasc Biol 1994;14:1990-98.

Kagan VE, Savov VM, Didenko VV, et al. Calcium and lipid peroxidation inmitochondrial and microsomal membranes in the heart. Bull Exp Biol Med 1982;95:459-461.

Kinscherf R, Claus R, Wagner M, et al. Apoptosis caused by oxidized LDL is manganese superoxide dismutase and p53 dependent. FASEB J 1998;12:463-67.

Knight JA. Laboratory Medicine and the Aging Process. Chicago. ASCP Press; 1996:89-143.

Li PF, Dietz R, von Harsdorf R. Differential dffect of hydrogen peroxide and superoxide anion on apoptosis and proliferation of vascular smooth muscle cells. Circulation 1997:96:3602-09.

Maggi E, Chiesa R, Melissano G, et al. LDL oxidation in attients with severe carotid atherosclerosis: A study of invitro and in vivo oxidation markers. Aterioscler Thromb 1994;14:1892-99,

McCord JM, Fridovich I. The reduction of cytochrome c by milk xanthine oxidase. J Biol Chem 1968;243:5753-60.

McCord JM. Free radicals and myocardial ischemia: An overview and outlook. Free Radical Biol Med 1988;4:9-14.

McGinnis JM, Goege WH. Actual causes of death in the United States. JAMA 1993;27-:2207-12.

Mehta J. Intake of antioxidants among American cardiologists. Am J Cardiol 1997;79:1558-60.

Mitsos SE, Fantone JC, Gallagher KP, et al. Canine myocardial reperfusion injury: protection by a free radical scavenger, N-2-mercaptopropionyl glycine. J Cardiovas Pharm 1986;8:978-98.

Miwa K, Miyagi Y, Igawa A, et al. Vitamin E deficiency in variant angina. Circulation 1996;94:14-18.

Murphy E, Aitcon JF, Horres Cr, Lieberman M. Calcium elevation in cultured heart cells: Its role in cell injury. Am J Physiol 1983;245:C316-321.

Nigdikar SV, Williams NR, Griffin CD, Howard AN. Consumption of red wine polyphenols reduces the susceptibility of low-density lipoproteins to oxidation in vivo. Am J Clin Nutr 1998;68: 258-65.

NyyssonenK, Parviainen MT, Salonen R, et al. Vitamin C deficiency and risk of myocardial infarction: Prospective population study of men from eastern

Finland. Br Med J 1997;314:634-38.

Oliver CN, Starke-Reed PE, Stadtman ER, et al. Oxidative damage to brain proteins, loss of glutamine synthetase activity, and production of free radicals during ischemia/reperfusion-induced injury to gerbil brains. Proc Natl Acad Sci USA 1990;87:5144-47.

Packer L, Tritschler HJ, Wessel K. Neuroprotection by the metabolic antioxidant alpha-lipoic acid. Free Radical Biol Med 1997;22:359-378.

Quinn MT, Parthasarathy S, Steinberg D. Endothelial cell-derived cgenitactuc activity for mouse peritoneal macrophages and the effect of modified forms of low density lipoprotein. Proc. Natl Acad Sci USA 1985;82:5949-53.

Rangan U, Bulkley GB. Prospects for treatment of free radical-mediated tissue injury. Br Med Bull 1993;49:700-18.

Regnstrom J, Nilsson J, Moldeus P, et al. Inverse relation between the concentration of low-density-lipoprotein vitamin E and severity of coronary artery disease. Am J Clin Nutr 1996;63:77-85.

Retsky KL, Freeman MO, Frei B. Ascorbic acid oxidation product(s) protect human low density lipoprotein against atherogenic modification. J Biol Chem 1993;268:1304-09.

Rimm EB, Katan MB, Ascherio A, et al. Relation between intake of flavonoids and risk for coronary heart disease in male health professionals. Ann Intern Med 1996;125-:384-89.

Ross R. The pathogenesis of atherosclerosis: A perspective for the 1990s. Nature 1993;362:801-09.

Stampfer MJ, Malinow MR, Willett WC, et al. A prospective study of plasma homosyst(e)ine and risk of myocardial infarction in U.S. physicians. JAMA 1992;268:877-81.

Steinberg D. Modified forms of low-density lipoprotein and atherosclerosis. J Intern Med 1993;233:227-32.

Steinbrecher UP, Parthasarathy L, Leake DS, et al. Modification of low density lipoprotein by endothelial cells involves lipid peroxidation and degradation of low density pipoprotein phospholipids. Proc Natl Acad Sci USA 1984;83:3883-87.

Stephens NG, Parsons A, Schofield PM, et al. Randomised controlled trial of vitamin E in patients with coronary disease: Cambridge Heart Antioxidant Study (CHAOS). Lancet 1996;347:781-86.

Sun J, Giraud DW, Moxley RA, Driskell JA. Beta-carotene and alpha-tocopherol inhibit the development of atheroxclerotic rabbits. Int J Vitam Nutr Res 1997;67:155-63.

Thaulow GE, Sandvik L, Stormarker H, Erikssen J. Hematocrit: A predictor of cardiovascular mortality? J Intern Med 1993;234:493-99.

Westhuyzen J. The oxidation hypothesis of atheroxclerosis: An update. Ann Clin Lab Sci 1997;27:1-10.

Witztum JL. The oxidation hypothesis of athersclerosis. Lancet 1994;344:793-95.

Diabetes

Cowden WB, Lewis-Hughes PH, Clark IA. Protection against alloxan-induced diabetes in mice by the free radical scavenger butylated hydrox-yanisole. Biochem Pharmacol 1985;34:3601-03.

Fisher IJ, Hamburger SA. Inhibition of alloxan action in isolated pancreatic islets by superoxide dismutase, catalase, and a meta chelator. Diabetes 1980;29:213-16.

Matkovics B, Kotormanm, Varga IS, et al. Oxidative stress in experimental diabetes induced by streptozotocin. Acta Physiol Hung 1997-98;85:29-38.

Nishigaki I, Hagihara M, Tsunekawa H, et al. Lipid peroxide levels of serum lipoprotein fractions of diabetic patients. Biochem Med 1978;25:373-78.

Oberley LW. Free radicals and diabetes. Free Radical Biol Med 1988;5:113-24.

Palmer AM, Thomas CR, Gopaul N, et al. Dietary antioxidant supplementa-tion reduces lipid peroxidation but impairs vascular function in small mesen-teric arteries of the streptozotocin-diabetic rat. Diabetologia 1998;41:148-56.

Rerup CC. Drugs producing diabetes through damage of the insulin secreting cells. Pharmacol Rev 1970;22:485-518.

Slonim AE, Surber ME, Page DE, et al. Modification of chemically induced diabetes in rats by vitamin E: Supplementation minimizes and depletion enhances developmental diabetes. J Clin Invest 1983;71:1282-88.

Uzel N, Sivas A, Uysal M, Oz H. Erythrocyte lipid peroxidation and glu-tathione peroxidase activities in patients with diabetes mellitus. Horm Metab Res 1987;19:89-90.

Lung Disease

Bast A, Haenen GRMM, Doelamn CJA. Oxidants and antioxidants: State of the art. Am J Med 1991;91:2S-13S.

Behr J, Maier K, Degenkolb B, et al. Antioxidative and clinical effects of high-dose N-acetylcysteine in fibrosing alveolitis: Adjunctive therapy to mainte-nance immunosuppression. Am J Respir Crit Care Med 1997;156:1897-1901.

Binger CAL, Faulkner JM, Moore RL. Oxygen poisoning in mammals. J Exp Med 1927;45:849-64.

Borek C. Antioxidants and cancer. Sci Med 1997;Nov/Dec:52-61.

Britton JR, Pavord ID, Richards KA, et al. Dietary antioxidant vitamin intake and lung function in the general population. Am J Respir Crit Care Med 1995;151:1383-87.

Euler DE, Dave SJ, Guo H. Effect of cigarette smoke on pentane excretion in alveolar breath. Clin Chem 1996;42:303-08.

Freeman BA, Crapo JD. Hyperoxia increases oxygen radical production in rat lungs and lung mitochondria. J Biol Chem 1981;256:10986-92.

Fung H, Kow YW, Van Houten B, Mossman BT. Patterns of 8-hydroxy-deoxyguanosine formation in DNA and indications of oxidative stress in rat and human pleural mesothelial cells after exposure to crocidolite asbestos. Carcinogenesis 1997;18:825-32.

Gadek JE, Fells GA, Crystal RG. Cigarette smoking induces functional antiprotease deficiency in the lower respiratory tract of humans. Science 1979;202:1315-16.

Guyer B, Strobino DM, Ventura SJ, et al. Annual summary of vital statistics – 1995. Pediatrics 1996;98:1007-1019.

Hamid Q, Springall DR, Riveros-Moreno V, et al. Induction of nitric oxide synthase in asthma. Lancet 1993;342:1510-13.

Hatch GE. Asthma, inhaled oxidants, and dietary antioxidants. Am J Clin Nutr. 1995;61 (Suppl):625S-630S.

Hautamaki RD, Kobayashi DK, Senior RM, Shapiro SD. Requirment for macrophage elastase for cigarette smoke-induced imphysema in mice. Science 1997;277:2002-04.

Janoff A. Elastases and emphysema: Current assessment of the protease antiprotease hypothesis. Am Rev Respir Dis 1985;132:417-33.

Leff JA, Wilke CP, Hybertson BM, et al. Postinsult treatment with N-acetyl - L-cysteine decreases IL-1 induced neutrophil influx and lung leak in rats. Am J Physiol 1993;265:L501-06.

Leff JA, Parsons PE, Day CE, et al. Serum antioxidants as predictors of adult respiratory distress syndrome in patients with sepsis. Lancet 1993;341:777-780.

Lykesfeldt J, Loft S, Nielsen JB, Poulsen HE. Ascorbic acid and dehy-droascorbic acid as biomarkers of oxidative stress caused by smoking. Am J Clin Nutr 1997;65:959-63.

MacNee W, Wiggs B, Belzberg AS, Hogg JC. The effect of cigarette smoking on neutrophil kinetics in human lungs. N Engl J Med 1989;321:924-28.

McElroy MC, Postle AD, Kelly FJ. Catalase, superoxide dismutase and glu-tathione peroidase activities of lung and liver during human development. Biochim Biophys Acta 1992;1117:153-58.

Nash G. Blennerhassett JB, Pontoppidan H. Pulmonary lesions associated with oxygen therapy and artificial ventilation. N Engl J Med 1967;276:368-74.

Olusi SO, Ojutiku OO, Jessop WJE, Iboko MI. Plasma and white blood cell ascorbic acid concentrations in patients with bronchial asthma. Clin Chim Acta 1979;92:161-66.

Owen S, Pearson D, O'Driscoll R, et al. Evidence of free radical activity in asthma. N Engl J Med 1991;325:586-87.

Rahman I, Morrison D, Donaldson K, MacNee W. Systemic oxidative stress in asthma, COPD, and smokers. Am J Respir Crit Care Med 1996;154:1055-60.

Rahman I, Skwarska E, MacNee W. Attenuation of oxidant/antioxidant imbalance during treatment of exacerbations of chronic obstructive pulmonary idsease. Throax 1997;52:565-68.

Repine JE, Beehler CJ. Nurtrophils and adult respiratory distress syndrome: Two interlocking perspectives in 1991. Am Rev Respir Dis 1991;144:251-52.

Ryfeldt A, Bannenberg G, Moldeus P. Free radicals and lung disease. Br Med Bull 1993;49:588-603.

Sibile Y, Reynolds HY. Macrophages and polymorphonuclear neutrophils in lung disease and injury. Am Rev Respir Dis 1990;141:471-501.

Smith JL. Pathological effects due to increase of oxygen tension in air breathed. J Physiol 1899;24:19-35.

Taylor CG, McClutchon TL, Boermans HJ, et al. Comparison of Zn and vitamin E for protection against hyperoxia-induced lung damage. Free Radical Biol Med 1997;22:543-550.

Terpstra GK, Wassink GA, Hudiekoper HJ. Changes in the broncho-alveolar lavage fluid in smoker and patients with chronic obstructive pulmonary disease. Int J Clin Pharmacol Res 1987;7:357-61.

Turrens JF, Crapo JD, Freeman BA. Protection against oxygen toxicity by intravenous injection of liposome-entrapped catalase and superoxide dismutase. J Clin Invest 1984;73:87-95.

White CW, Jackson JH, Abuchowski A, et al. Intravenous treatment with polyethylene glycol (PEG)-conjugated superoxide dismutase (SOD) and catalase (CAT) prolong survival of rats exposed to hyperoxia. J Clin Res 1984;32:60A.

Liver and Kidney Disease

Albano E, Lott KAK, Slater TF, et al. Spin-trapping studies on the free-radical products formed by metabolic activation of carbon tetrachloride in rat liver microsomal fractions isolated hepatocytes and in vivo in the rat. Biochem J 1982;204:593-603.

Baud L, Ardaillou R. Involvent of reactive oxygen species in kidney damage. Br Med Bull 1993;49:621-29.

Borek C. Antioxidants and cancer. Sci Med 1997;Nov/Dec:52-61,

Cahill A, Wang X, Hock JB. Increased oxidative to mitochondrial DNA following chronic ethanol consumption. Biochem Biophys Res Commun 1997;235:286-90.

Ceballos-Picot I, Witko-Sarsat V, Merad-Boudia M, et al. Glutathione antioxidant system as a marker of oxidative stress in chronic renal failure. Free Radical Biol Med 1996;21:845-53.

Cederbaum AI. Role of lipid peroxidation and oxidative stress in alcohol toxicity. Free Radical Biol Med 1989;7:537-39.

Chen H, Tappel A. Protection by multiple antioxidants against lipid peroxidation in rat liver homogenate. Lipids 1996;31:47-50.

de la Asuncion JG, Millan A, Pla R. et al. Mitochondrial glutathione oxidation correlates with age-associated oxidative damage to mitochondrial DNA. FASEB J 1996;10:333-338.

Falk FJ, Terrell RS, Charles RA, et al. Anti-neutrophil cytoplasmic auto-antibodies induce neutrophils to degranulate and produce oxygen radicals in vitro. Proc Natl Acad Sci 1990;87:4115-19.

Fantone JC, Ward PA. Role of oxygen-derived free radicals and metabolites in leukocyte-dependent inflammatory reactions. Am J Pathol 1982;107:397-418.

Ferrario F, Castiglione E, Colasanti G, et al. The detection of monocytes in human glomerulonephritis. Kidney Int 1985;28:513-19.

Hartley DP, Kroll DJ, Petersen DR. Proxidant-initiated lipid perodication in isolated rat hepatocytes: Detection of 4-hydroxynonenal- and malondialdehyde-protein adducts. Chem Res Toxicol 1997;10:895-905.

Holdworth SR, Neale TJ, Wilson CB. Abrogation of macrophage-dependent injury in experimental glomerulonephritis in the rabbit. Use of an anti-macrophage serum. J Clin Invest 1981;68:686-98.

Kaneko T, Tahara S, Matuso M. Retarding effect of dietary restriction on accumulation of 8-hydroxy-2-deoxyguanosine in organs of Fischer 344 rats during aging. Free Radical Biol Med 1997;23:76-81.

Kashem A, Endoh M, Yamauchi F, et al. Superoxide dismutase activity in human glomeralonephritis. Am J Kidney Dis 1996;28:14-22.

Kelly GS. Clinical applications of N-acetylcysteine. Altern Med Rev 1998;3:114-27.

Kone BC. Nitric oxide in renal health and disease. Am J Kidney Dis 1997;30:311-333.

Kurose I, Higuchi H, Kato S, et al. Oxidative stress on mitochondria and cell membrane of cultured rat hepatocytes and perfused liver exposed to ethanol. Gastroenterology 1997;112:1331-43.

Leonarduzzi G, Scavazza A, Giasi F, et al. The lipid peroxidation end product 4-hydroxy-2,3-nonenal up-regulates transforming growth factor beta 1 expression in the macrophage lineage: A link between oxidative injury and fibrosclerosis. FASEB J 1997;11:851-57.

Lieber CS. Pathogenesis and treatment of liver fibrosis in alcoholics: 1996 Update. Dig Dis 1997;15:42-46.

Lieber CS. Biochemical and molecular basis of alcohol induced injury to liver and other tissues. N Engl J Med 1988;319:1639-50.

Nath KA, Paller MS. Dietary deficiency of antioxidants exacerbates ischemic injury in the rat kidney. Kidney Int 1985;28:513-19.

Oh SI, Kim CI, Chun HG, Park SC. Chronic ethanol consumption affects glutathione status of rat liver. J Nutr 1998;128:758-63.

Polavarapu R, Spitz DR, Sim JE, et al. Increased lipid peroxidation and impaired antioxidant enzyme function is associated with pathological liver injury in experimental alcoholic liver disease in rats fed diets high in corn oil and fish oil. Hepatology 1998;27:1317-23.

Poli G, Albano E, Dianzani MU. The role of lipid peroxidation in liver damage. Chem Phys Lipids 1987;45:117-42.

Poli G. Liver damage due to free radicals. Br Med Bull 1993;49:604-20.

Porta EA. Dietary modulation of oxidative stress in alcoholic liver disease in rats. J Nutr 1997;127:(5 Suppl):912S-915S.

Rajbala A, Sane AS, Zope J, et al. Oxidative stress status in children with nephrotic syndrome. Panminerva Med 1997;39:165-68.

Recknagel RO. Minireview: A new direction in the study of carbon tetrachloride hepatotoxicity. Life Sci 1982;33:401-08.

Rehan A, Johnson KJ, Wiggins RC, et al. Evidence for the role of oxygen radicals in acute nephortoxic nephitits. Lab Invest 1984;51:396-403.

Rehan A, Johnson KJ, Dunkel RG, Wiggins RC. Role of oxygen radicals in phorbol myristate acetate-induced glomerular injury. Kidney Int 1985;27:503-11.

Shah SV. Oxidant mechanisms in glomerulonephritis. Sem Mephrol 1991;11:320-26.

Slater TF. Free-radical mechanisms in tissue injury. Biochem J 1984;222:1-15.

Slattery JT, Wilson JM, Kalhorn TF, Nelson SD. Dose dependent pharmacokinetics of acetaminophen: Evidence of glutathione depletion in humans. Clin Pharmacol Ther 1987;41:413-18.

Zhang D, Okada S, Yu Y, et al. Vitamin E inhibits apoptosis, DNA modification, and cancer incidence induced by iron-mediated peroxidation in Wistar rat kidney. Cancer Res 1997;57:2410-14.

Neurodegenerative Disease

Adams JD, Odunze IN. Oxygen free radicals and Parkinson's disease. Free Radical Biol Med 1991;10-161-69.

Akama KT, Albanese C, Pestell RG, Van Eldik LJ. Amyloid beta-peptide stimulates nitric oxide production in astrocytes through an NFkappaB-dependent mechanism. Proc Natl Acad Sci USA 1998;95:5795-5800.

Anggaard E. Nitric oxide: Mediator, murderer, and medicine. Lancet 1994;343:1199-1206.

Ambani IM, Van Woert MH, Murphy S. Brain peroxidase and catalase in Parkinson's disease. Arch Neurol 1975;32:114-18.

Barbeau A. Etiology of Parkinson's disease. Can J Neurol Sci 1984;11:24-28.

Barker JE, Heales SJ, Cassidy A, et al. Depletion of brain glutathione results in a decrease of glutathione reductase activity: An enzyme susceptible to oxidative damage. Brain Res 1996;716:118-22.

Beckman JS, Carson M, Smith CD, Koppenol WH. ALS, SOD and peroxynitrite. Nature 1993;364:584.

Bostanjopoulou S, Kyriazis G, Katsarou Z, et al. Superoxide dismutase activity in early and advanced Parkinson's disease. Funct Neurol 1996;12:63-68.

Brown RH. Superoxide dismutase and familial amytrophic lateras sclerosis: New insights into mechanisms and treatments. Am Neurol 1996;39:145-46.

Brown BH. Clinical implications of basic research: A transgenic-mouse model of amyotrophic lateral sclerosis. N Engl J Med 1994;331:1091-92.

Bowern N, Ramshaw IA, Doherty PC. Inhibition of autoimmune neuro-pathological process by treatment with an iron chelating agent. J Exp Med 1984;160:1532-43.

Calabrese V, Ragusa N, Antico A, et al. Cysteine-induced enhancement of lipid peroxidation in substantia nigra: Comparative effect of exogenous administration of reduced glutathione. Drugs Exp Clin Res 1997;23:25-31.

Cardoso SM, Pereira C, Oliveira CR. The protective effect of vitamin E, idebenone and reduced glutathione on free radical mediated injury in rat brain synaptosomes. Biochem Biophys Res Commun 1998;246:703-710.

Cassarino DS, Fall CP, Swerdlow RH, et al. Elevated reactive oxygen species and antioxidant enzyme activities in animal and cellular models of Parkinson's disease. Biochim Biophys Acta 1997;1362:77-86.

Clemens JA, Phebus LA. Dopamine depletion protects striatal neurons from ischemia-induced cell death. Life Sci 1988;42:707-13.

Cooper RL. Multiple sclerosis: An immune legacy? Med Hypothesis 1997;49:307-11.

Dexter DT, Wells FR, Agid F, et al. Increased nigral iron content in post-mortem parkinsonian brain. Lancet 1987;2:1219-20.

Dowson JH. Neuronal liposuscin accumulation in ageing and Alzheimer's dementia: A pathogenic mechanism? Br J Psychiatr 1982;140:142-48.

Evans PH. Free radicals in brain metabolism and pathology. Br Med Bul 1993;49:577-87.

Ferrante RJ, Browne SE, Shinobu LA, et al. Evidence of increased oxidative damage in both sporadic and familial amyotrophic lateral sclerosis. J Neurochem 1997;69:2064-74.

Forster MJ, Debey A, Dawson KM, et al. Age-related losses of cognitive function and motor skills in mice are associated with oxidative protein damage in the brain. Proc Natl Acad Sci USA 1996;93: 4765-69.

Frey WH II, Emory CR, Wiebenga ME, et al. Inhibitor of antagonist binding to the muscarinic receptor is elevated in Alzheimer's brain. Brain Res 1994;655:153-60.

Frey WH, Najarian MM, Kumar KS, et al. Endogenous Alzheimer's brain factor and oxidized glutathione inhibit antagonist binding to the muscarinic receptor. Brain Res 1996;714:87-94.

Gurney ME, PuH, Chiu AY, et al. Motor neuron degeneration in mice that express a human CU,Zn superoxide dismutase mutation. Science 1994;264:1772-75.

Gurney ME, Cutting FB, Zhai P. et al. Benefit of vitamin E, riluzole, and gabapentin in a transgenic model of familial amyothrophic lateral sclerosis. Ann Neurol 1996;39:147-57.

Halliwell B, Gutteridge JMC. Oxygen toxicity, oxygen radicals, transition metals and disease. Biochem J 1984;219:1-14.

Harman D. The aging process. Proc Natl Acad Sci USA 1981;78:7124-28.

Hensley K, Carney JM, Mattson MP, et al. A model for beta-amyloid aggregation and neurotoxicity based on free radical generation by the peptide: Relevance to Alzheimer's disease. Proc Natl Acad Sci USA 1994;91:3270-74.

Hooper DC, Spitsin S, Kean RB, et al. Uric acid, a natural scavenger of peroxynitrite, in experimental encephalomyelitis and multiple sclerosis. Proc Natl Acad Sci USA 1998;95:675-80.

Hung HC, Lee EH. MPTP produces differential oxidative stress and antioxidative responses in the nigrostriatal and mesolimbic dopaminergic pathways. Free Radical Biol Med 1998;24:76-84.

\Ihara Y, Hayabara T, Sasaki K, et al. Free radicals and superoxide dismutase in blood of patients with Alzheimer's disease and vascular dementia. J Neurol Sci 1997;153:76-81.

Jeandel C, Nicolas MB, Dubois F, et al. Lipid peroxidation and free radical scavengers in Alzheimer's disease. Gerontology 1989;35:275-82.

Karlhuber GM, Bauer HC, Eckl PM. Cytotoxic and genotoxic effects of 4-hydroxynonenal in cerebral endothelial cells. Mutat Res 1997;381:209-16.

Katzman R. Alzheimer's disease. N Engl J Med 1986;314:964-73.

Kisby GE, Milne J, Sweatt C. Evidence of reduced DNA repair in amyotrophic lateral sclerosis brain tissue. Neuroreport 1997;8:1337-40.

Knight JA. Reactive oxygen species and the neurodegenerative disorders. Ann Clin Lab Sci 1997;27:11-25.

Konat GW, Wiggins RC. Effect of reactive oxygen species on myelin membrane proteins. J Neurochem 1985;45:1113-18.

Korpela H, Kinnunen E, Juntunen J, et al. Serum selenium concentration, glutathione peroxidase activity and lipid perosides in a co-twin control study on multiple sclerosis. J Neurol Sci 1989;91:79-84.

Lan J Jiang DH. Excessive iron accumulation in the brain: A possible potential risk of neurodegeneration in Parkinson's disease. J Neurol Transm 1997;104:649-60.

LeVine SM. The role of reactive oxygen species in the pathogenesis of multiple sclerosis. Med Hypotheses 1992;39:271-74.

Lieberman A. Emerging perspectives in Parkinson's disease. Neurology 1992;42(Suppl 4):5-7.

Lyras L, Perry RH, Perry EK, et al. Oxidative damage to proteins, lipids, and DNA in cortical brain regions from patients with dementia with Lewy bodies. J Neurochem 1998;71:302-12.

Marcus DL, Thomas C, Rodriguez C, et al. Increased peroxidation and reduced antioxidant enzyme activity in Alzheimer's disease. Exp Neurol 1998;150: 40-44.

Markesbery WR, Lovell MA. Four-hydroxynonenal, a product of lipid peroxidation, is increased in the brain in Alzheimer's disease. Neurobiol Aging 1998;19:33-36.

Naidoo R, Knapp ML. Studies of lipid peroxidation products in cerebrospinal fluid and serum in multiple sclerosis and other conditions. Clin Chem 1992;38:4349-54.

Nakamura K, Wang W, Kang UJ. The role of glutathione in dopaminergic neuronal survival. J Neurochem 1997;69:1850-58.

Odunze IN, Klaidman LK, Adams JD. MPTP toxicity in the mouse brain and vitamin E. Neurosci Lett 1990;108:346-49.

Offen D, Zif I, Sternin H, et al. Prevention of dopamine-induced cell death by thiol antioxidants: Possible implications for treatment of Parkinson's disease. Exp Neurol 1996;141:32-39.

Packer L, Tritschler HJ, Wessel K. Neuroprotection by the metabolic antioxidant alpha-lipoic acid. Free Radical Biol Med 1997;22:359-78.

Pappolla MA, Chyan YJ, Omar RA, et al. kEvidence of oxidative stress and in vivo neurotoxicity of beta-amyloid in a transgenic mouse model of Alzheimer's disease: A chronic oxidative paradigm for testing antioxidant therapies in vivo. Am J Pathol 1998;152:871-77.

Perrig WJ, Perrig P, Stahelin HB. The relation between antioxidants and memory performance in the old and very old. J Am Geriatr Soc 1997;45:718-24.

Perry TL, Godin DV, Hansen S. Parkinson's disease: A disorder due to nigral glutathione deficiency? Neurosci Lett 1982;33:305-10.

Poirer J, Kogan S, Gauthier S. Environment, genetics and idiopathic Parkinson's disease. Can J Neurol Sci 1991;18:70-76.

Poulin JE, Cover C, Gustafson MR, Kay MMB. Vitamin E prevents oxidative mofification of brain and lymphocyte band 3 proteins during aging. Proc Natl Acad Sci USA 1996;93:5600-03.

Przedborski S, Donaldson D, Jakowee M, et al. Brain superoxide dismutase, catalase and glutathione peroxidase activities in amyotrophic lateral sclerosis. Ann Neurol 1996;39:158-65

Raine CS. Demyelinating diseases. In: Davis RL, Robertson DM, eds. Textbook of Neuropathology, 2nd ed. Baltimore, MD: Williams & Wilkins;1991:535.

Ravindranath V, Shivakumar BR, Anandatheerthavarada HK. Low glutathione levels in brain regions of aged rats. Neurosci Lett 1989;101:187-90.

Reiter RJ. Oxidative processes and antioxidative defense mechanisms. BASEB J 1995;9: 526-33.

Rivett AJ. Preferential degradation of the oxidatively modified form of glutamine synthetase by intracellular mammalian proteases. J Biol Chem 1985;260:300-05.

Rodriquez M. Multiple sclerosis: Insights into molecular pathogenesis and therapy. Mayo Clin Proc 1997;72:663-64.

Rosen DR, Siddique T, Patterson D, et al. Mutations in Cu/Zn superoxide dismutase gene are associated with familial amyotrophic lateral sclerosis. Nature 1993;362:59-62.

Sadovnick AD, Ebers GC, Dyment DA, Risch NJ. Evidence for genetic basis of multiple sclerosis. Lancet 1996;347:1728-30.

Seaton TA, Cooper JM, Schopira AH. Free radical scavengers protect dopaminergic cell lines from apoptosis induced by complex 1 inhibitors. Brain Res 1997;777:110-18.

Smith CD, Carney JM, Starke-Reed PE, et al. Excess brain protein oxidation and enzyme dysfunction in normal aging and in Alzheimer's disease. Proc Natl Acad Sci USA 1991;88:10540-43.

Smith MA, Hirai K, Hsiao K, et al. Amyloid-beta deposition in Alzheimer's transgenic mice is associated with oxidative stress. J Neurochem 1998;70:2212-15.

Smith MA, Richey-Harris PL, Sayre LM, et al. Widespread peroxynitrite-mediated damage in Alzheimer's disease. J Neurosci 1997;17:2653-57.

Spina MB, Cohen G. Dopamine turnover and glutathione oxidation: Implications for Parkinson's disease. Proc Natl Acad Sci USA 1989;86:1398-1400.

Spina MB, Cohen G. Exposure of school synaptosomes to L-dopa increases levels of oxidized glutathione. J Pharm Exp Ther 1988;247:502-07.

St George-Hyslop PH, Tanzi RE, Polinsky RJ, et al. The genetic defect causing familial Alzheimer's disease maps on chromosome 21. Science 1987;235:885-90.

Toshniwal PK, Zarling EJ. Evidence for increased lipid peroxidation in multiple sclerosis. Neurochem Res 1992;17:205-207.

Van ees Vliet A, Smith D, O'Neill CA, et al. Interactions of peroxynitrite with human plasma and its constituents: Oxidative damage and antioxidant depletion. Biochem J 2994;303:295-301.

Volicer L, Crino PB. Involvement of free radicals in dementia of the Alzheimer's type: A hypothesis. Neurobiol Aging 1990;11:567-71.

West MJ, Coleman PD, Flood DG, Troncoso JC. Differences in the pattern of hippocampal neuronal loss in normal ageing and Alzheimer's disease. Lancet 1994;344:769-72.

Wisniewski KE, Wisniewski HM, Wen GY. Occurrence of neuropathological changes and dementia of Alzheimer's disease in Down's syndrome. Am Neurol 1985;17:278-82.

Zaman Z, Roche S, Fielden P, et al. Plasma concentrations of vitamins A and E and carotenoids in Alzheimer's disease. Age Ageing 1992;21:91-94.

Inflammatory Disease & the Immune System

Anderson R, Lukey PT. A biological role for ascorbate in the selective neutralization of extracellular phagocyte-derived oxidants. Ann NY Acad Sci 1987;498:229-233.

Babior BM. Oxidants from phagocytes: Agents of defense and destruction.

Blood 1984;6a4:959-60.

Babior BM. The respiratory burst of leukocytes. J Clin Invest 1984;73:599-601.

Bach J-F, Dardenne M, Pleau JM, Bach M-A. Isolation, biochemical characteristics, and biological activity of a circulating thymic hormone in the mouse and in the human. Ann NY Acad Sci 1975;249:186-210.

Beck FWJ, Prasad As, Kaplan J, et al. Changes in cytokine production and T cell subpopulations in experimentally induced zinc-deficient humans. Am J Physiol 1997;272:E1002-E1007.

Beck MA. Increased virulence of coxsackievirus B3 in mice due to vitamin E or selenium deficiency. J Nutr. 1997;127:966S-970S.

Beck MA. The influence of antioxidant nutrients on viral infection. Nutr Rev 1998;56:S140-S146.

Becker IL, Ward P. Chemotaxis. In Parker CW, ed. Clinical immunology. Philadelphia:WB Saunders;1980:272.

Berr C, Nicole A, Godin J et al. Selenium and oxygen-metabolizing enzymes in elderly community residents. A pilot epidemiological study. J Am Geriatr Soc 1993;41:143-48.

Biemond P, van Eijk HG, Swaak AJG, Koster JF.Superoxide dependent iron release from ferritin in inflammatory diseases. Free Radical Biol Med 1988;4:185-88.

Blake DR, Hall ND, Treby DA, et al. Protection against superoxide and hydrogen peroxide in synovial fluid from rheumatoid patients. Clin Sci 1981;61:483-86.

Blaylock B. The ageing immune system and common infections in elderly patients. J ET Nurs 1993;20:63-67.

Bogden JD, Bendich A, Kemp FW, et al. Daily micronutrient supplements enhance delayed-hypersensitivity skin test responses in older people. Am J Clin Nutr 1994;60:337-347.

Boxer LA, Yoder M, Bonsib S, et al. Effects of a chemotactic factor, N-formylmethionyl peptide, on adherence, superoxide anion generation, phagocytosis, and microtubule assembly of human polymorphonulcear leukocytes. J Lab Clin Med 1979;93:506-14.

Burkhardt H, Schwingel M, Menninger H, et al. Oxygen radicals as effectors of cartilage destruction. Arthritis Rheum 1986;29:379-387.

Ceballos-Picot I, Trivier J-M, Nocole A, et al. Age-correlated modifications of copper-zinc superoxide dismutase and glutathione-related enzyme activities in human erythrocytes. Clin Chem 1992;38:66-70.

Chandra RK. Effect of vitamin and trace-element supplementation on immune responses and infection in elderly patients. Lancet 1992;340:1124-27.

Chaudiere J. Wilhelmsen EC, Tappel AL. Mechanism of selenium-glutathione peroxidase and its inhibition by mercapto-carnoxylic acids and other mercaptans. J Biol Chem 1984;259:12043-12050.

Chew BP. Role of carotenoids in the immune response. Symposium on Antioxidants, Immune Response and Animal Function. J Dairy Sci 1993;76:2804-11.

Cunningham-Rundles S, Bockam RS, Lin A, et al. Physiological and pharmacological effects of zinc on immune response. Ann NY Acad Sci 1990;487:113-22.

Daniel LR, Chew BP, Tanaka TS, Tjoelker LW. In vitro effects of beta-carotene and vitamin A on peripheral blood mononuclear cell proliferation. J Dairy Sci 1991;74:911-15.

Dardenne M, Boukaiba N, Gagnerault M-C, et al. Restoration of the thymus in aging mice by in vivo zinc supplementation. Clin Immunol Immunopathol 1993;66:127-135.

Daynes RA, Araneo BA. Prevention and reversal of some age-associated changes in immunologic responses by supplemental dehydroepiandrosterone sulfate therapy. Aging Immunol Infect Dis 1992;3:135-54.

Droge W, Eck HP, Mihm S. Oxidant-antioxidant status in immunodeficiency virus infection. In: Packer L, ed. Oxygen radicals in biological systems, Part C. SanDiego, CA: Academic Press 1994;594-601.

Duchateau J, Delepesse G, Vrijens R, Collet H. Beneficial effects of oral zinc supplementation on the immune response of old people. Am J Med 1981;70:1001-04.

Effros RB, Casillas A, Walford RL. The effect of thymosin 0:1 on immunity to influenza in aged mice. Aging Immunol Infect Dis 1988;1:31-40.

Fidelus RK, Tsan M-F. Enhancement of intracellular glutathione promotes lymphocyte activation by mitogen. Cell Immunol 1986;97:155-63.

Fortes C, Forastiere F, Agabiti N, et al. The effect of zinc and vitamin A supplementation on immune response in an older population. J Am Geriatr Soc 1998;46:19-26.

Frei B, England L, Ames BN. Ascorbate is an outstanding antioxidant in human blood plasma. Proc Natl Acad Sci USA 1991;88:11003-06.

Gillis S, Kozak R, Durante M, Weksler ME. Immunological studies of aging from aged humans. J Clin Invest 1981;67:937.

Gillis S, Kozak R, Durante M, Weksler ME. Immunological studies of aging: Decreased production of, and response to, T cell growth factor by lymphocytes from aged humans. J Clin Invest 1981;67:937.

Gilman SC, Rosenberg JS, Geldman JD. T lymphocytes of young and old rats. II. Functional defects and the role of interleukin-2. J Immunol 1982;128:644-50.

Goldstein IM, Roos D, Kaplan HB, Weissmann G. Complement and immunoglobulins stimulate superoxide production by human leukocytes independently of phagocytosis. J Clin Inves 1975;56: 1155-63

Good RA, Yunis E. Association of autoimmunity, immunodeficiency and aging in man, rabbits, and mice. Fed Proc 1974;33:2040-50.

Goso C, Frasca D, Doria G. Effect of synthetic thymic humoral hormone factor (THF-gamma2) on T cell activities in immunodeficient aging mice. Clin Exp Immunol 1992;87:346-51.

Goya RG, et al. Effects of growth hormone and thyroxine on thymulin secretions in aging rats. Neuroimmunology 1993;58:338-43.

Grimble RF. Nutritional antioxidants and the modulation of inflammation: Theory and practice. New Horizons 1994;2:175-85.

Gutteridge JMC. Iron promoters of the Fenton reaction and lipid peroxidation can be released from haemoglobin by peroxides. BEBS Lett 1986;139:169-73.

Hirokawa K. Reversing and restoring immune functions. Mech Age Dev 1997;92:119-24.

Hirokawa K. Understanding the mechanism of the age-related decline in immune function. Nutr Rev 1992;50:361-66.

Hirokawa K, Sato K, Makinodan T. Restoration of impaired immune function in aging animals. V. Long-term immunopotentiating effect of combined young bone marrow and newborn thymus grafts. Clin Immunol Immunopathol 19776;22:297-304.

Hilliquin P, Borderie D, Hernvann A, et al. Nitric oxide as S-nitrosoproteins in rheumatoid arthritis. Arthritis Rheum 1997;40:1512-17.

Kayanoki Y, Jujii J, Islam KN, et al. The protective role of glutathione peroxidase in apoptosis induced by reactive oxygen species. J Biochem Tokyo 1996;119:817-22.

Keen CL, Gershwin ME. Zinc deficiency and immune function. Ann Rev Nutr 1990;10:415-31.

Kirwood TB, Ritter MA. The interface between ageing and health in man Age Ageing 1997;26-S4:9-14.

Knight JA, Blaylock RC, Searles Da. The effect of vitamins C and E on lipid peroxidation in stored erythrocytes. Ann Clin Lab Sci 1993;23:51-56.

Kumar V, Cotran RS, Robbins SL. Acute and chronic inflammation. In Basic Pathology. Philadelphia: WB Saunders; 1992:31.

Lipschit DA, Udupa KB. Influence of ageing and protein deficiency on neutrophil function. J Gerontol 1986;41:690-94.

Lunec J, Blake DR, McCleary SJ, et al. Self-perpetuating mechanisms of immunoglobulin G aggregation in rheumatoid inflammation. J Clin Invest 1985;76:2084-90.

Luster AD. Chemokines – Chemotatic cytokines that mediate inflammation. N Engl J Med 1998;338:436-45.

Makinodan T, Day MMB. Age influence on the immune system. Adv Immunol 1980;29:287-330.

Mandell GL. Bactericidal activity of aerobic and anaerobic polymorphonuclear nueutrophils. Infect Immun 1974;9:337-41.

Meeker HC, Eskew ML, Scheuchenzuber W, et al. Antioxidant effects on cell-mediated immunity. J Leuk Biol 1985;38:451-58.

Meydani SN, Hayek M. Vitamin E and the immune response. In: Chandra RK, ed. International Conference on Nutrition, Immunity, and illness in the Elderly, St. Johns, Newfoundland: ARTS Biomedical Publishers and Distributors 1992:105-28.

Meydani SN, Meydani M, Blumberg JB, et al. Vitamin E supplementation enhances in vivo immune response in healthy elderly: A dose-response study. J Am Med Assoc 1997;277:1380-86.

Meydani M, Martin A, Bibaya-Mercado JD, et al. Beta-carotene supplementation increases antioxidant capacity of plasma in older women. J Nutr 1994;124:2392-2403.

Michal JJ, Chew BP, Wong TS, et al. Modulatory effects of dietary beta-carotene in blood and mammary leukocyte function in periparturient dairy cows. J Dairy Sci 1994;77:1408-22.

Murata T, Tamai H, Morinobu T, et al. Effect of long-term administration of beta-carotene on lymphocyte subsets in humans. Am J Clin Nutr 1994;60:597-602.

Niki E. Interaction of Ascorbate and alpha-tocopherol. Ann Ny Acad Sci 1987;498:186-99.

Palozza P, Krinsky NI. Antioxidant effects of carotenoids in vivo and in vitro: an overview. In: Packer L, ed. Methods in enzymology, Carotenoids. San Diego, CA: Academic Press; 1992:403-39.

Penn ND, Purkins I, Kelleher J, et al. The effect of dietary supplementaion with vitamins A, C, And E on cell-mediated immune function in elderly long-stay patients: A randomized controlled study. Age Ageing 1991;20:169-74.

Peterhans E. Oxidants and antioxidants in viral diseases: Disease mechanisms and metabolic regulation. J Nutr 1997;127:962S-65S.

Rosseau EJ, Davison AJ, Dunn B. Protection by beta-carotene and related compounds against oxygen-mediated cytotoxicity and genotoxicity: implications for carcinogenesis and anticarcinogenesis. Free Rad Biol Med 1992;13:407-33.

Samuelsson B. Leukotrienes: Mediators of immediate hypersensitivity reactions and inflammation. Science 1983;220:568-75.

Schmidt K. Antioxidant vitamins and beta-carotene: Effects on immunocompetence. Am J Clin Nutr 1991;53:383S-85S.

Schreck R, Rieber P, Baeuerle PA. Reactive oxygen intermediates as apparently widely used messenges in the activation of the NFkB transcription factor and HIV-1. EMBO J 1991;10:2247-58.

Selvaraj RJ, Sbarra AJ. Relationship of glycolytic and oxidative metabolism to particle entry and destruction in phagocytosing cells. Nature 1966;211:1272-76

Senator GB, Muirden KD. Concentration of iron in synovial fluid, and serum in rheumatoid arthritis and other joint diseases. Ann Rheum Dis 1968;27:49-53.

Shi HN, Scott ME, Stevenson MM, Koski KG. Energy restriftion and zinc deficiency impair the functions of murine T cells and antigen-presenting cells during gastrointestinal nematod infection J Nutr 1998;128:20-27.

Silverstein SC, Steinman RM, Cohn ZA. Endocytosis. Annu Rev Biochem 1977;46:669-722.

Simchowitz L, Atkinson JP, Spilberg I. Stimulus-specific deactivation of chemotatic factor-induced cyclic AMP response and superoxide generation by human neutrophils. J Clin Invest 1980;66:736-47.

Sun E, Xu H, Liu Q, et al. The mechanisms for the effect of selenium supplementation on immunity. Biol Trace Element Res 1995;48:231-38.

Smyth MJ. Glutathione modulates activation-dependent proliferation of human peripheral blood lymphocyte populations without regulating their activated function. J Immunol 1991;146:1921-27.

Suthanthiran M, Anderson ME, Sharma UK, Meister A. Glutathione regulates activation-dependent DNA synthesis in highly purified normal human T lymphocytes stimulated via CD2 and DC3 antigens. Proc Natl Acad Sci USA 1990;87:3343-47.

Thoman ML, Weigle WO. Cell-mediated immunity in aged mice: An underlying lesion in IL2 synthesis. J Immunol 1982;128:2358-61.

Umeki S, Sumi M, Niki Y, Soejima R. Concentrations of superoxide dismutase and superoxide anion in blood of patients with respiratory infection and compromised immune system. Clin Chem 1987;33:2230-33.

Utsuyama M, Hirokawa K. Hypertrophy of the thymus gland and restoration of immune functions in mice and rats by gonadectomy. Mech Age Dev

1989;47:175-85.

Weimann BJ, Weiser H. Effects of antioxidant vitamins C, E, and beta-carotene on immune functions in MRL/pr mice and rats. Ann NY Acad Sci 1992;669:390-92.

Weinberg JB, Granger DL, Pisetsky DS, et al. The role of nitric oxide in the pathogenesis of spontaneous murine autoimmune diaease: Increased nitric oxide production and nitric oxide synthase expression in MRL-lpr/pr mice, and reduction of spontaneous glomerulonephritis and arthritis by orally administered NG-monoethyl-L-arginine. J Exp Med 1994;179:651-60.

Weiss J, Victor M, Standhal O, Elsbach P. Killing of gram-negative bacteria by polymorphonuclear leukocytes: Role of an oxygen-independent bactericidal system. J Clin Invest 1984;69:959-70.

Weksler ME. Immune senescence and adrenal steroids: Immune dysregulation and the action of edhydroepiandrosterone (DHEA) in old animals. Eur J Clin Pharm 1993;45(suppl 1):521-33.

Wikby A, Johansson B, Fergunson F, Olsson J. Age-related changes in immune parameters in a very old population of Swedish people: A longitudinal study. Exp Gerontol 1994;5:531-41.

Winrow VR, Winyard PG, Morris CJ, Blake DR. Free radicals in inflammation: Second messengers and mediators of tissue destruction. Br Med Bull 1993;49:506-22.

Yasmineh WG, Kaur TP, Blazar BR, Theologides A. Serum catalase as a marker of graft-vs-host disease in allogenic bone marrow transplant recipients: A pilot study. Clin Chem 1995;41:1574-80.

Yim C-Y, Hibbs JB, McGregor JR, et al. Use of N-acetyl cysteine to increase intracellular glutathione during the induction of antitumor responses by IL-2. J Immunol 1994;152:5796-5805.

Young JD-E, Peterson CGB, Venge P, Cohn ZA. Mechanism of membrane damage mediated by human eosinophil cationic protein. Nature 1986;321:613-16.

Section VI: Total Health

Balch JF. The Super Antioxidants. New York: M Evans and Co, Inc, 1998.

Cooper R, Cooper L. Low Fat Living. Emmaus, Penn: Rodale Press Inc, 1996.

Dement WC, Vaughn C. The Promise of Sleep. New York: Random House Inc, 1999.

Firshein R. The Neutraceutical Revolution. New York: Riverhead Books, 1998.

Hauri P, Linde S. No More Sleepless Nights. New York: John Wiley & Sons Inc, 1996.

Kune S. Stressful events and cancer. Epidemiology 1993;4:395-97.

Looker T, Gregson O. Managing Stress. Chicago:Contemporary Pub. Co, 1997.

Mason L. Guide to Stress Reduction. Berkeley, CA: Celestial Arts, 2001.

Packer L, Colman C. The Antioxidant Miracle. New York: John Wiley & Sons Inc, 1999.

Pressman A, Buff S. The GSH Phenomenon. New York: St. Martin's Press, 1997.

Smoking and Health – A National Status Report. A Report to Congress. Publication No. HHS/PHS/CDC 87 – 8396. Washington, DC: Department of Health and Human Services; 1987.

Weisburger JG. Dietary fat and risk of chronic disease: Mechanistic insights from experimental studies. J Am Dietetic Ass 1997;97(suppl 7):16-23.

Index

Epilogue

Are We Finding The Fountain Of Youth?

Are we really getting any closer to the chance of stopping the aging process? Countless scientists are working at the inevitable ending to each of our times spent on this planet. As physicians, many of us hope for improvement in quality of life and not just a life extension. Of course there will be many proponents of a longevity medicine rationale but there will be many that will be detractors that will profess to know that anti-aging treatments are unlikely because humans are too complicated to be affected by simple supplements, diet and exercise programs. Yet, elegant simplicity is the fundamental principle that we strive for in the best of scientific endeavors. Some scientists are disgusted by the glut of health products that are sweeping the world, offering possibilities to protect the body and brain from the ravages of age deterioration. Whenever there is a flurry of interest, the businessmen are sure to follow. This has been the standard in modern times and of course, if there is some way to improve health and longevity, then everyone wants to know about it and the entrepreneurs want more, to be involved in the growth of this industry. Please don't blame the entrepreneurs and don't blame the scientists and health care professionals that continue to investigate the claims made by their friends and patients. Hopefully the investigators that we have placed our faith in to lead the way, will direct our attention away from the placebos and red herrings that have pervaded science for centuries. No more so than today with scandals pervading the most august of scientific journals. The truth always wins out and with the attention given to longevity science, we personally feel that many of the exciting theories and treatments that we study now are leading the way into a new and superlative branch of preventative medicine. This will be foreign and threatening to the establishment that has thrived on a disease based system that has only recently accepted the use of supplements for health (folate for heart health and prevention of fetal abnormalities for example).

It is well known that many diseases are related to aging. Diseases like Parkinson's, osteoarthritis, Alzheimer's, atherosclerosis with heart disease, diabetes, osteoporosis, cancer and macular degeneration. If these problems could be delayed or prevented, most of us would have a more pleasant time in our senior years. Many of these diseases are helped and prevented by medications and supplements. Hormones and antioxidants have been shown to alter the course of many of these diseases with the subsequent rationale that aging may be influenced as well. Scientists and clinicians have been fed all the essentials to weigh theory by experiment. Many of the standard medicines "proven" to be effective years ago have fallen by the wayside and many of the medicines used have been discontinued because they didn't work or they were harmful. Many of the treatment protocols proposed for optimal health and longevity may also be dropped in the future due to poor results but time will tell. Unfortunately the ultimate proof requires long term studies and many of us are using our "common sense" and scientific principles to guide us in this new branch of medicine. As physicians, we all remember our special pledge to our patients to "first cause no harm" and hopefully bring health and happiness to our patients. Progress is slow but we must be very careful and methodical in our quest for evidence to back our treatments.

Some of us have been slow to profess "proper" nutrition and exercise because there have been no studies to prove the benefits on longevity or even well being. Doctors are often concerned by the multitude of trauma seen as our older patients try to participate in fitness programs and sports with their frail bodies. Some doctors use "common sense" and limited studies to encourage exercise and diets that reduce obesity and inactivity. Calorie restriction has certainly helped in animal models to improve health and longevity and antioxidants have helped worms and rats live much longer with less disease. So does hormone replacement and antioxidant therapy with human health and aging. The majority of scientists would take the natural jump to humans from the animal model but with caution. The therapies when used properly with careful attention paid to concomitant diseases are relatively safe. There is no doubt that the therapies that are used will be blamed for problems since everyone will have different requirements for supplementation. It has taken many years for us to deplore the use of cigarettes until proper studies proved the health risk even though we all had anecdotal evidence that it was our smokers that got the lung cancer, emphysema, osteoporosis and heart problems early. Many groups including the American Academy of Anti-Aging Medicine (A4M) and the Canadian Longevity And Anti-Aging Academy (CLA4) are gathering data from clinicians slowly. Judging the treatment practices that are common today and streamlining the protocols will make the best current information available to everyone for their own personal use.

Longevity medicine is here to stay. It will be considered common sense in the future and humans will continue to strive for the best health for as long as possible as they age. The advances are fast and furious and some information will be distorted but progress marches on. Physicians will continue to weigh the pros and cons of Hormone Replacement therapies (HRTs) and the use of various antioxidants for good health but hopefully will recommend a better diet and exercise plan for their patients.

For the moment, though, readers who are interested in anti-aging treatments would be well-advised to seek out physicians interested in anti-aging medicine for further advice and recommendations. A primary source for those individuals would be through the American Academy of Anti-Aging Medicine (A4M) in the U.S., or in Canada, the Canadian Longevity and Anti-Aging Academy (CLA4). Web sites that may be of interest are listed below:

http://www.cla4.com

http://www.healthandlongevitycentre.com

http://www.worldhealth.net

Dr. McLeod's and Dr. White's next exciting new book dealing with everything you wanted to know about Testosterone and Andropause, entitled.

"Testosterone Power"

will be available in the spring of 2003.

CANADIAN LONGEVITY AND ANTI-AGING ACADEMY

A team of professionals that are dedicated to slowing the onset of degenerative diseases and promoting a healthy lifespan by utilizing the latest scientific research in the quest for longevity.

CLA4 MISSION STATEMENT

VISION: We are advancing toward a new era of increasingly powerful and sophisticated technology. The Canadian Longevity and Anti-Aging Academy, which is a non profit organization of Physicians, scientists, health researchers and interested individuals, proposes to bring the best of anti-aging therapies to Canada to allow us each to make a choice about how we age.

MISSION: Members of the Academy believe that aging and disability from degenerative disease including cardiovascular disease, cancer, diabetes and neurological deterioration is not inevitable. The Academy provides a public forum for discussion, development and promotion of medical practice, technology and therapeutics that retard or even reverse the deterioration of the human body resulting from the physiology of aging.

GOALS: To promote changes in the medical curriculum so that future physicians will be well informed in the developments in anti-aging medicine. To raise awareness among the public and to disseminate evidence based information to physicians to apply the clinical application of longevity medicine. To act as an information source for anti-aging science and to act as a liaison for government in future studies of longevity.

DISCLAIMER

The contents of this book are the opinions of the authors and may not represent the consensus of opinion of the medical profession at this time. The contents of this book are not intended to be used to treat, cure, mitigate or diagnose any medical condition. The readers should consult their doctors before embarking on any changes that could affect their health.